Praise for
The SparkPeople Cookbook

"Everything you need to know for cooking and eating healthy—and losing weight in the process. Packed with easy recipes for breakfast, lunch, and dinner; techniques for maximizing flavor and cutting fat; and tips for stocking a healthy kitchen, this is an indispensible guide to getting good-for-you meals on the table fast."

—Betty S. Wong, editor in chief, *Fitness* magazine

"As our country faces both an obesity epidemic, as well as a hunger and nutrition crisis in many communities, it is more important than ever that we all learn how to eat less expensive but more nutritious alternatives to fast food and 'junk' food. This book offers great tips, tools, and recipes; and proves that we can all enjoy eating good food, while getting healthier."

—Dan Glickman, former Secretary of Agriculture

"Meg is one of the leading voices for putting sound nutrition into practice. Her commonsense approach to cooking, eating, and activity is one every physician and parent can easily embrace."

—Christopher F. Bolling, M.D., pediatrician, Pediatric Associates; program chairman, American Academy of Pediatrics, Provisional Section on Obesity

"When Meg cooks for her family, she serves a large helping of sensibility. She believes in cooking and eating good food, and eating it together. This book will appeal to anyone who wants to embark on a journey of better health through the door of the kitchen."

—Maggie Green, LD, RD; author of *The Kentucky Fresh Cookbook*

"The SparkPeople Cookbook *is inspirational, motivational, and informational. And best of all, it features real feedback about healthy living from real people—people I can trust because they've been there and done that. I particularly love how each recipe comes with a handy chart so you can tell, at a glance, how many servings of veggies or fruit are in the dish or whether the recipe would be great for a dinner party. No gimmicks, no tricks—just healthy, fresh food and concrete advice from the wonderful members of SparkPeople."*

—Caitlin Boyle, blogger of HealthyTippingPoint.com, editor of OperationBeautiful.com, and author of *Operation Beautiful*

*"**The SparkPeople Cookbook** is unlike any other cookbook I've read. It gives you the knowledge and know-how to make permanent lifestyle changes to your eating habits. Healthy eating should be simple—and even fun—and **The SparkPeople Cookbook** provides straightforward, interesting, and satisfying recipes that will help you lose weight without leaving you feeling deprived."*

—Tina Haupert, author and blogger, Carrots 'N' Cake

THE

SPARKPEOPLE
COOKBOOK

Love Your Food, Lose the Weight

ALSO FROM SPARKPEOPLE.COM

Books

The Spark: The 28-Day Breakthrough Plan for Losing Weight, Getting Fit, and Transforming Your Life

CD

The Spark: The Breakthrough Plan for Losing Weight, Getting Fit, and Transforming Your Life

DVDs

The Spark: Fit, Firm, & Fired Up, with Coach Nicole

SparkPeople Cardio Blast, with Coach Nicole

THE
SPARKPEOPLE COOKBOOK

Love Your Food, Lose the Weight

MEG GALVIN
and STEPFANIE ROMINE

Food photographs by Randall Hoover Photography

HAY HOUSE, INC.
Carlsbad, California • New York City
London • Sydney • Johannesburg
Vancouver • Hong Kong • New Delhi

Published and distributed in the United States by: Hay House, Inc.: www.hayhouse.com • *Published and distributed in Australia by:* Hay House Australia Pty. Ltd.: www.hayhouse.com.au • *Published and distributed in the United Kingdom by:* Hay House UK, Ltd.: www.hayhouse.co.uk • *Published and distributed in the Republic of South Africa by:* Hay House SA (Pty), Ltd.: www.hayhouse.co.za • *Distributed in Canada by:* Raincoast: www.raincoast.com • *Published in India by:* Hay House Publishers India: www.hayhouse.co.in

Project Editor: Marisa Bulzone
Indexer: Jay Kreider
Interior design: Tricia Breidenthal

Library of Congress Cataloging-in-Publication Data

Galvin, Meg.
  The SparkPeople cookbook : love your food, lose the weight / Meg Galvin and Stepfanie Romine ; food photographs by Randall Hoover Photography. — 1st ed.
     p. cm.
  Includes index.
   ISBN 978-1-4019-3132-2 (hardback)
 1. Low-calorie diet—Recipes. 2. Low-fat diet—Recipes. 3. Cooking, American. 4. Cookbooks. I. Romine, Stepfanie. II. Title.
  RM222.2.G345 2011
  641.5'6384—dc22
                              2011015662

Hardcover ISBN: 978-1-4019-3132-2
Digital ISBN: 978-1-4019-3134-6

14 13 12 11   4 3 2 1
1st edition, October 2011

Printed in China

To SparkPeople members everywhere, and
to anyone who thought they had to give up
the foods they love in order to be healthy.

CONTENTS

APPENDICES

Note to readers of E-books:
Any page numbers referred to (e.g., *see page* xv)
correspond to the printed version of the book.

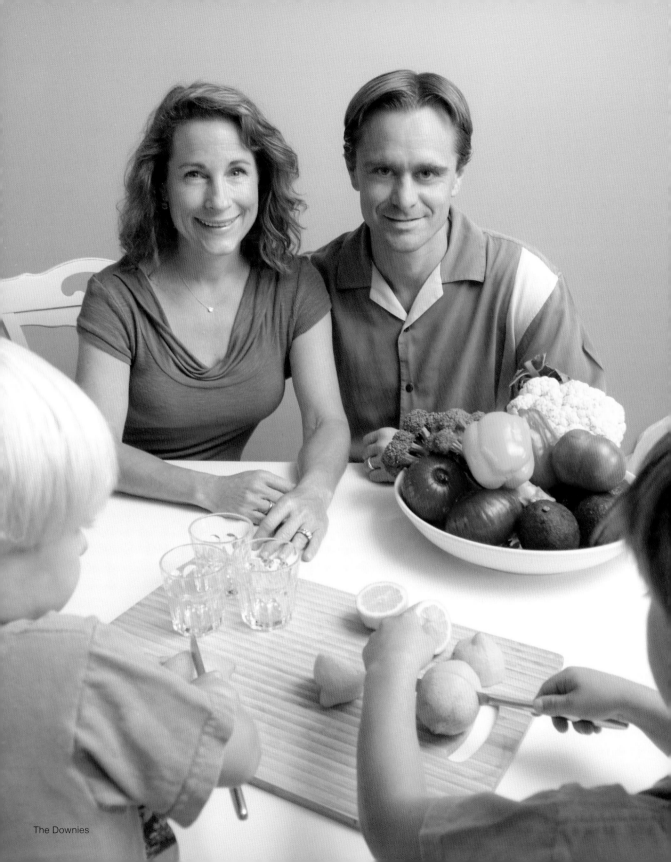

The Downies

INTRODUCTION

by Chris Downie, Founder, CEO, and Motivation
Expert of SparkPeople.com, and best-selling author of
The Spark

Back in 2007, the scale was inching closer to 300 pounds for Birdie Varnedore. Her closet was filled with sizes 26, 28, and 30, with some 24s for her "skinny days." (Though she admits: "The 26s only fit on a good day!") Despite living in Orlando, Florida, where temperatures in winter can top 80 degrees, she owned no clothing that came above the knee or elbow.

She was tired. She was obese. She was tired of being obese.

Birdie ate up to 6,000 calories a day, mostly in the form of simple carbs and junk food: cookies, cakes, ice cream, chocolate. "My meals were giant heaps of spaghetti, multiple dinner rolls with butter, large servings of rice and beans," she says.

As if medical school and then her fledgling career as a physician weren't hard enough, Birdie and her husband, Nick, were also building their family and today have five children. At night, when she studied, her appetite raged. To deal with the stress, she ate. Cartons of Chinese takeout, bags of Snickers candy bars, entire pizzas.

I'm a smart woman, a doctor, a neurologist! So why am I abusing my body? she thought. *As a physician, science and math are supposed to be my strengths! It's just calories in versus calories out. What's my problem?*

She was unhappy with her body and knew she was abusing herself, but she reasoned, "How else was I going to cope with the pressures of medical school, being broke, and raising a family? I kept piling on stress when I knew I couldn't handle it, but I didn't want to change, didn't want to give up my drug." Birdie's drug? Food.

Then, on July 23, 2007, she took the first step—after downing half a sheet cake at her youngest child's first birthday party. For a few weeks, she struggled on her own. Then she found SparkPeople, shed 140 pounds, and became the wife, mother, and physician she always knew she could be. It wasn't easy, but through

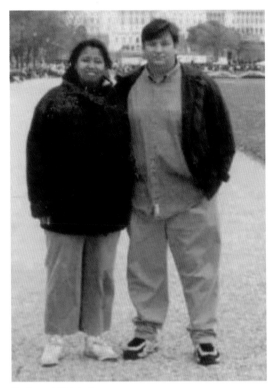

Birdie and Nick before

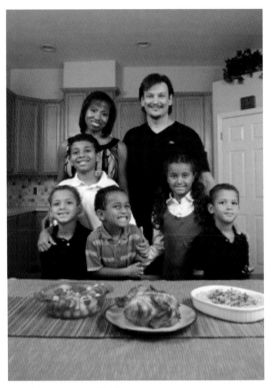

Birdie, Nick, and family after

exercise, calorie counting, hard work—and sheer determination—she reached her goal, even posing in a size 8-bikini in *People* magazine.

Despite her initial success with weight loss, there was an area of healthy living she had yet to tackle, one that she knew could be the key to keeping her weight off and staying healthy for the long run: cooking. Birdie has plenty of reasons to grab takeout or rip open a box at mealtime. But, as you might have guessed, she isn't a woman who gives up easily.

Saving money and improving her family's health—not to mention monitoring her sodium and saturated fat intake—are the driving forces behind her culinary education. And once again she has turned to SparkPeople and our

healthy-cooking site, SparkRecipes, for help. Meal by meal, and step by step, she and Nick are making the time to cook and becoming more comfortable in the kitchen. Their dinners aren't always gourmet, and they're not always eaten together, but they're healthy, made with love, and budget friendly. Most important, they're quick to prepare.

"I make the time," Birdie says. "Sometimes I prepare dinner very late in the evenings and the kids have to eat separately because I can't expect them to wait for me. I'm still trying to balance it all."

We all are.

Long before I started SparkPeople, I was an eager new graduate with an enviable first job: staff accountant for Procter & Gamble. But despite my success, I was stressed. My life revolved around work. I was certain I needed to make healthy living a priority. As I wrote in our first book, *The Spark: The 28-Day Breakthrough Plan for Losing Weight, Getting Fit, and Transforming Your Life,* "I realized there had to be a better way to fulfill my life. During lunch breaks I began reading goal-setting and leadership books, speckling the pages with ketchup. For the first time I made myself seriously focus on what I wanted for my future—to specifically name and visualize it." I knew the answer was a combination of things that are good for your body, like exercise and healthy food, and things that are good for your mind, like stress management, goal setting, leadership, and community support. I developed a program to help me reach my goals using these principles, and I soon began to thrive.

Using my newfound energy and confidence, I left my job and then began an online company called Up4Sale.com with three friends. Eventually, after a couple of years of working 100 hours a week and struggling along the way, that company was sold to eBay just before it went public. The stock from our sale exploded, and we were all millionaires many times over.

A few years later when I was ready to leave eBay, I returned to my dream of sharing my own program with others since it had worked so well for me, I started SparkPeople, using these same principles that had helped me gain momentum in my own journey to be happy and healthy: 10-minute bursts of fitness, small goals set along the way to achieve larger ones, a tight-knit network to offer support, and healthy, easy-to-prepare food to fuel an active life.

As SparkPeople grew, we realized that our members loved to eat but needed help tracking their favorite recipes and finding healthy new ones. SparkRecipes, which is now the web's largest healthy-recipe site, was born. In the tens of millions of comments on the site, we've been told that, to fit into a weight-loss plan, a recipe must meet some key criteria: it must be easy to make, it must be delicious, and it must be healthy enough to fuel your body and hearty enough to keep hunger at bay for a few hours. In 2008, to further expand SparkRecipes, we brought healthy-cooking expert Meg Galvin on to our team. Her "Healthy Home Cooking" recipes, videos, and blogs were an instant hit with members.

Not too long after, we published *The Spark,* along with our groundbreaking Secrets of Success survey. In it, we learned that cooking has a profound effect on members' weight-loss success, bolstering what they'd been telling us anecdotally for years. The findings prompted us to write *The SparkPeople Cookbook.* It's unlike any cookbook you've ever read.

Like the site that inspired it, this cookbook is intended to guide you, step by step and goal by goal, to become a healthier you. We don't expect you to become a gourmet healthy chef overnight. Instead, you can take it at your own pace and find ways to improve your diet by cooking one meal at a time. It's an approach that's worked for countless members, including Leah Reed, aka SPRING4FAL, who was featured in our first book.

Back then, Leah was struggling to get comfortable in the kitchen. Now 60 pounds lighter and armed with quick and easy healthy recipes from Chef Meg and SparkRecipes, she says she's made great progress and actually enjoys cooking.

Though Leah, a marathon runner, doesn't cook every night and sometimes reaches for low-sodium frozen meals supplemented with extra vegetables, she sees healthy cooking as an ongoing goal. She says, "The biggest lesson I have learned in the kitchen is to continue to try and don't give up!" She can't wait to try more recipes in the book.

Written by our very own Chef Meg, SparkRecipes editor Stepfanie Romine, and the SparkPeople team, this cookbook shows that healthy eating can be simple and fun. Even better, it shows that eating for health and weight loss can be delicious and satisfying—that you can eat to lose weight but still absolutely love your food. In fact, it proves it! While developing the cookbook, we conducted a formal taste test and follow-up pilot program to show that if people ate flavorful, satisfying foods, prepared to optimize taste but minimize fat and calories, they could eat fewer calories without even realizing it, yet be more satisfied while losing weight! (You might be shocked to know this, but we learned that 68 percent of "dieters" still believe you have to eat bland foods you don't like in order to lose weight—and of course, SparkPeople had to prove them wrong!)

If you haven't yet tried one of Chef Meg's healthy and satisfying recipes, you're in for a treat. We call her "Chef Meg," but in the culinary world she's known as Meg Galvin, one of only 20 women with the designation of World Master Chef. Chef Meg is an instructor at the renowned Midwest Culinary Institute at Cincinnati State Technical and Community College, where she teaches classes in both classical cooking and healthy cooking. She is classically trained, with a certificate from Le Cordon Bleu in London and several awards from prestigious culinary associations. At first one might think it ironic that a healthy-cooking expert trained as a French chef, learning to make the perfect hollandaise sauce and the flakiest pastries with gobs of real butter! But, once you taste Meg's healthy foods, you then understand that the classic training and primary focus on flavor and taste have given her an arsenal of tips and tricks to get the most flavor and pleasure from foods—without all the fat and calories. Cooking this way allows you to eat the foods you most love, without the guilt or extra pounds. It *has* to taste good or Meg isn't satisfied!

Chef Meg's cooking philosophy—a result of her upbringing on a farm, her classic culinary training, and her passion for health and fitness—and SparkPeople's nutritional guidelines, which our head dietitian Becky Hand outlines in Chapter 2, perfectly align: an abundance of *real foods* like fruits and vegetables; plenty of whole grains, lean protein, and low-fat dairy; and salt, fat, and sugar used in moderation. No food group is excluded (she even uses ingredients long-considered taboo for dieters like butter and bacon!), and our plates are full of colors, flavors, and textures. Even better: our "diet" (really a healthy eating plan) bans bland diet foods, meager portions, and growling bellies. Our recipes replace extra fat with added flavor, extra calories with great tastes. You'll learn to love the food you eat, ditch the diet forever, and still lose weight.

My own family follows this same philosophy, with some modifications because of my oldest son's severe food allergies. Finding a diet that works for us all has been difficult, but my wife, Karina, has been amazing in meeting this challenge. She has fun transforming ordinary recipes into dishes that are both healthy and flavorful, and one of our favorite moments as a family is coming together for a meal—especially the Honey-Ginger Salmon on page 227. This experience has helped us focus on real foods, and best of all, our son's allergies have improved. We believe Karina's healthy, delicious cooking is at least partly responsible for that.

Karina and I are a great team. She helps me stay on track with nutrition, and I help motivate her with fitness. Our collaboration highlights one of the most important reasons for cooking this way: in addition to the pleasure of eating good food, we want to experience the most out of life. Fueling our bodies the right way lets us have energy to really live life! As parents, we also feel the responsibility to give our kids a great start since what they eat now can have a tremendous impact on their future. (If you're struggling with the same concerns for your children's eating habits, see Raising Kids to be Healthy Eaters on page 389.)

Because of my experiences both with my own family and my SparkPeople family, I'm so excited to share this cookbook with you. I hope it helps you learn to love the food *you* eat and reach your most important goals in life. Spark-People is America's largest healthy-living website because we deliver straightforward advice, manageable steps toward a better you, and support that really works. This book takes the same approach. We believe that once you're armed with the knowledge and the recipes that let you eat what you want most, you can optimize your health and lose weight without deprivation! Best of all, it's an approach that works for everybody. You don't need expensive kitchen gadgets, special foods, or a culinary degree—just a willingness to learn to cook the food you love.

GET READY

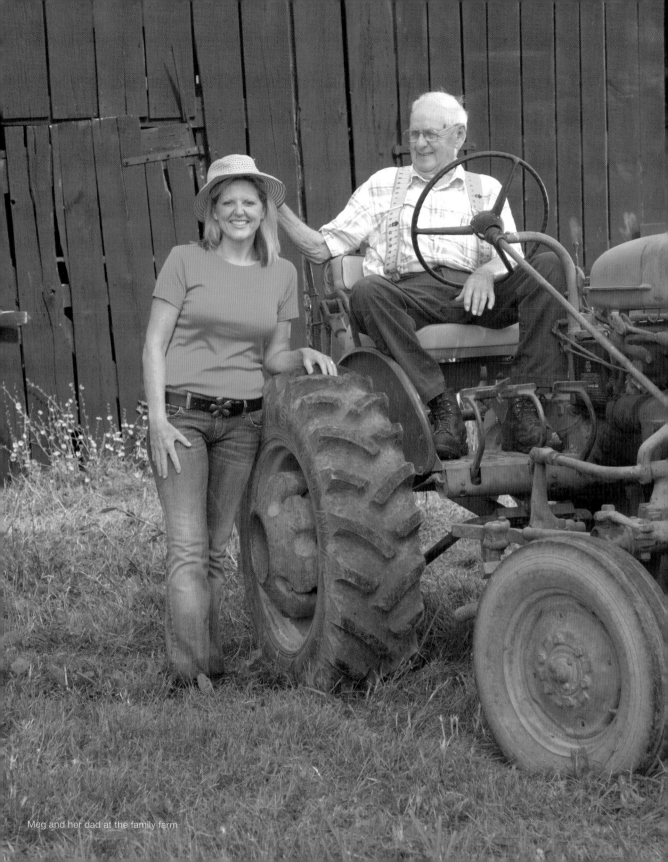

Meg and her dad at the family farm

SATISFYING, SUSTAINING, AND STRESS-FREE EATING

I'm Meg Galvin, otherwise known as Chef Meg. I'm a culinary instructor, decorated chef, and healthy-cooking expert at SparkPeople .com. Healthy living is a deep passion of mine, but so is good food. I fell in love with cooking partly because of the warm, happy memories of life on my family's farm—with fresh, abundant food always at the center. Today I'm also a distance runner and a mom. Those two roles steer my palate and my passion away from the heavy "mother sauces" and rich meats I learned to prepare in culinary school, toward delicious food that provides pleasure for all who eat it—without adding pounds to anyone's waistline.

"How do you do it?" friends, neighbors, and colleagues ask. "How do you cook like this and look like that?" Simple. I've found a way to cook the food I love to eat in ways that satisfy me without breaking the calorie budget. I pack flavor and nutrition into every bite, without adding

excess fat, calories, or carbs; which means I'm never deprived and I enjoy everything I eat. By adopting this attitude and cooking and eating only foods that *you* love, you'll feel satisfied at every meal, and when you're satisfied, you're less tempted to overeat or graze later on.

As the country's largest health and fitness website, we encourage everyone to make life an adventure, set goals and reach them, one step at a time. After *The Spark* became a *New York Times* bestseller, we heard from people that our quick bursts of fitness and endless motivation were helping them change their lives—but they still needed help in the kitchen. Money, knowledge, but, most important, time were keeping them from fully reaching their nutrition and health goals.

Twenty-something Alexa is down 90 pounds, thanks in large part to the healthy attitudes and affinity for "real food" she's developed over the last four years on SparkPeople. Living in San Francisco means she has access to fresh and interesting ingredients, but her fast-paced life can leave her with limited time to cook them. For Alexa, any recipe "needs to be simple, fit my nutritional needs, and most of all, it must taste good."

This sentiment also echoes Birdie and Nick's experiences as they adopt cooking at home as a new way of staying fit.

AN EDUCATION IN HEALTHY COOKING

We wrote this book for Alexa, Birdie, Nick, and everyone else we know who's trying to balance healthy living with real life. After months of testing and tasting, we've created what will become your new favorite cookbook. It's more than a collection of recipes; it's an education in how healthy recipes can taste great *and* let you lose weight. SparkPeople is decidedly of the "teach a man to fish" school of thought, so we viewed each recipe as a learning experience, a chance to practice a healthy-cooking technique and integrate it into your everyday life. Soon, you'll be removing the training wheels and creating healthy recipes of your own.

While calorie counts, ingredient lists, and nutrition info can make healthy eating seem like a great deal to digest, after cooking just a few of our recipes, you'll soon find that healthy eating really involves a natural, common-sense approach—real foods in the right proportions, packed with great taste and nutrition. For me, food has always had to taste good *and* fuel me throughout my busy life—and it has to satisfy my family as well. These recipes have all been

tested by my three teen sons and my husband. With few exceptions, they never would think of what they were eating as "diet" recipes or "health food."

And, as a chef, I really have to be committed to eating well and not overeating because gaining weight is a real hazard in my line of work! I battled my weight while in culinary school and after my sons were born, so I have learned first-hand how to balance eating to live and living to eat! I also weaned myself away from baking and then eating as an emotional outlet. What works for me—aside from my regular early-morning workouts—is creating food that is every bit as delicious as it is good for me. I'm a chef; I love food! So, I can't do deprivation. Instead, I've committed to making healthy food taste good and making every bite count. I have some other tricks to keep the weight off, like sampling little bites of lots of fabulous foods rather than eating whole platefuls and "saving" room in my calorie budget by eating less at some meals so that I can indulge at others.

But strategy No. 1 is eating foods I love so that I don't feel deprived, and loving the food I eat so much that I will be satisfied with a meal that fits my diet plan.

How do I create such great food that helps keep me slim? I draw heavily from my training. I rely on simple swaps of nutrient-dense ingredients; low-calorie, flavor-maximizing cooking techniques; food choices and combinations that complement the other tastes in the dish; plus plenty of spices, herbs, and seasonings that make food irresistible without excess fat or calories. Coupled with my use of whole, fresh, hearty foods that have innate qualities that satisfy us, these techniques yield meals that are healthy and delicious. While some low-fat products are fantastic, I steer clear of overprocessed "diet" foods because they don't satiate me and I end up eating more. Instead, I cut calories and fat by choosing low- or non-caloric cooking techniques and save room for some rich and savory ingredients like a little bit of butter, cream, bacon, or full-fat cheese—the ones that make your taste buds quiver with excitement. If you use those ingredients in the right amounts, you get the benefit of their flavors and satisfaction without breaking the calorie bank.

From family favorites like Dark Chocolate Cake (page 360) and Slimmer Sloppy Joes (page 221) to exciting flavor combinations like Grilled Shrimp with Jicama-Grapefruit Slaw (page 119) and Baked Sunburst Fries (page 319), we have dishes for every mood and every night. Because we believe in flexibility, we've included tips to help you fit these dishes into your budget and schedule. SparkPeople members share how they've adapted these recipes, and we've added my chef secrets that streamline the cooking process. Whether you're a novice cook taking the first steps to improve your health, or just looking for new, nutritious recipes to add to your repertoire, this cookbook can help you. This will become your healthy-cooking bible.

In *The SparkPeople Love Your Food, Lose the Weight Cookbook* you'll find:

- More than 160 recipes, plus hundreds of variations—all guaranteed to be satisfying, sustaining, and stress-free!

- "Slim It Down" options for dozens of the recipes, so that those of us who are on stricter weight-loss plans can eat well on even fewer calories.

- Full nutrition info for each recipe.

- "Make It a Meal" features—quick and tasty suggestions to turn every main dish into a well-balanced meal in just minutes.

- A full 150 meal ideas and recipes that take 30 minutes or less to prepare—plus dozens of other, more elaborate meals for days when you have more time to cook.

- Expert tips and tricks to increase flavor and satiety while cutting unnecessary calories, fat, and salt.

- A healthy pantry checklist, a list of cheap but nutritious foods, and sidebars on new-to-you "superfoods."

- Two weeks of meal plans—with breakfast, lunch, dinner, and two snacks—all for 1,400–1,600 calories.

- Stories of how real people like you used these recipes and our plan to lose weight and eat the foods they love.

- Step-by-step guides to all the healthy cooking techniques you'll need, plus a list of equipment for a healthy kitchen.

You'll also read all about our "Ditch the Diet" Taste Test, which proved once and for all that you don't have to eat boring and tasteless food to lose weight. In the taste test, we saw that many yo-yo dieters think that to lose weight, they have to deprive themselves and eat the blandest or most stripped-down foods possible. Some dieters will even choose foods they don't like eating because they believe they'll lose weight faster!

We proved to them that our tasty foods were not only more nourishing but also contained fewer calories.

In the follow-up pilot program, participants raved about our recipes—and were shocked to discover the meal we served them had 100 calories less than a typical diet meal. Not only did they say they felt satisfied, they still felt sustained when they went home three hours later.

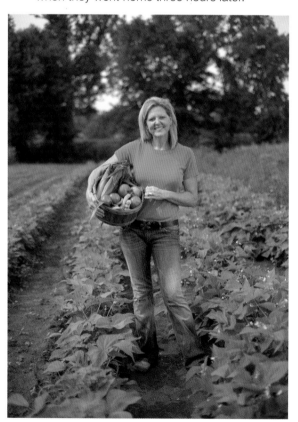

Meg and the summer harvest

Once they cooked these recipes for themselves, they raved about how stress-free the dishes were. Turned loose with a few more of our recipes and two weeks to try them at home, our eager taste-testers reported impressive results. Renee lost 6½ pounds—and broke through a plateau—while Tara (you'll meet her later in the book) came within one pound of her goal weight, which she reached one week after that.

CHANGING LIVES, ONE FAMILY DINNER AT A TIME

This cookbook—and the SparkRecipes that inspired it—has already changed lives. By focusing on satisfaction and flavor, our healthy recipes can sway even the diehard meat-and-potatoes crowd, as SparkPeople member REVELATIONGIRL learned. She lost 30 pounds and changed the way her family eats forever:

"I love to cook, but I am a country cook— big, heavy, full-course meals to feed an army. We always loved our salad, as long as it was accompanied by meat, mashed potatoes and gravy, creamy veggies, and dessert. Through SparkPeople, I've made one little change after another until my suppers today really do not resemble those of the last 25 years. I've dropped the sauces, and my family has discovered that they love roasted veggies. The meat is more often a lean chicken cooked with a recipe I've found on the site. I have introduced things like whole-wheat pasta, whole-grain breads, and low-fat cheeses, which have become staples.

"Using SparkPeople has made me very aware now of what we are lacking and how many empty or unhealthy calories my family was consuming. My family is everything to me and feeding them well, instead of feeding them too much, has become the goal. My younger son has also lost 30 pounds with the changes we've made in the last six months. My daughter-in-law has lost 25 pounds and is very close to her goal weight. Although my husband and older son are at healthy weights, I am pleased knowing they are eating properly now and getting the nutrition they need."

In contrast to diet programs that expect perfection, focus on deprivation, and set you up for long-term failure and disappointment, Spark-People's recipes fit into your real life and allow you to enjoy food without feeling guilty. We want you to eat what you love and never feel deprived! We hope that you'll add these recipes to your daily life, and that they'll help you be healthier, happier, more satisfied, and less stressed at mealtime.

MAINTAINING A SATISFYING, SUSTAINING, AND STRESS-FREE DIET

These days, everyone keeps saying we've forgotten how to eat. But if you look around you'll see that, with waistlines expanding and life expectancies decreasing, we're actually quite good at eating. In fact, what we've forgotten how to do is taste. The good news is that retraining your palate is not as hard as it seems, as REV-ELATIONGIRL and her family learned.

Food That's Satisfying. To lose weight, get healthy, and forge a healthy relationship with food, you need to like the food you're eating. It's not enough for the food to just be nutritious. It must also be delicious, or eating will feel like punishment. Unlike most diet recipes, which strip away ingredients and flavor, SparkPeople recipes focus on adding ingredients and layers of flavor so that every bite is satisfying.

Close your eyes and think about the most memorable meals of your life.

I think first about my mom's homemade chicken pot pie, made from scratch and at my request, on all special occasions: flaky crust, made with real butter, that she'd rolled out by hand. Tender, juicy chicken we'd raised ourselves, crisp and sweet vegetables from the garden, and just enough rich, creamy sauce to bind it all together.

I remember watching her in the kitchen as she made enough to feed six growing kids and her hard-working farmer husband. Her food was simple, but it was made with love and it lingers in my memory more than 35 years later.

My mind travels 15 years forward, across the ocean, to a little Indian restaurant called the Bombay Brasserie. It was my mom's last night in London, and we dined with my two uncles, who would be looking after me while I was in culinary school. Tandoori spices tickled my throat and brought tears to my eyes. The raita, a balance of cool, acidic cucumber and creamy yogurt, soothed my mouth, while the perfect simplicity of the lentil soup that accompanied it made my mind race. The next day I would begin training to become a chef, but tonight, I was still a farm girl from Kentucky, with a palate more accustomed to Swiss steak and roast chicken than to the spicy garam masala that lay before me.

Years later, I had another standout food moment, this one with no remarkable environmental influences. I remember the most perfect apple, impulsively grabbed to quiet a rumbling stomach while grocery shopping for my own family.

The Granny Smith's taut skin gave way to the crisp flesh, with just the right balance of sweet and sour. Juices ran down my hand as I closed my eyes and enjoyed a moment of pure peace, sitting in my car, giving in fully to the experience of smelling, tasting, and feeling that simple, flawless piece of fruit.

We all have meals that conjure memories, but when we delve deeper, we realize that there's more to those experiences than eating. It helps to understand that it's not just the food—it's what (and who) surrounds the food that counts.

Food That's Sustaining. How many times have you eaten at a restaurant, only to come home hungry? When was the last time you were "on a diet" yet ended up gaining weight because you couldn't stop eating? How often do you find yourself staring mindlessly into the fridge or the pantry after dinner, looking for something that hits the spot?

We've all been there. Diet foods are bland (we proved that while writing this book—and we'll tell you all about it in the next chapter) and the portions are too small. If you are lucky enough to find a healthy restaurant option, it's usually as lacking in substance as it is in flavor.

Healthy living doesn't have to be that way. SparkPeople never would have grown into America's largest healthy-living community if that were the case. We believe that eating right is not about deprivation. It's not about the word "no." It's definitely not a time to be a food martyr, sacrificing all flavor and joy for the sake of a few measly pounds.

With the help of a few key principles like heart-healthy fats, lean proteins, fiber-rich whole grains, and voluminous fruits and vegetables, these meals will keep you—and your entire family—comfortably full and happy until the next one. No growling bellies, no meager portions, and no bland food—we promise!

Food That's Stress-Free. This cookbook is not part of a fad diet that will help you achieve the perfect body. It isn't about standing over a hot stove for hours on end. And it isn't about spending your whole paycheck on obscure ingredients and expensive products. (If I couldn't find an ingredient at my neighborhood supermarket in northern Kentucky, it didn't make it in the book.) It's about finding that balance between food and the rest of your life, about eating the way we were meant to eat, and about making the right choices for you and your family. It's about eating more but being satisfied with fewer calories. It's about using fat, sugar, and salt judiciously; appreciating the natural flavors of food; and reaching for other flavor-enhancing ingredients and techniques whenever possible.

At our SparkPeople conventions, our head dietitian, Becky Hand, delivers a presentation about determining your eating style. Before she starts speaking, she hands out a small packet of trail mix (find the recipe on page 338). A snack during a talk on nutrition? Members aren't sure what to expect.

She asks them to open the packet, select a piece, and place it in their mouths. Then they chew, closing their eyes, allowing all of their senses to take over. Instead of reaching immediately for a second piece, they pause, reflecting on the bite they ate. Those almonds, peanuts, raisins, and chocolate candies have a lingering effect, and they're eating with full awareness and enjoying single bites and moderate portions more than ever before.

Successful SparkPeople members apply that principle to their own meals and their own lives. They allow their senses to really experience the food. They eat, but they don't overeat because what they eat satisfies them. They don't turn down dessert, and they don't skimp on flavor. They indulge at times and abstain at others—and make sure every bite counts.

The effects of healthy eating permeate members' entire lives, to which SASSYBEAN1 can attest. At almost 50, the hospice nurse from Austin has been overweight her entire life, but that's changing "10 percent at a time" with the help of SparkPeople.

"I feel so positive about everything, and I *love* to exercise (never thought I'd say that!). My tastes have changed so much that I am putting less sweetener in my coffee or tea, and I have a feeling that eventually I'll stop sweetening it. Fruits are the sweetest things I've ever tasted now. I reach for fruits and vegetables for snacks, and high-fat foods leave a layer of sludge on my tongue."

Because eating is only half of the equation, let's take a look at how the simple act of cooking (and cooking simply) can help you lose weight, feel better, and become a healthier person.

These recipes will help you recapture the joy of eating, retrain your palate to appreciate food's natural goodness, and resurrect the family meal. In each chapter, you'll learn how to make over a meal with healthy and easy-to-follow recipes that load up on flavor in the right proportions. We delve into the science of satisfaction, introduce new and nutritious ingredients, teach you the basics of cooking, and help you integrate healthy habits into your life so you can love your food, lose the weight, and ditch the diet forever. Like the SparkPeople plan upon which this cookbook is based, we rely on small steps to achieve great results—and change lives forever.

THE SCIENCE
OF SATISFACTION

Molière told us we should eat to live, but most of us live to eat—grabbing unhealthy foods on the run, munching mindlessly when we're stressed out, overeating at mealtime and in between. Food, as the source of energy and nutrition for our bodies, is what allows us to get off the couch, run a 5K, and chase after our kids all day. It's also, as we know, a source of pleasure. As much as we might try to dissociate food and emotions, the two are inextricably linked. How do you strike a balance so that you can celebrate and enjoy food without overdoing it or obsessing about it? The trick is the right food in the right proportions, prepared to taste great and satisfy you on every level. Each bite you take should bring you joy, without any feeling of guilt or remorse. Food should also satisfy us, body and mind. It should provide real pleasure *and* nutrients that keep us fueled and prevent us from that incessant sense of never getting enough to eat. Food is so very fundamental to our lives, loving the food you eat without feeling deprived is the only way to live.

We suspected that anyone stuck in a diet rut wasn't eating food they loved. So we asked members: have you ever eaten foods you don't like in an effort to lose weight or improve your health? The answers poured in by the thousands, and the consensus was a resounding "Yes": 68 percent have eaten foods they don't like to try to shed pounds or get healthy.

Comeka, a SparkPeople member from Texas, was among them.

"When I believed in 'dieting,' I ate all kinds of foods I didn't like because I thought that was the only way to lose weight—cottage cheese, plain tuna, grapefruit, and that nasty cabbage soup come to mind in particular," she said. "Luckily, I found SparkPeople and now know that there are many, many tasty foods that I love that will work well in my healthy-eating plan. No more forcing myself to eat stuff I don't love!" In our Ditch the Diet Taste Test, designed with SparkPeople's Head Dietitian Becky Hand and conducted at the Midwest Culinary Institute, we saw firsthand that breaking the cycle of yo-yo dieting, trusting your taste buds, and starting to take pleasure in healthy eating is possible. To understand how, let's examine the basics behind the science of satisfaction, starting with the science of hunger.

THE SCIENCE OF HUNGER

Hunger describes the escalating, physiological sensations you experience when your body actually needs food: beginning with rumbling, unpleasant stomach contractions (hunger pangs), mild lightheadedness, difficulty concentrating, irritability, and finally faintness and headaches. For most people who regularly eat a balanced diet with adequate calories, hunger will set in about four hours after the last meal and will escalate after about five hours.

Feelings of fullness or satiety will occur when your stomach reaches a certain level of fullness (about 75 percent of its maximum capacity). These sensations also escalate from mild fullness, to "stuffed," to bloated and uncomfortable.

Ignoring all other emotional and environmental signals, your brain will tell you when you've had enough to eat, though it takes about 20 minutes for the message to travel from your stomach.

That's what happens in a perfect world.

In reality, we don't eat because we're hungry, and we don't eat foods as Mother Nature intended. We eat away from home; out of boxes, cans, and pouches; in front of the TV; and in the car. We eat on the run, and we snack instead of eating meals. Our food is oversalted, underspiced, overspiced, watered-down, condensed, dehydrated, rehydrated, hydrogenated, crusted, filled, and stuffed—and so are we.

There's no balance, and society's bad eating habits have made "Goldilocks eaters" out of all of us. At restaurants, we're served oversized portions that are often brimming with salt, sugar, and fat. Food makers tempt us with snacks, desserts, and "diet" foods that fill our bodies with empty calories without filling us up. Between our busy lives and the convenience of these creations, we fall prey to the drive-thru and processed foods.

We leave the table wanting more, never satisfied. Like our flaxen-haired fairy-tale heroine, we're constantly on the hunt for that proverbial perfect bowl of porridge, for that food that's "just right."[1]

It boils down to the fact that we've lost our sense of taste, and we've forgotten how truly *good* good food is. Food should nourish and satisfy, comfort and nurture. All hope isn't lost, and there's a movement afoot to reclaim food's rightful place at the center of the family. Food unites us, it excites us, it gives a reason to gather together. SparkPeople members, who have a love for food, who eat at home or as a family whenever possible, who value homemade over processed, are at the center of a healthy-eating revolution

*AMBER512, who has lost more than 90 pounds, describes how she and her husband's relationship with food has changed. "We can't wait to get back to normal after we go on vacation. It feels great at first to be a little lax on healthy eating, but we arrive home and can't wait to get right back on track."

Since committing to healthy eating in September 2008, MIEZEKATZE's relationship with junk food has completely changed. "The biggest difference for me is that it doesn't take nearly as much food as it used to for me to feel full! I eat pretty healthy 90 percent of the time, but when I indulge a bit on that other 10 percent, I find I cannot eat very much of it or else I'll feel 'bleh.' Before, I had no problem wolfing down bad-for-you foods."

Another member wrote to us about a recent trip to a buffet. That time, she chose lean turkey breast, broccolini, green salad, and roasted root vegetables. She says, "I noticed the difference in my plate and others'. My tastes have definitely changed. My meal was delicious and I enjoyed every bite. As I looked at what others had put on their plates, it didn't even look appetizing to me."

After shedding more than 100 pounds, Frances says she now craves vegetables—which she previously had to choke down. She loves the taste of pure, unadulterated veggies, which surprised her at first.

REAL FOOD TASTES GOOD

Real food tastes good, but only if you take the time to enjoy it, to slow down and savor it, not just get it to your stomach as quickly as possible. Chewing your food thoroughly is actually the first step in the complex process of digestion, and if you glaze over it, just chewing the minimum amount of times necessary to get the food down your esophagus, you're actually compromising this process and depriving your taste buds of maximum satisfaction. And it's a mistake many people make.

What effect does all of this have on weight loss and satisfaction? Eating is about more than fueling your body and chewing and swallowing your food. The routines, environment, and even the company you keep while eating can affect your weight, according to researchers.

Eating more slowly gives your body a chance to tell your mind that it's full, so that you stop eating before you go overboard. In a preliminary study presented at the North American Association for the Study of Obesity's Annual Scientific Meeting in 2004, study subjects ate less when they were instructed to eat more slowly.[2]

We see a lot in the news these days about the importance of the family dinner table—and with good reason. A 2006 Census Bureau statistic cites a 25 percent drop in the number of parents and children who eat both breakfast and dinner together between early childhood and adolescence.

What kind of damage are we doing to our children by not making mealtime a priority? The evidence is clear:

- A September 2009 study found that the more often children have dinner with their parents—free from distractions like cell phones, laptops, and TVs—the less likely they are to smoke, drink, or use drugs.[3]

- A study published in the March 2010 issue of the journal *Pediatrics* found that children who regularly ate dinner as a family, had regular and adequate sleep, and had limited access to "screen" media such as television and computers, were less likely to be obese than peers who didn't follow the same habits.[4]

- In 1975, 25 percent of all money spent on food in the United States was on meals and snacks consumed at restaurants. By 2008, that figure had risen to 50 percent.[5]

We've set out to compile a collection of recipes that puts flavor at the center of the plate. Having delicious, satisfying food to eat gives us a great reason to slow down and love every bite! It's what helps us ditch our diets forever, love our food, and still lose the weight and keep it off.

A PRACTICAL AND FUN APPROACH TO NUTRITION

It's terrifying stats like those above that motivate and encourage Becky Hand, SparkPeople's head dietitian. Becky, who has a bachelor's degree in food, nutrition, and dietetics from Marian College, a master's degree in health promotion and education from the University of Cincinnati, and more than 25 years of nutrition experience in hospital and community settings, knows that counting calories and dieting can be dull. That's why she makes nutrition fun and practical.

She and I share similar passions for family and food. Becky lives on a farm with her husband and son in southern Indiana. (She also has a daughter in college.) The closest fast-food restaurant is 20 minutes away, and the nearest shopping mall is an hour's drive away, but she prefers to tend her vegetable garden and create new recipes. Like me, she uses her family as guinea pigs—and they love the healthy dishes she creates.

Becky says, "My children will tell you that I am fixated on eating meals together as a family at the kitchen table. This is often the only chance we have to connect and catch up. It is a time to comfort the pains of the day and celebrate the joys of living."

She's also passionate about helping people. A licensed and registered dietitian, she teaches weight-management classes for children and adults, conducts cooking classes and food demonstrations, assists school districts in implementing wellness policies—and presents at SparkPeople conventions.

Whether she's talking to schoolchildren, a Scout troop, college students, high-school athletes, a women's club, church group, or corporate America, she wants nutrition to be practical, easy to apply, and fun!

PROOF YOU'LL BE SATISFIED

Here's how Becky applies the Science of Satisfaction to real life:

Satiety (suh-TIE-uh-tee) is that wonderfully pleasant feeling of fullness you get as you eat, when you're no longer hungry but aren't overly stuffed or uncomfortable. You are just satisfied beyond desire. The more satisfied you feel after a meal, the less you'll eat later. So how do you increase satiety without eating more?

When making food choices, it's still important to meet the nutrition recommendations outlined later in this chapter. But our No. 1 tip to stay fuller longer is to lean on low-density foods. Calorie density refers to the number of calories per gram of food. Foods that are high in calorie density contain a high number of calories per gram; foods that are low in calorie density contain a low number of calories per gram. Calorie density is the key to feeling full without overeating.

When you eat too many calorie-dense foods, you end up consuming a lot of calories to fill your belly. If you focus on low calorie density foods, such as those used in our recipes, you can fill up on fewer calories because low-density foods contain a lot more water, which adds weight and volume to the food, but no calories.

Just drinking a glass of water along with the meal does not provide the same degree of satiety. Research, including a yearlong study at Penn State University, has shown that to reduce hunger and boost fullness, *the water has to be in the food*.[6] Why? Because there are separate mechanisms in the brain to control hunger and thirst. If the food you eat contains the water, it will stay in the stomach longer while the food is being digested. Beyond that, there is also the psychological component of eating food versus drinking water. When you eat food, even water-rich food, you get more sensory stimulation because you have more food going through your mouth and you're eating for a longer period of time, both of which help you feel more satisfied with your meal.

The following water-rich food choices contain about 90-percent bound water and can have a great impact on the calorie density of your diet.

- *EAT MORE broth-based soups.* (See Chapter 6 for plenty of soup recipes.)

- *EAT MORE leafy greens* like lettuce, baby spinach, and mixed salad greens with low-fat dressing. (We have more than a dozen green-salad recipes in Chapter 5.)

- *EAT MORE fruits* like apples, blueberries, cantaloupe, grapefruit, oranges, peaches, strawberries, and watermelon. (Try our Fruit Salad with Poppy Seed Dressing on page 346.)

- *EAT MORE nonstarchy vegetables* like asparagus, broccoli, carrots, cauliflower, celery, cucumbers, tomatoes, and winter squash. (Chapter 10 is chock full of vegetable recipes, but 30 of our recipes contain more than one serving of fruits and/or vegetables!)

Fill Up on Fiber

Fiber contains only 1.5 to 2.5 calories per gram, while other carbohydrates contain 4 calories per gram. Fiber-rich foods also necessitate more chewing and slow the passage of food through the digestive tract. The fiber in carbohydrates helps prevent those peaks and valleys in blood-sugar levels that can cause cravings and poor food choices. They also may stimulate a satiety hormone in the brain.

- *EAT MORE fiber* from whole grains, fruits, and vegetables with skins, beans, lentils, and legumes. Aim for 25 to 35 grams each day to help reduce your calorie intake and increase your satiety level. Read more about carbohydrates—and the importance of getting your 25 to 35 grams of fiber daily—in Chapter 9.

Lean on Protein

Studies suggest that protein appears to help prolong satiety more than carbohydrates or fat can. Meeting your protein needs is important, but eating more protein than your body needs will *not* boost your metabolism.

- *EAT MORE lean protein* from meats, chicken, seafood, low-fat dairy, legumes, lentils, and soy products. For meat, poultry, and seafood recipes, check out Chapter 7. We cover meat-free recipes in Chapter 8.

Fit In the Fat

Cutting fat intake reduces the calorie density of a food. In other words, you get a bigger portion of food for the same calories when it has fewer fat grams. However, if you go too low in fat you won't enjoy the flavor, texture, or satiety of your food. Plus dietary fat is essential for staying healthy.

- *EAT ENOUGH fat* (20 percent to 35 percent of your daily calories). This will bring the pleasure and satisfaction back to your meals so you're less likely to overeat later. We've eliminated fat where you don't need it and opted for reduced-fat and healthier sources wherever possible. Fat-free diets were a passing fad, but many people still attempt to adhere to them, we learned in our Ditch the Diet Taste Test. Later in this chapter, we'll debunk them.

Drink Up!

Drinking water can help with your weight-management program, especially if you are substituting it for high-calorie beverages. Drinking water throughout the day also keeps hands busy so that you're less likely to eat out of habit or boredom. SparkPeople recommends 8 cups a day.

THE BASIS OF OUR SPARKPEOPLE "DIET"

So why are we unable to achieve that perfect level of satiety? Because most of us are overfed but undernourished. Though we're eating more than we should, obtaining good nutrition can be a challenge. For optimum health, we recommend a balanced diet filled with a variety of good, whole foods that will contribute the more than 45 different nutrients that your body needs each day. These can be divided into two classes: macronutrients (carbohydrates, proteins, and fat) and micronutrients (minerals such as iron, calcium, and zinc and vitamins such as A, B_{12}, and D).

Each nutrient has a particular job to perform in the building, maintenance, and operation of your body. Some jobs require that nutrients work together as a team. These jobs are nutrient-specific and cannot be done by other nutrients; an extra supply of one nutrient cannot make up for a shortage of another. That's why a balanced diet that includes a variety of foods from all food groups is so essential. Your body requires all these nutrients, not simply a few. Some must be replenished every day from food, while others can be stored in the body for future use.

To eat a healthy, nutrient-packed diet, choose a wide variety of foods using these guidelines:

PORTION SIZES		
EXAMPLE	ONE SERVING	LOOKS LIKE
Grains: 6 to 11 Servings Daily		
Bread	1 ounce (1 small slice, ½ bagel, ½ bun)	Index card
Cooked grains	½ cup cooked oats, rice, pasta	Billiard ball
Dry cereal	½ cup flakes, puffed rice, shredded wheat	Billiard ball
Vegetables and fruits: 5 to 9 servings daily		
Fruit	½ cup fresh, canned, frozen fruit	Billiard ball
Dried fruit	¼ cup raisins, prunes, apricots	An egg

PORTION SIZES		
EXAMPLE	ONE SERVING	LOOKS LIKE
Juice	6 ounces 100% fruit or vegetable juice	Hockey puck
Raw vegetables	1 cup leafy greens, baby carrots	Baseball
Cooked vegetables	½ cup cooked broccoli, potatoes	Billiard ball
Protein: 2 to 3 servings daily		
Meat & Tofu	3 ounces cooked beef, poultry, fish, tofu	Deck of cards
Beans	½ cup cooked beans, split peas, legumes	Billiard ball
Nuts & Seeds	2 tbsp nuts, seeds, nut butters	Ping-Pong ball
Dairy: 2 to 3 servings daily		
Cheese	1 ounce or 1 thin slice of cheese	A pair of dice
Milk	1 cup milk or yogurt (or calcium-fortified nondairy equivalents)	Baseball
Fats: Use sparingly		
Fat & Oil	1 tsp butter, margarine, oil	One die

While all foods found in nature offer at least some health benefits, some are better than others. Following the philosophy of making every bite count, we've created a healthy pantry checklist—full of foods that pack a powerful nutrient punch, from fruits and vegetables to proteins and grains. For a full list of these foods, see Appendix B on page 409.

Turn on the morning news or flip open a magazine, and you're likely to read about the latest fad diet. Whether it's high-protein or low-carb, those diets don't work, but that doesn't seem to prevent them from being hyped. The truth is that any diet that excludes a food group or macronutrient should be avoided. With very few exceptions, SparkPeople doesn't prohibit any food, and when it comes to losing weight from healthy eating, we are of the "tortoise" school of philosophy. Fad diets, like the hare in the fable, lose in the long run. As we established in *The Spark,* our "diet" plan is a lifestyle change that has helped our millions of members lose weight and keep it off.

We adhere to generally accepted ranges for carbohydrates, fat, and protein intake, which we believe help to ensure that a person is receiving a sufficient intake of other essential nutrients, vitamins, and minerals. These ranges are supported by years of research that have examined the relationship between nutrient intake and disease prevention. The recommendations from the Food and Nutrition Board of the Institute of Medicine of the National Academies are:

- 45 to 65 percent of calories eaten should come from carbohydrates (169 to 244 grams based on a 1,500-calorie meal plan).

- 20 to 35 percent of calories eaten should come from fat (33 to 58 grams).

- 10 to 35 percent of calories eaten should come from protein (60 to 131 grams for women and 75 to 131 grams for men).

(**Note:** Because our members are striving to meet weight-loss goals through calorie restriction, we also recommend a minimum level of protein—at least 60 grams daily for women and 75 grams daily for men—to promote feelings of fullness and help prevent muscle loss.)

SparkPeople takes a middle-of-the-road approach with these ranges. Our specific breakdown is approximately 50 percent carbohydrates, 30 percent fat, and 20 percent protein, all of which fall into the healthy ranges above. The table below converts these percentages into grams needed each day based on overall calorie intake:

Nutritional Guidelines for Meals
Based on a 1,500-calorie meal plan
Breakfast: 300 calories
Lunch: 400 calories
Dinner: 400 calories
Two Snacks: 200 calories each
<ul><li>Meals should have 15 to 20 grams of protein; snacks should have 5 to 10.</li><li>Meals should be 25% whole grains or starchy vegetables, 25% lean meat or protein alternatives, and 50% fruits and vegetables.</li><li>Meals should have no more than 700 mg sodium.</li></ul>

Your actual intake of carbohydrates, fat, and protein may be somewhat higher or lower than our range, because of your taste preferences, cooking style, culture, fitness routine, health conditions, and day-to-day changes in diet. We created our recipes to follow these guidelines as well. Because each recipe has been created with the SparkPeople philosophy in mind, each ingredient adds a layer of satisfaction to the dish.

The recipes use "right-sized" portions, and we focus on volume.

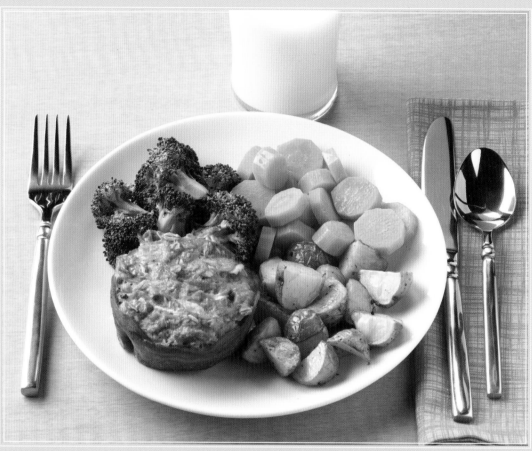

This 9-inch plate shows a meal in perfect proportion: one half filled with nonstarchy vegetables, one quarter filled with lean protein, and one quarter with grains or a starchy vegetable.

Begin with a plate that has a 9-inch eating surface. As shown in the photo above, your plate should be divided into four quadrants: Half of the plate should be filled with nonstarchy vegetables; one quarter should be filled with lean meat or a vegetarian protein, such as legumes or tofu; and one quarter should be grains or a starchy vegetable. Round out the meal with a small serving of fruit and a glass of low-fat milk. Your plate will be full, and you will be satisfied, without overeating!

As you study the photographs throughout the book, you'll see that the plates reflect the *actual portion size* given in our recipes. Notice that the food is colorful and appealing to the eye—and you won't find any bare spots on the plate! Those full plates really threw our taste-test participants for a loop!

THE GREAT "DITCH THE DIET" TASTE TEST

Over the past decade, SparkPeople has managed to rewrite the rules of weight loss through sound advice from experts like Becky, endless support from our community, and tools that make tracking your goals simple and fun. We've unmasked fad diets; explained why starvation doesn't lead to rapid weight loss; and exposed the world of gadgets, pills, and quick fixes. We didn't just rewrite the rules; we wrote a book, one that appeared on numerous bestseller lists.

But we found out that some of our most successful members had lost their weight without changing much about how they cooked and ate their food. Sure, they were controlling portions and making smarter menu choices, but many were still eating their meals on the run or in front of the TV—and their food came from a bag or box. They weren't cooking at home or eating at the table with family. And that worried us.

Sure, they had great excuses:

Birdie, whom we met at the beginning of the book, has five young children and is a physician. Frozen entrées and healthier fast food formed the backbone of her meal plans.

Tara—down almost 40 pounds—was training to run a marathon. She had swapped Froot Loops for high-fiber flakes but still snacked her way through a large container of cereal each day at work.

Amber, who battled stomach issues as she shed 96 pounds, reached for fat-free, tasteless foods with lengthy ingredient lists. She wasn't satisfied, but she was skinnier.

If our Success Stories were going to remain successful, we knew they needed some help in the kitchen. Even though these members eventually—with SparkPeople's vast resources, some of my recipes, and sheer determination—changed their cooking and eating habits, we knew that they weren't isolated cases. We knew that others were still stubbornly clinging to their old ways of eating—bland diet foods, ordering takeout, and using their ovens for storage.

Thus, the "Ditch the Diet" Taste Test was conceived.

We believed 100 percent in our satisfying way of cooking and eating, but we wanted to put our beliefs to the test. We conducted the Ditch the Diet Taste Test to prove once and for all that healthy foods can be satisfying, sustaining, and stress-free, and that you can love your food and still lose weight!

The taste test had two parts. To start, we recruited about 50 people to join us for a blind taste test at the Midwest Culinary Institute, where I teach here in Cincinnati. As we hadn't yet revealed to anyone we were writing this cookbook, we told the participants—a third of them yo-yo dieters and the rest SparkPeople members—that they would be trying new healthy recipes made by my students. That much was true; what they didn't know was that the two meals they would eat were remarkably different.

PART ONE: THE TASTE TEST

We sent each potential participant an online survey with 33 questions, asking about their weight-loss histories, fitness and eating practices, and food preferences. We also asked them five nutrition questions, each aimed at debunking a different diet myth.

Before our participants even walked through the door, we knew most of them:

- Had tried between one and five diets in five years (almost half were currently on a diet).

- Wanted to lose at least five pounds.

- Ate in front of the TV or computer, with friends, or at their desk more than once a day.

- Have gained weight in the past five years.

When asked to describe a typical day of eating, we learned that plenty of them were ignoring guidelines that SparkPeople considers crucial to a healthy lifestyle. Skipping breakfast, little protein, few fruits and vegetables—some participants were ignoring all of the Secrets of Success, the keys to long-term weight loss and better health that we found when we surveyed our most successful members for *The Spark*.

So we knew that our participants, while they have established healthy habits, hadn't yet broken the cycle of yo-yo dieting. Though they had the desire to cook, obstacles (like time, money, and know-how) blocked their path to a healthier life.

When they showed up for lunch one day in May, we were armed and ready to challenge their long-held dieting beliefs. We fed them equal, half-size portions of two meals.

Meal A comprised typical "diet" foods: poached chicken, steamed carrots, steamed white rice, iceberg salad with fat-free dressing, and a "healthy" muffin made with artificial sweetener, whole-wheat flour, applesauce, and no salt. Nutritional value of Meal A: 272 calories, 4 grams fat, 3 grams fiber.

We chose those foods deliberately. Poached chicken is healthy but often bland, as are steamed carrots and plain rice. Fat-free dressing contains nothing to temper the acidity of vinegar, and without fat, your body isn't able to fully metabolize the vitamins in the salad. The muffin employs several low-fat baking techniques that, when combined, yield a dense and flavorless product. These diet foods are low in fat and calories—but totally lacking in flavor.

Meal B was made of recipes from the book: Lemon Herb-Roasted Chicken, Sautéed Cumin Carrots, Baked Lemon-Spiced Rice, Mixed Greens with Tomato-Basil Vinaigrette, and a Spring Cupcake with Citrus Icing. Nutritional value of Meal B: 268 calories, 9 grams fat, 4 grams fiber.

Roasting the chicken, sautéing the carrots, and adding herbs and spices to the rice and dressing added flavor without much extra fat, while the lower-fat cupcake was in fact a zucchini and carrot–based muffin. The cooking methods are still healthy and easy, but they are designed to add flavor, as you'll read in the next chapter.

We asked participants to compare and rate the foods individually and as a meal, judging taste, appearance, texture, and satisfaction levels. In addition, they told us which meal they would prefer to eat again and which meal they thought was healthier.

The Results Across the board, they loved the recipes from this book and scored them higher on average in the categories of appearance, taste, and satisfaction. They did suspect that some of the "diet foods" were healthier but noted they had less flavor. The astounding success of our recipes, compared with the high number of votes that those tasteless "diet foods" were "healthier," proved to us that dieters fear flavor. They were suspicious that we were sneaking in way too much fat, sugar, and salt—and sabotaging their health goals.

The predominant adjectives they used to describe that "healthy" meal were "bland" and "boring." Fifteen people chose the diet meal as the healthier meal, but less than half of them wanted to eat it again. All of them want to lose at least 10 pounds. Hmm . . . if you're trying to lose weight but keep failing, could it be that you're relying on bland and boring foods?

Tara, the veteran SparkPeople member we introduced earlier, was one of those who believed the diet meal was healthier—but wanted to eat our recipes again.

"Overall, Meal B was way better tasting," she wrote. "I think Meal A is healthier only because the other tasted so good, something in it probably was bad! Please tell me Meal B was healthier."

As we sorted through the responses, a trend emerged. Of the diet meal, participants wrote: "less interesting"; "nothing was bad but a lot of simple and bland dishes"; and "no flavor." Yet they believed it was healthier.

The results confirmed what we believed: Dieters think healthy food cannot be tasty or satisfying. They don't believe they can eat the food they love and still lose weight.

That's why we invited about a dozen of them to come back for a cooking class and follow-up taste test.

PART TWO: THE COOKING CLASS

After work one Monday night, a select group of participants joined us for Part Two of the study, which included dinner, an interactive "Debunk the Diet" presentation, and a hands-on cooking class—with leftovers to provide them with at least two healthy meals.

This time, we divided the group into two, with half eating our meal and half eating a "diet" meal that had more fat and calories. Little did they know that though the portion sizes were comparable, our meal had 100 fewer calories than the bland and boring diet foods!

Group A ate a low-carb, high-fiber tortilla filled with steamed broccoli, poached chicken, fat-free ranch dressing and fat-free cheddar cheese, alongside a plain baked sweet potato topped with light margarine. Nutritional value: 459 calories, 8 grams fat, 16 grams fiber.

Group B ate Chicken Kebob Pitas with Creamy Cucumber Sauce, plus Baked Sunburst Fries with Spicy Yogurt Sauce for dipping. Nutritional value: 356 calories, 7 grams fat, 6 grams fiber.

After they ate, we again asked them to rate their meals. And once again, Meal B rated higher across the board. They loved it!

Then Mary, a SparkPeople member whose biggest challenge is balancing work, school, and life, tried some of the Spicy Yogurt Sauce that others were raving about. "We were robbed," she exclaimed. "This (yogurt sauce) was an event. The other was just to sustain us for a meal."

The meal and the subsequent class were meant to debunk more diet myths:

- Low-carb, low-cal breads are the best choice. (See Breaking Down Bread, page 279.)

- You should always choose fat-free versions of your favorite foods. (See Proof You'll Be Satisfied, page 15.)

- Plain vegetables are better for you. (See Dress It Up, page 107.)

- When you're watching your weight, you have to eat less. (See Proof You'll Be Satisfied, page 15.)

- Baking and steaming are the only cooking methods you need to know. (See Chapter 3, The New Healthy Kitchen.)

- When you cut back on salt and fat, you forgo all flavor in food. (See Chapter 12, Herbs, Spices & Seasonings.)

You'll learn more about these myths throughout the book, but that night we asked participants to try for themselves. We passed out samples of bread and cheese to combat the first two myths. When tasting fat-free processed Cheddar alongside a sharp Vermont Cheddar, the difference was clear.

Jack, a retiree who's passionate about food and looking to lose 20 pounds, gave a real-life example: "I made grilled cheese for lunch twice last week," he said. "The first day I used a sharp Vermont Cheddar, and the next day I used a diet yellow cheese. It was a world of difference between the two. The sharp Cheddar had interest, and it had flavor. The other—why bother?" His

sample of the fat-free cheese went uneaten, as did several others' portions.

We then asked them to compare "light" and low-carb bread against a whole-wheat bakery-style bread. Notice the texture, the flavor, the feel in the mouth, we advised them. Several people complained that the low-carb bread stuck to the roof of their mouths and felt gummy. That's because of the refined carbs with added fiber, we told them.

From there, we moved on to the kitchen. We set to work making Better-For-You Beef Stroganoff (see page 214) and Easy Steamed Vegetable Packets (see page 323), with some modifications so they could finish the meal at home and serve it the next day.

During exit interviews, we asked each participant what they had learned.

Remember Tara, our cereal addict, marathon runner, and most enthusiastic participant? Tara told us: "I'm still a newbie when it comes to eating healthy, so it's amazing to me to see all the things I can eat."

She continued:

"I was excited about this class because my eating habits are still out of the box, literally. You open the box . . . granted they're healthier foods—like whole grains and nonsugary cereals, but they're still out of the box. I knew I needed to incorporate more vegetables.

"In this class I learned that you can have a healthy meal, and it will taste excellent. You will clean your plate. I learned that the (unfamiliar) vegetables you see in the store, you can cook with them. Everyone can do it. I'm not really a person who's eaten much more than carrots and celery. Now I can cut up a leek, and I can cut up a pepper—the proper way. I can have all these vibrant colors that will make my meal not only appealing to my eye but to my sense of smell."

Will the Real Strawberry Milkshake Please Stand Up!

My family rarely eats fast food, but when we do, I can tell you that my kids love it! Actually, scratch that. They used to love it. Was it the prize that came with the meal, the playground in the restaurant, or the actual food that made them beg for a trip to see the clown? I think all three.

Now that they are getting older, they realize that the foods there are loaded with salt, and, while they might have stronger flavors, the "commercially" manufactured foods don't taste as good as Mom's.

We so often grab these fast foods and gulp them down, we don't stop to think about what we're actually ingesting. Take, for example, a strawberry milkshake. I love to make ice cream for the kids as a treat, and in the spring when we can go to the garden and pick the berries, it's even better.

My strawberry milkshake contains: cream, milk, sugar, homemade vanilla extract, and strawberries. Now compare that to one I could get at a burger joint, which contains:

> Milk, sugar, cream, nonfat milk solids, corn syrup solids, mono- and diglycerides, guar gum, dextrose, sodium citrate, artificial vanilla flavor, sodium phosphate, carrageenan, disodium phosphate, cellulose gum, vitamin A palmitate, sugar, water, corn syrup, strawberries, high-fructose corn syrup, natural (botanical source) and artificial flavors, pectin, citric acid, xanthan gum, potassium sorbate (preservative), caramel color, calcium chloride, red 40

Really whets the appetite, doesn't it? When you look at and smell the two milkshakes, there are two very distinct differences. Mine is pale in color and the aroma is subtle. The fast-food version is bright pink, with a strawberry scent that's detectable from 20 paces. The fast-food version wins points for "in-your-face" color and smell, and the homemade version pales in comparison—literally—only because it doesn't contain "red 40."

For some people, it's been so long since they've had the real, homemade, from-scratch thing—whether it's cinnamon rolls, strawberry milkshakes, or spaghetti with meatballs—that they think the real stuff is boring and bland. Our taste buds are overstimulated and trained to expect the exaggerated flavors of salt, fat, and artificial ingredients. But when you're accustomed to the real thing, the artificial version overwhelms your palate. It's too sweet, unnaturally thick, and smells fake. Once you reconnect with real food, we promise you, you won't miss those artificial ingredients. This book is going to help you retrain your taste buds and learn to love real, healthy food again!

And Mary, the outspoken one who felt "robbed"? Well, as a culinary student and food stylist, she's no stranger to the kitchen, but she struggles to find time to cook for her family.

"What I learned today I can take and use in my daily life," she said, suddenly soft-spoken. "If you don't serve just a whole piece of chicken, if you cut it up, you can extend it and it can be prepared ahead of time and ready for you."

She had always envisioned that the plate had to be very traditional: meat at the center, a heaping helping of starch, and sometimes vegetables on the side. This changed her mind.

After turning them loose with a folder full of recipes, a two-week meal plan, the leftovers from the cooking class, and even a grocery-store gift card to help them get started, we sent them home for two weeks. Then we checked in.

The Results Across the board, our participants started cooking more and started losing some long-held beliefs about how they should eat that were just plain wrong. Just two weeks later, they had already made changes in their lives. Renee reached the halfway point of her weight-loss journey and is on track to meet her goal of losing 100 pounds.

"Before attending the workshop and using the Ditch the Diet plan, I had fallen into some bad eating habits," said the single mother. "I thought I was too busy to cook, so I'd either grab a bowl of cereal or bagel for dinner, or more often I'd head to a fast-food drive-thru. When I cooked, it almost always involved the use of prepackaged convenience foods. The food I did prepare from scratch was often bland or unappealing because of the cooking methods I used (baking, boiling, etc.) so I'd add lots of salt. The result was an unbalanced diet loaded with sodium, sugar, and preservatives."

Newlyweds Jeff and Lauren Anderson, already healthy eaters, realized they could share cooking duties and have fun in the process.

"I learned that I don't always have to rely on her because cooking can be easy, fun, and quick," said Jeff. "I need to not be afraid of the kitchen."

Lauren added: "We're trying to eat more whole foods—fruits, vegetables, and things without additives."

Most reported some significant changes.

Whether they shed their "fat phobias" like Renee, found confidence in the kitchen like Jeff, or felt more motivated to eat right because of weight loss like Tara, all of our participants told us we had opened their eyes to how easy, satisfying, and delicious healthy eating could be.

THE NEW
HEALTHY KITCHEN

Before you can learn to love the food you eat, you have to learn to *cook* the food you eat. Drive-thrus, frozen meals, grab-and-go sections at supermarkets, and take-out menus make it too easy to avoid the kitchen and rely on someone else to make your meals. But the thing is, when you consistently let someone else control what goes into your food, it's hard to maintain control of your weight and your health. When you're in charge, you'll know exactly how much fat, sugar, and salt are in everything you're eating, thus taking control of your weight loss. You'll be able to plump up your meals with extra servings of low-calorie, high-volume foods like fruits and vegetables. And you'll be able to make everything to *your* liking.

Even if you don't know the difference between poaching and steaming, or if the idea of roasting a chicken makes you break out in a sweat, you can cook every one of the recipes in this cookbook. I have a culinary degree, but all *you* need is this cookbook, a bit of time, and the desire to learn to cook food that is both good for you and just plain good! When I approach a recipe, I break it down to its most basic components, analyze how I can boost the flavor of each part, then put it back together again. I focus on changing one or two aspects of the dish: boosting the fiber, cutting the fat, lowering the sodium, or adding more fruits or vegetables. I also think about which aspects of the dish I want to keep, and I choose my cooking techniques, ingredients, and seasonings accordingly. Though it sounds very scientific, it's actually quite fun—and the techniques, tips, and tools laid out in this chapter and throughout the book will help you learn to do the same thing to your favorite recipes. But for now, you can just use our recipes and get cooking!

Let's take our Tuna Noodle Casserole on page 231 as an example. The traditional version is made with white noodles, condensed soup, processed cheese product, buttered breadcrumbs, and sometimes a few vegetables. One serving can have 470 calories, 29 grams fat, 708 milligrams sodium, and almost no fiber.

To make a lighter, healthier, but still delicious tuna casserole, I wanted to lower the fat and sodium while boosting the fiber. I wanted to make this a meal unto itself, with protein, whole grains, and a serving of vegetables while still keeping the creamy rich cheese sauce. The first things to go were the processed cheese and condensed soup, which are full of artificial ingredients, fat, and salt. Instead, I created a lower-fat cream sauce with Swiss cheese, and I used *full-fat* Swiss for its sharp flavor and creamy texture. From there, I made an easy swap: whole-wheat noodles (the "no yolks" variety) for the white ones. Finally, I bulked up the dish with one cup of vegetables per portion: onions, peas, carrots, and mushrooms. Sweating the onions and mushrooms in butter added a layer of flavor, and the butter served double duty; it and the vegetables were cooked with flour to make a thickening agent for our sauce. Thyme and pepper added spice and freshness, while the milk and cheese finished the rich, mouthwatering sauce. Finally the whole-wheat breadcrumbs form a crispy crust—and a contrast to the creamy casserole beneath.

Take one bite of this casserole and you'll learn a great deal about textures, flavors, and techniques. When you create a dish, it's important to have contrasts in all three. In this case the creamy sauce and soft tuna contrast the crisp vegetables and crunchy topping. Baking creates a crust that wouldn't have been present if we had served this dish from the stovetop (which you could do). Sweating adds a softness to the onions and mushrooms that baking them raw wouldn't attain.

In the end, I created a casserole that has 307 calories, 6.5 grams total fat, 234.5 milligrams sodium, 36.4 grams total carbs, and 6 grams dietary fiber—a big improvement in terms of nutrition without sacrificing flavor.

And did I mention this meal was ready in just 35 minutes? That's the same time as the original. This method of reworking a recipe is the basis of my approach to healthy cooking— the right balance of flavors and ingredients that keep the components that satisfy us most, but swap out other ingredients that just add fat and calories.

THE LOVE YOUR FOOD, LOSE THE WEIGHT COOKING SCHOOL

Learning to cook is like learning to dance. Once you know the basics, you'll be able to walk onto the dance floor and know immediately whether you should waltz, tango, or jitterbug to a particular piece of music. Try to tap dance at a wedding reception or waltz to a bluegrass band. It doesn't feel right, does it? The same goes for cooking. Learn the classic methods, and you'll be able to walk into any farmers' market or grocery store, pick up any ingredient, and cook it with pretty good results. There are reasons you don't steam pot roast or sauté muffins. Below are the techniques I use most often to create healthy and delicious foods. Learn these techniques, and you'll be whipping up meals you love to eat—with and *without* a cookbook—in no time!

Basically, methods of cooking are broken down into two categories: those using dry or moist heat. Dry heat methods promote browning of foods. Browning occurs as water in the foods evaporates. This is particularly evident in sautéing and roasting as the natural sugars in the food caramelize. With moist heat, the foods are cooked in or over liquids, which will prevent browning. Moist heat methods seal in food's natural flavors and nutritional benefits. Both have a place in the new healthy kitchen and will yield satisfying, nutritious results.

DRY HEAT COOKING METHODS

Roasting

When we roast, we surround foods with hot air. Roasting does not require fat for cooking, though a small amount is sometimes added for flavor and moistness. At home, I prefer to roast meats and vegetables using herbs and citrus with minimal oil to add flavor. Roasting brings out the natural sugars in vegetables, and it creates a lovely, satisfying brown exterior on meats. This is one of my favorite cooking techniques for bringing out full flavor with little to no added calories or fat.

The temperature for roasting can range from 325 degrees to 475 degrees Fahrenheit. The rule is, the larger the pieces of food, the lower the temperature to avoid undercooked interiors and burned outsides. Roasting vegetables, proteins, or starches at a high heat like this is a great way to "faux fry" your food. I use this method for everything from potatoes to chicken tenders.

Sometimes members write to us asking how they can learn to like vegetables. I tell them to try roasting everything from radishes to broccoli. Start today with the Roasted Beet and Apple Salad (page 116), which yields tender and sweet beets that pair well with tangy Granny Smith apples. And next Thanksgiving, instead of spending all that time running back and forth to

the oven to baste the turkey, make the self-basting Herb-Roasted Turkey (page 198) and spend more time catching up with family and watching the game.

Guidelines for successful roasting:

- Always preheat your oven and wait until it reaches the desired temperature. Most ovens will go to a higher temperature than selected when turned on and then regulate down. My oven takes a full 25 minutes to regulate to the desired temperature.

- Heat rises in your oven like it does in your home. For roasting, place items in the center.

- When roasting, give the foods space and privacy. Don't open the door unless necessary to turn vegetables or test the temperature of meat. Opening the door releases hot air, which will affect the cooking times. If you want to watch your food cook, turn on the oven light.

- Use a heavy-bottomed pan that's large enough to hold all the ingredients in a single layer. If you pile the food up on the pan, it will steam and not create the crispy exterior you want. For meat, choose a pan with a raised center so the fat can drain off.

- Don't use disposable roasting pans for heavy cooking. The thin aluminum does not conduct heat well, and they can buckle in the center, which can lead to dangerous spills of hot pan juices.

- You don't need much fat when it comes to roasting. You can use just a teaspoon or two of oil for an entire pan of vegetables. Avoid using nonstick cooking spray when roasting, as the emulsifiers it contains will burn and create a sticky, brown coating on your pans.

Grilling and Broiling

Grilling cooks with heat below the food, and broiling uses heat from above. We usually think of burgers and steaks when we think of grilling and broiling, but vegetables, pizza, and even fruits love the dry heat of a grill as well.

In general, tender cuts of meat are used for grilling or broiling. If the meat is not tender, a marinade made with herbs, an acid such as vinegar or citrus, and some oil will help break down the tough connective tissues. Grilled Southwest Flat-Iron Steak (page 220) is a great example of this.

I like to create a hot and cool spot on the grill so that I can move foods around if they are getting overcooked. On a gas grill, set one burner on a lower temperature; if using coals, move the hot coals to one side of the grill.

Hone your grilling skills with Grilled Shrimp with Jicama-Grapefruit Slaw (page 119) and the Grilled Veggie Sandwiches with Fresh Mozzarella (page 145).

Guidelines for successful grilling:

- Preheat the grill or coals to desired temperature before adding foods.

- Once hot, scrape the grates with a wire brush to remove any dried-on foods, which can cause flare-ups.

- *Never* spray a nonstick cooking spray on a hot grill. This is extremely dangerous! Also avoid pouring oil or flammable alcohol on the grill. Let your meat talk to you. You're not crazy—when a protein is ready to be turned, it will release itself from the grill and turn easily. If it is not ready, you'll feel some hesitation when you try to turn it. You'll also risk ripping it open or losing meat in the grill.

- For those lovely grill marks, leave your food in place until it's ready to flip. Constantly moving it means the foods won't have time to develop those lines.

Guidelines for successful broiling:

- Move an oven rack to the highest position before preheating the oven.

- Preheat the broiler to high and let it reach the desired temperature before placing food under the heat.

- Never broil foods on parchment paper or silicone liners.

- Always leave the oven door ajar while broiling to allow smoke to escape and to keep an eye on your food. Broiling occurs quickly and is quick to burn, too!

Sautéing and Sweating

Cooking over high or low heat with minimal oil. In the healthy kitchen, these methods are workhorses because they require little to no fat. In French, *sauté* means "to jump." The translation is perfect: If the pan and oil are hot, the food will jump and not just sit in the oil. The other benefit to sautéing is that foods are cooked quickly over high heat, so the loss of nutrition is minimal. Sweating is basically the same cooking technique, but it takes place over lower heat to prevent browning.

Sautéing is a great cooking technique when you want crisp, flavorful vegetables or protein that has a nice brown crust. Stir-fries use the sautéing technique to yield healthy, quick meals. Sautéing is a versatile cooking technique, and it's a great way to impart flavor with minimal effort. This is a perfect example of a simple change that really amplifies your satisfaction. As an experiment, try steaming your favorite vegetable, then the next night, try sautéing it. Which one had more flavor? The sautéed vegetable, right? That's because the high heat sealed in juices and nutrients while caramelizing the natural sugars and creating that savory brown exterior.

Sweating is used with aromatic vegetables such as garlic, onions, peppers, and carrots to temper their strong flavor. You want them to be background singers not the diva in most dishes. For example, onions are sweated before being added to the Black-Bean Burgers with Lime Cream (page 139) to remove their harsh taste and soften them. If you added raw onions to the dish, they would overpower the other ingredients. Sweating levels the playing field in a dish. It mutes louder flavors and gives the timid ones a chance to be heard.

Guidelines for successful sautéing:

- Choose an appropriate-sized pan. If you are sautéing only a cup of onions you don't need a 16-inch sauté pan. But don't crowd your pan, either. If you try to cook, say, a pound of chicken in a 6-inch sauté pan, the water that needs to release from the protein will not have room to evaporate. The chicken will steam instead of sauté and that tasty browning will not occur. Your food should fit comfortably in a single layer with space in between pieces. It's better to sauté food in batches if you don't have a large enough pan.

- Heat the pan, heat the oil, then add the food. Adding food to a cold pan or cold oil will cause it to absorb more oil and prevent browning. If you aren't adding oil, add the food to the hot pan.

- Minimal if any oil should be used. As often as possible, use nonstick pans and rely on the water in foods to help transfer the heat. Mushrooms and spinach are perfect examples. They're high in water, so they won't stick to the pan, even if no oil is used.

Guidelines for successful sweating:

- Sweating is primarily used for vegetables. Cook over low heat so that the foods exude some of their own juices and don't brown.

MOIST HEAT COOKING METHODS

Poaching

Immersing foods in a liquid, usually a seasoned one, and simmering on the stovetop or in the oven. Poaching is a gentle and easy way to cook tender cuts of meats and fish. The resulting food will be moist and tender. The foods are completely covered by a flavorful liquid: a stock or water mixed with herbs, spices, aromatic vegetables, and sometimes wine. Because the foods are immersed in the liquid, they don't brown. The flavors are very subtle and refined, perfect for eggs, fish, and poultry.

Poaching is a prime example of how cooking is teamwork. Each ingredient has a role to play, and if it steps out of place, it throws off everything else. Just as raw onions would have overwhelmed the Black-Bean Burgers, grilled chicken would do the same to the Crunchy Chicken Salad (page 127). The neutral flavor of the chicken provides a tender, moist addition to the salad without overpowering the other flavors.

Guidelines for successful poaching:

- The oven temperature should never exceed 350°F. In a convection oven, turn the fan to low or off.

- Poaching liquid should reach no more than 160°F to 180° F, just a simmer. You shouldn't see anything more than tiny bubbles around the edge of the pan.

- Use the smallest pan possible. If you are poaching one egg, there is no need to fill a 4-quart saucepan with a gallon of water.

Braising and Stewing

Essentially the same technique, a combination of dry and moist heat. Food is first browned, then liquid is added to finish the cooking process. The term "braise" is used when cooking a large cut of meat (like a pot roast), while stews incorporate small pieces of protein and vegetables.

These methods of cooking really make me feel warm inside: They're long, slow cooking processes that fill the kitchen with savory smells. And since both make tender work of tougher, usually less-expensive cuts of meat, these techniques are easy on the pocketbook, too.

The beauty of braising and stewing is that the nutrients are trapped in this low-heat method and remain in the dish. The food is first browned, then placed with a flavored liquid into a heavy saucepan with a fitted lid (or a Dutch oven) and cooked slowly in the oven or on the stove. Braised Mexican Beef with Crispy Corn Tortillas (page 219) turns a chuck roast into a rich and tender dish. Ratatouille (page 258) is an amazingly rich and healthy vegetable dish that relies on stewing for its flavors.

Guidelines for successful braising:

- Meats should be seared on the stovetop first.

- Once seared, add liquids only halfway up the sides of the meat. Occasionally check the liquid to make sure it has not evaporated.

- Use a heavy enameled cast-iron pan or heavy saucepan with a lid to braise, and make sure the handles and knobs are oven safe. To trap the steam and seal in flavor, the lid should not have any vents.

- The oven temperature should not exceed 350° F. In a convection oven, turn the fan to low or off.

- Place braised dishes in the center or lower part of the oven.

- You don't need to test the temperature of braised meats; they are done when they're fork tender.

- Sturdy root vegetables such as hard-fleshed squash, potatoes, and carrots, stand up well to braising. So do celery and fennel.

Guidelines for successful stewing:

- Meats and vegetables should be cut into uniform-sized pieces.

- All of the food should be submerged entirely in the liquid.

Steaming

Using steam from heated liquid to cook foods indirectly, sealing in flavor and nutrients. I saved the best for last! Healthy cooking and steaming are a perfect marriage. Steaming uses no fat, and is a quick cooking method, which keeps the vitamins and minerals in the foods where they belong. Food is placed on a rack, which is then placed above a pan of boiling water, and covered to seal in the steam.

Although this is, in my opinion, the best method for healthy cooking, it is because of that lack of fat that little additional flavor is created from steaming. This is where I really rely on my salt-free seasoning blends (see Chapter 12) and fresh herbs. They don't overpower the food or add many calories but give the foods an added flavor boost. Broccoli and Spaghetti Squash with Lemon Pepper (page 243) relies on the microwave for a quick and flavorful vegetarian meal.

Another foolproof way to steam foods is to cook it *en papillote,* as the French say. Fish, thin cuts of chicken, or vegetables are placed in packets of folded cooking parchment with a bit of liquid and herbs and spices, then sealed, and placed in an oven to cook. As the liquids heat, they turn to steam and the foods are delicately cooked. Plus, they make for a beautiful presentation when you cut the packets open at the table—and there's little to clean up. You can use foil for these, but the packets cook faster, so pull them out a couple of minutes earlier to prevent tough fish and soggy vegetables. (Note that chicken takes up to an extra 10 minutes longer than fish to cook.)

Guidelines for successful steaming:

- Vegetables should be chopped into even pieces for even cooking; choose thin fish fillets for best results.

- Make sure the liquid is boiling to produce steam before you add the foods.

- Check the liquid level during steaming and add more if necessary. If it completely evaporates, you could burn your food and the pan.

- Add flavor to steamed foods with herb and spice blends or low-fat vinaigrettes.

STOCKING THE NEW HEALTHY KITCHEN

You won't find mango slicers, shrimp deveiners, or egg separators in my kitchen. I'm just not that kind of cook. At Le Cordon Bleu in London, I was taught to cook anywhere and any time. My workspace was about as wide and as tall as I am, with no room for gadgets or fancy equipment. Cramped spaces, limited ingredients, and minimal tools are no excuses for a cook. I have carried this style with me today and try to impress the same philosophy on my students. Most of the tools that I have in my kitchen today have been around for years. I still have the same knives that I received from Le Cordon Bleu 25 years ago!

Guests are surprised when they watch me cook at home. Large and spacious, with plenty of windows that overlook our garden and the woods out back, the kitchen is uncluttered yet fully stocked. As I pull out my favorite pan, eyebrows raise. It's a cast-iron skillet, passed down from my grandmother. My skillet is so well-seasoned that food develops better flavor and doesn't stick to the pan as it would in new pans.

When you purchase quality goods and care for them properly, they will last a lifetime. You'll spend less money in the long run and keep clutter from overtaking your kitchen. What should you have in your healthy kitchen?

- *A chef's knife with a steel:* Purchase a high-carbon stainless steel knife and keep it sharp! High-carbon stainless steel will not corrode or discolor. You don't need a 12-inch knife. I prefer the control of a smaller knife, like a 6- or 8-inch knife. Chopping vegetables with a dull knife not only takes longer, but you run the risk of injuring yourself. Whether you're prepping all those green vegetables for Spring Garden Stir-Fry (page 216) or chopping mushrooms for your morning frittata, a sharp knife will ease the task.

    Honing your knife is very important. To do this, run the blade of the knife along the steel at a 20-degree angle three times on each side. Remember to draw the blade along the entire length of the steel. The steel keeps the blade straight and keeps an edge on it. Leave actual sharpening to professionals. If you're afraid to handle a sharp knife, don't be. A dull knife is more dangerous than a sharp one because you have to apply more pressure to cut foods when a blade is dull.

To keep your knife sharp, hone it with steel before each use, never wash it in the dishwasher, always hand dry it, and store it away from other objects. A steel is long piece of slightly abrasive steel that usually comes with most knife kits but can be purchased separately.

- *Wooden cutting board:* Buy the largest wooden cutting board your kitchen can accommodate. A larger board means more room to chop and prep your ingredients. Instead of pulling out several bowls to hold your ingredients as you prepare them, you can keep them on the board, which means fewer dirty dishes. Many of the recipes in the book include several different vegetables, fruits, or herbs that need to be chopped, so a big board will come in handy.

Hard plastic boards are a fine substitute, but please don't use a glass cutting board. (Who in the heck thought that one up?) Cutting on glass will ruin your knives, and it makes a dreadful racket. The reason I prefer wood is that if it gets nicked you can sand out the spot, which is not the case with plastic. I am not crazy about those color-coded thin plastic boards that are meant to keep foods separate. Who has the kitchen space? If you keep your board clean, by washing it with hot water and soap, you don't need special boards for different products.

Be sure to always use a moist paper or cotton towel or a rubber cabinet liner to secure your board to the counter so it doesn't slip.

- *Nonstick 8- or 10-inch sauté pan:* Nonstick pans enable you to use less oil, and they've come a long way in terms of quality. For beginners, they can't be beat. Never use a metal utensil (use wood or plastic instead) or a scouring pad on them—you'll rough up or scratch the coating. And to prevent the nonstick surface from flaking, don't stack nonstick pans on top of each other. While I love my cast-iron skillet, you can't beat a nonstick one when it comes to cooking eggs, pancakes, or anything else that tends to stick. When using nonstick cooking spray in these pans, only spray the area where the food will be, not the entire pan. And don't let these pans sit over a high flame; as soon as they reach the desired temperature, add oil or food. (These pans should not be heated above 350 degrees Fahrenheit.)

- *Pots and pans:* I recommend buying one 10-inch sauté pan, one cast-iron skillet, one 2-quart saucepan with a lid, one 4-quart saucepan with two handles and lid, and one enameled cast-iron Dutch oven.

You don't need a fancy brand-name set of pots and pans. Choose them based on weight. The heavier the saucepan, the better conductor of even, steady heat it will be. Choose pans that will go from the stovetop to oven: look for handles that are sturdy and heatproof. They hold heat and make cooking a breeze. They also give you a good arm workout because they are heavier than heck. For braised dishes and soups, I love my cast-iron Dutch oven. That and my cast-iron skillet are the workhorses in my kitchen.

And remember, you can be a bargain hunter and search anywhere, from department stores on down to church resale stores when you're looking for pots and pans. Compare prices, do your research, and search for coupons before you make a major investment.

- *Baking dishes:* Two aluminum, nonstick baking sheets, a 9- x 13-inch glass baking dish, and a round, deep casserole dish with a lid are all great to have in the kitchen. The baking sheets are perfect for roasting vegetables, the baking dish can double as a cake pan, and the casserole dish is useful for one-dish meals. Also helpful for those who

bake are a deep 9-inch pie plate and two round cake pans.

When using these baking dishes, opt to use a very small amount of oil, parchment paper, or silicone baking liners. This will help you avoid the sticky coating that is left by nonstick cooking sprays.

- *A fork:* There's no need to go out and buy a special fork. Just grab one from your silverware drawer. Or seek a fancy one out at a thrift store. Any fork will replace a half-dozen single-use gadgets in the kitchen. I use a lot of citrus flavor in my dishes to replace salt and sugar. A citrus reamer could do a fine job, but who needs one? Just cut the citrus fruit in half, insert a fork in the center, and, while squeezing the outside, twist the fork to work the juice free. You can also get rid of your carving forks and dough docker, which pricks holes in dough. A plain old fork can do the job.

- *Box grater or microplane:* A box grater will give you plenty of grating options but it does take up more space. (Look for a version that will fold up flat.) A microplane, a fine grating tool that chefs borrowed from a carpenter's workbench, is smaller but only has one size of grates. Either one can extract zest from citrus, grate cheese, or grate whole spices. Grating cheese with a microplane will help you stretch a small amount. Rather than a few thick shreds, you'll get a mound of fluffy shredded cheese.

But be careful! Graters like to eat knuckles and fingernails, so be sure to run the food into the grater, not the grater into the food, to prevent injury.

- *Immersion blender:* I love this tool because it makes life so simple. You can leave a soup or sauce in the saucepan and blend without having to transfer a hot liquid into a blender.

The whisk attachment makes whipping egg whites a breeze, and the mini chopping attachment that comes with most models is convenient for chopping nuts for morning oatmeal or making a small batch of pesto. Most come with a plastic measuring cup that is the perfect size for quick vinaigrettes—and its tall sides prevent splatters.

But do not blend directly in aluminum pots and pans. A chemical reaction can occur that will turn white sauces or soups an unsightly gray.

- *Coffee grinder:* Turn flax seeds into flax meal, bread into breadcrumbs, and whole herbs and spices into homemade seasoning blends with a few pulses of the grinder. Plain and simple, whole spices will last longer than ground, and freshly ground spices and herbs taste better.

To clean the grinder, don't use water. Wipe it with a dry towel, pulse salt or bread in the grinder to clean it, and then wipe it again. The salt or bread will cling to the bits of spices in crevices and help remove residue and neutralize lingering scents.

- *Rolling pin:* Have you looked at a boneless chicken breast lately? They are huge and usually thicker on one end. To ensure even cooking, you'll need to flatten it to a uniform thickness. My tool of choice: a rolling pin. Place the chicken breast between two sheets of plastic wrap and pound away with your rolling pin at the thicker end to even out the meat. By pounding chicken breasts, you'll also be able to better gauge a portion (about the size of a deck of cards). With chicken being such a popular protein choice, your rolling pin will get more use than you think!

Still think a rolling pin is an outdated gadget? Good for more than rolling dough, rolling pins can crush nuts or peppercorns, or smash crackers for breading. Whether you use a French style, which is just a long, thin wooden cylinder, or a variety with handles, a rolling pin is a versatile tool.

- *Measuring cups and spoons:* No matter how good of a cook you are or how long you've been baking, every kitchen should have a set of measuring spoons and dry measuring cups, and one liquid measuring cup (like the one that comes with your immersion blender). It is so important to use these tools if you are trying to count calories and prepare successful recipes. To this day, I use a measuring spoon to measure a teaspoon or tablespoon. These tools are important for accurate results. You should never measure liquids using a dry measuring cup or vice versa.

After I had the twins, I really had to watch what I ate to get back to my normal size. I was always amazed to see that what I thought was a one-cup serving was much larger. Hungry tummies make for big eyes.

Those tools are the absolute basics for a healthy kitchen, but to cut down on prep and cooking times, we asked members to help us devise a list of kitchen equipment that makes their lives a little easier. Even I take help where I can get it!

HEALTHY EATERS' KITCHEN "MUST-HAVES"

- *Microwave:* It's not just for frozen meals! Use it steam vegetables, heat healthy leftovers, and defrost meat for tonight's dinner.

- *Blender:* An immersion blender is wonderful, but it can't do everything. A regular blender is a

necessity for smoothies, among other healthy-food staples. But if you love smoothies as much as our members do, that is reason enough to buy one.

- *Slow cooker:* Birdie swears by hers, and mine is a lifesaver on busy nights. Spend a bit of time prepping dinner in the morning, and you'll be rewarded with a healthy, satisfying meal when you arrive home at night. It's a busy cook's best friend.

- *Countertop grill:* Grilled chicken is a staple in my house, usually rubbed with one of the spice blends in Chapter 12. In winter or when you only want to cook one piece of meat, a countertop grill is great. Plus, you can use it as a sandwich press.

- *Food processor:* There's no need to spend hundreds on a food processor. The cheaper versions will do the job just fine. Shredding, chopping, and mincing take no time at all when you use the food processor. You can have perfect carrot coins, fresh shredded cheese, and chopped nuts in far less time than it would take you and your trusty chef's knife.

- *Toaster oven:* A two-slice toaster is another single-use gadget, but a toaster oven can be used to reheat homemade pizza, warm rolls for dinner, broil, and, of course, toast

PANTRY STAPLES

The new healthy kitchen contains many of the staples you already rely on for quick and nutritious meals: fresh and frozen fruits and vegetables, lean proteins, and low-fat dairy. But there are 11 ingredients that might not make it into your shopping cart on a regular basis that will soon be atop your grocery list.

1. *Quinoa:* A seed that's categorized as a whole grain, full of protein, and quick to cook. Cook with broth, your favorite herbs, or a bit of lemon juice to add flavor. Use as a basis for casseroles, a higher-protein sub for morning oatmeal, or in place of rice.

2. *Greek yogurt:* Tangy, thick—even in low-fat or fat-free versions—this high-protein yogurt is great for breakfast. Use it to replace sour cream, heavy cream, and even mayo.

3. *Brown rice and brown pasta:* brown is the new white when it comes to grains, from rice to breads to pastas, because of the added fiber and other nutrients.

4. *Flaxseed:* This tiny seed packs mighty nutritional powers—fiber, protein, and several heart-healthy fats to name a few. It's a quick, nutty addition to dishes savory and sweet. Sprinkle it on cereal or oatmeal, stir it into yogurt, or mix it into your favorite nut butter. (**Note:** To preserve the delicate omega-3 fatty acids, eat your flaxseed raw most of the time.)

5. *Whole-wheat flour:* Like the aforementioned rice and pasta, brown is better for all your baked goods as well, and this flour is flavorful and versatile. To bake with whole-wheat flour, use half whole wheat and half white to start and gradually reduce the white flour, or choose whole-wheat pastry flour (available at most larger supermarkets).

6. *Beans and lentils:* Good for more than just chili, legumes add fiber and protein to any meal in a flash.

7. *Panko:* To satisfy a craving for crunchy coatings without frying, choose crispy and airy Japanese-style breadcrumbs. Also available in whole-wheat varieties, look for it in the Asian food aisle.

8. *Sweet potatoes and other colorful root veggies like parsnips, beets, and carrots:* While white potatoes' reputation has been restored, their sunnier counterparts boast impressive nutritional profiles that are a welcome addition to any meal.

9. *Herbs and spices:* This mighty duo takes over where fat and sugar left off, flavoring every food you make—with little to no calories and fat.

10. *Citrus:* Fresh and tangy juice and zest from lemons, limes, oranges, and grapefruit brighten and boost flavor when you cut down on salt.

11. *Stock:* Use salt-free or homemade chicken or vegetable stock to add flavor without any calories or fat. Use stock instead of water when cooking grains, and use it to steam vegetables for a boost of flavor.

bread. When you're only baking a single portion or don't want heat up the kitchen, turn to the toaster oven.

- *Fine-mesh strainer:* In addition to draining whole-grain pasta, it can be used to drain and rinse canned beans or vegetables to remove salt, or it can be used to strain a soup. Create your own Greek yogurt by lining the strainer with a coffee filter and pouring in regular yogurt. Store in the fridge over a bowl, and you'll have thick, creamy Greek yogurt by morning.

- *Steamer basket:* Whether you're cooking fish or vegetables, a steamer basket is a great way to cook with zero fat. Some people prefer the bamboo varieties; I like the new silicone ones that mold to the shape of any pot.

- *Storage containers in various sizes:* If you're going to cook healthy, delicious meals, you should reap the benefits—and take leftovers for lunch or store them for dinner the next day. Storage containers— I prefer glass, but plastic will do just fine—are a key component of kitchen organization. Be sure to stock up on various sizes. Big ones are great for salads; tiny ones hold just the right amount of dressing. Be sure to choose an appropriate-sized dish to keep portions in check.

- *Salad spinner:* For members who eat salads regularly, a salad spinner is a must. Your dressing will slide right off the greens if they're wet. A spinner ensures a perfect salad every time, and in a pinch, it can also serve as a colander or salad bowl. I also use mine to dry herbs before chopping them.

With these simple lists, you'll have a well-equipped kitchen and you'll be more than able to make any recipe in this book. And now that you have the equipment, find out how to keep it organized and minimize the time you actually spend in the kitchen.

ORGANIZATION: THE KEY TO QUICK, HEALTHY COOKING

The key to getting a nutritious and delicious dinner on the table in less than 30 minutes is not a culinary degree or a team of sous-chefs. It's one word: organization. Use these simple tips for preplanning your meals and organizing your ingredients and you'll never again ask the question "who has time to cook?"

- *Plan your meals for the week ahead and shop accordingly:* In Appendix A, we offer a step-by-step guide to weekly meal planning and shopping. Keep an inventory list of what is in your freezer, pantry, and refrigerator. When you are making your meal plans for the week, you'll know what you have so you don't waste food. It will encourage you to use up what is on hand instead of buying new. Always remember the saying, first in, first out. Let that be a reminder to date and label all your food.

- *Make every moment count:* If you have been saving stale bread for breadcrumbs and already have the food processor out, take a minute to make breadcrumbs. They'll come in handy for coating meats and topping casseroles, and it really doesn't take long at all. You'll be thankful on a busy school night when you need some to top Three-Cheese Macaroni (page 265). If you're waiting for dinner to finish baking, use that time to load the dishwasher, chop nuts for Nutty Fruity Granola (page 87), or prep tomorrow's dinner.

- *Set aside one afternoon a month for from-scratch projects:* Make homemade no-salt chicken and vegetable stocks (Chapter 6) and freeze for soups and sauces. Bake a batch of granola and some healthy muffins (see Chapter 4) for easy breakfasts on the go. Make Multigrain Rolls (page 302), and freeze them to use as sandwich buns or a quick dinner side.

- *Double up:* If you're already making one batch, make two. Roast two chickens instead of one and save the meat for sandwiches and salads throughout the week. Chop twice the vegetables for the stir-fry. Make two batches of Roasted Root Vegetables (page 315) if you have the

oven on anyway. This is also a good way to make the most of supermarket specials. And speaking of which . . .

- *Hoard like a pioneer!* When your garden or the farmers' market is overflowing, take time to put up food for the winter. Make pesto from mint, basil, and parsley; prepare tomato sauces for chili and stews; and blanch and chill corn, beans, and peppers for freezing. Roast tomatoes and peppers, and dry hot peppers and herbs. Enlist a friend or your partner to help you, and you'll have fun along the way. Knowing that the food was grown and prepared by you makes it taste that much better!

- *Unpack with purpose:* Don't just put groceries away wherever they fit. Group the condiments together on the fridge door. Place the vegetables in the produce drawer, the whole-wheat flour with the rest of the baking ingredients in the pantry, and the coriander in between the cardamom and cumin in the spice cabinet. A few minutes of organization prevents those frantic searches when you're making dinner.

- *Pre-chop your vegetables:* Whether you chop them ahead of time or buy them that way is up to you, but dinner seems like a much less daunting task when all you have to do is add ingredients to a pan. This is definitely something that helps me at home. Just because I show students how to perfectly dice an onion or julienne a carrot doesn't mean I want to do that every night when I come home!

- *Prepare spice blends in advance:* This is a great rainy day chore that will pay you back on a sunny day when you want to be outside. See Chapter 12 for recipes: having these blends on hand lets me add flavor without pulling several jars from the pantry and measuring. I save small jars to store these spice blends— they also make great hostess gifts.

Finally, when you're ready to cook, remember the short French phrase *mise en place*. In the kitchen, *mise en place* means everything in its place and a place for everything. Before you start any recipe, pull out all the ingredients. There's nothing worse than getting halfway through and realizing you're out of something! Complete any prep work as instructed: chop your vegetables, wash and mince herbs, measure out spices. Line up all your ingredients in advance and you'll find the cooking process will be smooth and stress-free.

BIG-BATCH COOKING

If time is your biggest hurdle when it comes to healthy cooking, I have a trick that will seem like a contradiction: big-batch cooking. You don't have time to cook one dinner every night, so how will you manage to cook several? Well, you'll need some time, but in the end you'll save precious minutes and hours throughout the week. Stepfanie, whose busy schedule necessitates such cooking most weeks, tells us how:

Confession: I often don't cook dinner during the week. Even though it's just the two of us, my boyfriend and I are busy. Neither of us is free until at least 8:30 P.M. many nights of the week. We don't always have time to cook at night, but we do crave a home-cooked meal.

We don't want to be standing over a stove until 10 P.M., but we enjoy a healthy, satisfying—and home-cooked—meal every night of the week. Plus we pack our lunches every day.

How? Big-batch cooking.

We have a Sunday evening routine that helps kick-start our week and wind down our weekend. He straightens up the house and tackles laundry, while I clean the kitchen and cook. Usually I prep and cook alone, but sometimes he helps me. Either way, I enjoy the time. I play music, sometimes pour a glass of wine, and tie on one of the aprons my mom made me for Christmas three years ago. Two hours or so later, we sit down to dinner. By then, we have lunches and dinners for at least another three days for both of us.

We clean up together and watch a movie, then turn in early. For the next few nights, we spend about 30 minutes a night on dinner, but that includes deciding what to eat, reheating it, eating, and cleaning up.

How do we do it? Organization and flexibility. We shop for ingredients each Sunday, eat the same meals a few times a week, and keep the kitchen clean and organized, which Meg has already told you is a chef's best-kept secret.

Why do we do it? We're on a budget, we like to cook, and most important, we like to eat tasty and satisfying food.

Step 1: Plan your meals

At some point during the weekend, usually over breakfast, we talk about the week's menu and our schedules. If we have dinner plans with friends or lunch meetings, we know we can cook less food. I ask my boyfriend for input, and I keep a mental inventory of what we have on hand. I include one meat meal for him, two vegetarian meals (for both of us), and a couple of side dishes that can be combined with fridge and pantry staples for a healthy meal. Here are some examples of how a typical week might go:

Week 1:

- *Entrée:* Stepfanie's Quinoa-Black Bean Casserole, page 248 (8 servings)

- *Entrée:* Black-Bean Burgers with Lime Cream, page 139 (8 servings)

- *Entrée:* Green Chicken Curry with brown rice, page 187 (4 servings)

- *Side dish:* Multigrain Rolls, page 302 (24 servings; half frozen, 4 used for Black Bean Burgers and 8 used for snacks with almond butter or hummus)

Week 2:

- *Entrée:* Lemon Herb-Roasted Chicken, page 184 (4 servings)

- *Entrée:* Spinach and Tomato Pasta Salad, page 255 (6 servings)

- *Side dish:* Herbed Bulgur and Lentil Salad, page 301 (8 servings)

For meal prep:

- Salad toppings

- Cannellini beans in the slow cooker

- Batch of wheat berries

- Thaw out remaining Multigrain Rolls

I check the pantry and fridge, choose recipes that use similar ingredients (such as cilantro and black beans in week 1), and write a shopping list.

In addition to the recipes, I always make a large batch of grains (about eight servings) and a large batch of dried beans (cannellini or black beans, or sometimes chickpeas), so I can add them to leftovers throughout the week.

Step 2: Prep your kitchen

Once home, with the kitchen cleaned, I read the recipes to determine what will take the longest. I pull out all the equipment I'll need, such as a cutting boards, measuring cups, and spoons, knives, spatulas, pans, etc. I fill pots of water, if necessary, assemble my food processor (my secret to fast recipe prep), and group recipe ingredients together.

Then I read through each recipe.

Step 3: Start cooking

Start with the recipes that will take the longest. While the dough rises, for example, for the Multigrain Rolls, I move on to the casserole. I start a pot of brown rice, then proceed to the curry while the casserole bakes. Once it's out of the oven, the rolls are ready to go in.

Take your time, and refer to recipes as you go along. I feel quite comfortable juggling several tasks in the kitchen at once. If you're a novice cook, start with one or two recipes and progress from there.

Some of my favorite time-saving tips are:

- Use the food processor whenever possible. The slicing blade makes perfect cucumbers for salads and keeps me tear-free when cutting onions, while I use the grating blade to shred carrots for salads and sweet potatoes for stir-fries and casseroles.

- Keep salad toppings chopped and ready to go for busy nights (I use my food processor for this, too). Salads are easy to prepare if you don't have to chop ingredients every night. Some favorites: hard-boiled eggs, shredded beets or carrots, chopped cucumbers, the aforementioned beans and grains I cook each week, plus anything else I have in the fridge.

Step 4: Divide your meals and eat!

We invested about $40 in 20 glass food-storage containers of various sizes. They're all different colors, so I can put all of my boyfriend's meals in the larger containers with blue lids, while all of my meals have red lids. I like to add extra vegetables to my meals and he prefers an extra serving of grains; we each have different condiment preferences. This way we always know whose food is whose.

Meals that have multiple parts are stored separately. With the Black-Bean Burgers, we store the rolls apart from the burgers so we can avoid soggy sandwiches. Meals we know we'll eat together later in the week are kept in larger containers.

Step 5: Relax!

Each morning, we each grab one of the containers in the fridge, then supplement it with a snack (usually carrots and hummus or almond butter and apples for me; peanut-butter-filled pretzels or crackers and cheese for him). I eat breakfast at work, so I usually prep that in the morning as well.

At night, we heat up whatever leftover dish appeals to us. If he's not feeling the green curry, he'll have the casserole or a bean burger. Sometimes we'll shake up the leftovers, adding extra spinach to the curry, serving the burgers chopped in a quesadilla, or eating the herbed chicken as a sandwich. We also add a serving of fruit (melon or berries in summer; citrus in fall and winter) and usually another vegetable (frozen broccoli with lemon juice, fresh spinach with homemade vinaigrette, and bell pepper strips are favorites) to the meal.

I confess that we do sometimes get tired of eating the same foods all week, but we love how much money we save by not resorting to take-out on busy nights. He has lost 10 pounds since we started dating, and I've maintained a 40-pound weight loss since 2006. We both feel healthier and happier when we eat meals we've made ourselves. We love the food we eat, and his co-workers are quite envious of his delicious, satisfying lunches!

On average weeks, I make two meals that equal three days' worth of food. The other nights of the week I cook meals for four, saving two servings for the next day's lunches.

Tips for using up big batches:

- *Take inventory midweek:* If we're running low on food by Wednesday, we make another meal. (He sometimes eats twice as much food as I do—this often happens to us!)

- *Don't waste it!:* If you made too much food, freeze it for those really busy weeks.

- *Enlist a friend:* In winter, my friend Sarah makes a huge batch of "gravy" (tomato sauce) or stuffed cabbage every Sunday. She is single, so she packs up a serving for several of our friends. In return, I give her homemade granola, my famous Turkish lentil soup, or Multigrain Rolls. We've also cooked together, with each of us taking home enough food for the week.

- *Surprise a co-worker with lunch:* My boyfriend carpools to work with a friend who usually eats take-out for lunch. Occasionally, he surprises him with a home-cooked lunch. It's a great way to brighten someone's morning and give them something to anticipate until noon!

- *Get the family involved:* Batch cooking is a great way to teach kids and partners to cook. Let kids do age-appropriate tasks such as grating carrots, washing vegetables, and assembling ingredients. Even better: have them help with the cleanup!

The Rules in Chef Meg's Kitchen

I hit the gym before dawn for a run or a strength-training session, then head back home to help my husband get our three teenage boys out the door. I'm in my office at the culinary school by 8:00 A.M., with a full day of lectures, kitchen lab classes, and meetings with students and faculty. After school, I shuttle the boys to their various activities and make dinner. Then there's grading assignments, creating recipes for SparkPeople, planning for my cooking show, and community work.

Truth be told, I've got no time to waste in the kitchen. Every minute and every bite counts.

I'm a chef and a farmer's daughter, and I'm committed to feeding my family nutritious and fresh foods: we eat breakfast and dinner together daily, and from-scratch healthy home cooking is always on the menu.

As our boys grew and our lives grew busier, it took a little more planning and a lot more flexibility to keep our family eating right. Through the years, I've learned to use my culinary training and my maternal instincts in tandem, developing tricks and tips to keep us organized and well-fed—on a budget and a schedule.

- *Forget perfection:* At school, I lecture about how to make the perfect béchamel, the right temperature at which to serve duck, and the myriad uses of chervil. In culinary school, there is no room for mistakes. At home, the no-nonsense chef who measures students' fingernails defers to the mom who has 30 minutes to prep a meal. Dinner can come from a slow cooker, consist of leftovers, or include some quality premade ingredients, as long as it's nutritious and well-balanced.

- *Be flexible:* There are days where I eat bites of 25 different soufflés, sample 16 variations of fried chicken, or taste every potato recipe known to man. There are nights where I'm sitting on the bleachers watching the boys' basketball games until 8:00 P.M. If I've had to taste rich foods at school all day, I'll eat a green salad or some fruit for dinner, or add an extra 10 or 20 minutes of cardio the next day. If the boys' activities have us on the road until after dark, I pack a small cooler of healthy snacks to tide us over and make omelets packed with vegetables or sandwiches on whole-wheat bread when we get home.

- *Stay organized:* The clerks at my local supermarket laugh when they see me coming each Friday. My cart is overflowing with food for school projects, SparkPeople recipe testing, as well as my family. I've got a binder of recipes, detailed lists, and an envelope of coupons. Once home, everything is put away in its proper place. Keeping my kitchen and pantry in order, along with weekly meal planning, eliminates much of the dinnertime stress.

A DOZEN STAPLE RECIPES

Ask a chef which recipes are her favorite, and like a mother, she'll answer, "I love them all equally." This cookbook was like a baby to me and, as a result, it's filled with recipes I love. While each and every one is satisfying and nutritious, here are a dozen I think will become staples in your household.

1. Slow-Cooker Salsa Chicken (page 181). There's a reason why this is the No. 1 recipe among SparkPeople members.

2. Lemon Herb-Roasted Chicken (page 184). Roasted chicken is like the little black dress of the kitchen.

3. Multigrain Rolls (page 302). Good for any meal, anytime. Make a couple of batches a month and freeze them. To reheat just pop them in the microwave for a few seconds, or leave them on the counter all day, then warm in a toaster oven.

4. Baked Lemon-Spiced Rice (page 288). A versatile whole-grain side that turns into great leftovers.

5. Quick Herbed Couscous with Vegetables (page 293). You'll have a whole-grain side and two vegetables in less than 15 minutes.

6. Black Bean and Corn Salad (page 121). Fast and full of fiber, serve it on the side or in a wrap to round out any meal.

7. Minestrone Soup with Parmesan Crisps (page 154). This soup is a great way to get kids to eat their veggies. We eat it all year round.

8. Tuna Noodle Casserole (page 231). I never thought I'd say it, but this one-dish meal is hearty and delicious. Even the pickiest kid will eat it.

9. Roasted Root Vegetables (page 315). Make two batches at a time and reheat these as omelet fillers, a quick side, or even a salad topper.

10. Egg-White Omelet (page 89). Full of protein and ready in just a few minutes, this is a fast breakfast favorite.

11. Baby Spinach Salad with Strawberries and Toasted Almonds (page 111). Ready in no time, it dresses up any meal. (Bulk it up with Lemon Herb-Roasted Chicken and Multigrain Rolls.)

12. Vegetable Chicken Soup (page 167). Comfort food that's perfect for even the busiest of nights.

At SparkPeople, we like to keep things simple, and the same is true of our first cookbook. We want to make it easy for you and your family to sit down and share healthy, satisfying, home-cooked meals. As you've seen, many of our most successful members credit their success to cooking the foods they love to eat—and they're a big part of this book, too. You'll find their advice, ideas, tips, and recipes on these pages (we use their online user names throughout the book), along with recipes from me, tips from Stepfanie, and nutritional advice from Becky.

Look to our icons to find the right recipe for you. You'll find a series of symbols at the start of every recipe to help you view what type of dish this is—and there's a handy index starting on page 437 so you can quickly find your favorites.

 Multiple Servings of Fruits and Vegetables: To help you get your "five a day," you'll quickly see which recipes give you more than ½ cup of a fruit or vegetable per serving.

 High Fiber: So important to your general health as well as a boon to weight loss, our icons point the way to fiber-rich dishes. Any dish that contains at least 5 grams of fiber per serving (between 14 and 20 percent of your daily recommended value) received this icon.

 30 Minutes or Less: Everyone cooks differently, but these are recipes that almost everyone can have on the table in a half hour or less.

 Freezes Well: To make the most efficient use of the time you spend in the kitchen, it's great to be able to cook two and freeze one. This symbol lets you know that the servings you freeze will reheat beautifully.

 Kid-Friendly: Ian, Josh, and Noah tested and approved! We've concluded this book with advice to help you introduce your children to the benefits of healthy eating (see page 389), but look for this symbol throughout the book to point you toward dishes we know kids of all ages will love.

 Member Makeovers: Our SparkPeople members love to share their recipes, so we've taken a number of their favorites and tweaked them just a bit to make them even healthier.

 Great for Company: Who says you can't entertain and feed your guests a healthy meal? Not us! Look for this symbol to find dishes that are elegant and easy, or fun for a crowd.

 Vegetarian: Whether or not you've chosen to make a complete lifestyle change, it's good for all of us to eat less meat. This symbol points to dishes that are meat-free.

continued on next page

Fit These Recipes into Any Meal Plan. Need to cut some calories? No problem. Throughout the book, you'll find "Slim It Down" suggestions, which will help you trim even more calories from our already healthy recipes.

Turn Any Dish into a Well-Balanced Meal. We've shared our favorite ways to prepare each recipe, often pairing up two or more dishes from this book. To help you save time and fit the recipes into even the busiest of nights, look for the "Make It a Meal" feature on all main dishes. You'll find quick tips to create two different meals—and we've listed the calories so you won't have to worry that you're eating too much. You'll note that serving sizes aren't included—that's because we based all our tips on the standard portion sizes as explained on page 17.

Online Bonus. SparkRecipes.com has an extensive video library of cooking demos. So if a recipe requires you chop an onion, segment an orange, or buy fresh fish, we've indicated that you can find a step-by-step video on our site to walk you through the process.

A Note about Time. Everyone cooks differently. Some of us might enjoy the relaxing rhythm of chopping mounds of vegetables for a stir-fry while others consider that the food processor's job—and still others will reach for the bag of pre-chopped vegetables bought at the supermarket. Whatever method you choose is the best method. Unless we've specifically indicated otherwise, the preparation times given for the recipes are based on handmade rather than pre-prepped ingredients. Look to our sidebars such as Member Tips, Variations, and Chef Meg's Secrets for suggestions and shortcuts.

Of course, the first time you make a recipe, it may take you a little longer. But as these recipes become family favorites (and we know they will!), you'll find your own variations and ways of saving time in the preparation—and we hope you'll share them with us on SparkRecipes.com, too!

Above all, make it easy on yourself. At SparkPeople, we encourage you to avoid pre-packaged, processed foods that tend to be high in fat, salt, and sugar, but that doesn't mean that all prepared foods are less than healthy—make use of whatever shortcut foods you find that fit into your budget, schedule, and nutritional profile. Need proof? Take a look at our recipe for Dark Chocolate Angel Food Cake with Rich Chocolate Glaze on page 359. We could have made an angel food cake from scratch, but why on earth would we want to separate a dozen eggs when a mix works perfectly fine?

Success Story:
I Now Enjoy My Life— and My Food

by Amber Kozera (AMBER512)
96 pounds lost

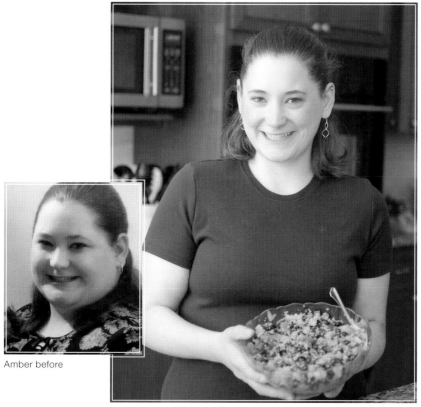

Amber before

Amber in her kitchen

Three years ago, Amber's definition of cooking was quite different than it is today. A rare activity in her life, cooking usually involved a few steps: Boil water, tear open packages, open jars, and stir together. No chopping, cutting, or prepping involved. For a "fancy" meal, she made spaghetti with jarred sauce and frozen garlic bread. Usually, it was mac and cheese with the orange powder, pizza pockets in the microwave, or ramen noodles.

> ## "Food provides me with strength for not only working out, but my daily life."

At 23, she tipped the scales at more than 245 pounds. She was happily married but knew she couldn't be the wife and, someday, the mother, she wanted to be if she continued on this unhealthy path. *If I'm not taking care of myself, I'm not going to be able to take care of a child*, she thought.

Two months after her life-changing decision, she hadn't made much progress. Then a friend recommended SparkPeople, and, 96 pounds later, she prides herself on her "clean" eating habits and profound love for fruits and whole grains. Amber eats more often than she did before, but she has little trouble keeping the weight off. Real food tastes better without spending hours in the kitchen, and she's satisfied without overeating.

Here, she shares her story.

I had my gallbladder out at 19, and the fatty, greasy foods I ate just killed my stomach, but they tasted good so I ate them anyway. When I started to cut back on the things that I knew irritated my stomach, I felt better. I had the energy to go for a walk, to go for a run, to get up and move.

Today I look for foods that taste good, that don't hurt my stomach—and are healthy for me and can help me have the energy to live my life. I didn't cook at all before SparkPeople, so cooking is definitely one of my tools to success. When I stopped eating so much processed junk, I started feeling a lot better.

My absolute favorite meals now combine a protein with a grain or starch and steamed vegetables (broccoli, Brussels sprouts, carrots, cauliflower, asparagus, etc.). Some examples:

- Black-bean wraps, brown rice, and steamed vegetables
- Homemade veggie burgers, roasted potato wedges, and steamed vegetables
- Spaghetti with a large vegetable salad with homemade ranch dressing

My palate has changed immensely. I had no idea that would happen! It is very rare for me to eat at a restaurant now—a huge change for me—because the food simply doesn't taste very good. Most of the food tastes like someone dumped a pile of salt on it.

I have learned to not just like, but *love* whole-wheat noodles, brown rice, and whole-wheat bread. I used to not eat a single whole grain. When I started swapping my usual food with whole-wheat versions, I found that they tasted so much better. And the texture is amazing, especially whole-wheat noodles.

When I first started learning about weight loss, I reached for fat-free, artificially sweetened "diet" foods. The more I learned about eating right, the more I started reading labels. One day, I flipped over my "light" yogurt and thought, *I've read books that are shorter than this.* That's not a good sign. Now I eat 2% Greek yogurt. It may be 130 calories compared with 80, but it's way creamier, it tastes better, and it doesn't have any junk.

Now I think, *Why did I ever eat this? It's horrible*. I'd rather lose weight in a nice slow fashion and enjoy life—and my food.

Success Story: Confessions of a Former Junk-Food Junkie

by Karen (ARCHIMEDESII)
55 pounds lost

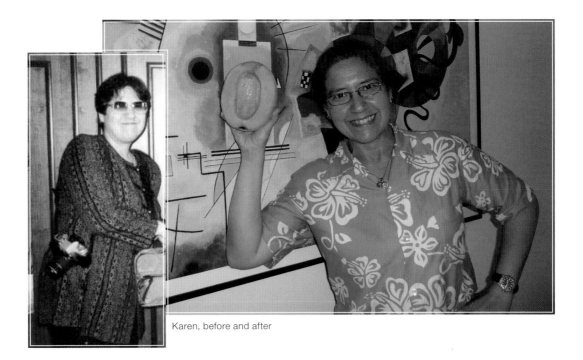

Karen, before and after

Seven years ago, Karen was a junk-food junkie. By her own admission, she drank a 2-liter bottle of Diet Coke a day, routinely ate one or two jumbo muffins as a mid-morning snack, and could eat a half a chicken for dinner. Her condiment of choice was ketchup; she put it on everything—even pizza.

But that's all in her past. By focusing on eating right and watching her portions, Karen lost 55 pounds over the course of a year—and she's kept it off. Embracing a healthy lifestyle led Karen to pursue her passion for kick-boxing, and she's now not only an instructor of the sport, but last year became a certified personal trainer.

Karen credits the most important part of her success to relearning her love of cooking.

I grew up in a family that loved to cook, and cooking has been an integral part of my life for as long as I can remember. But then there came a time when I stopped cooking for myself, and that's when I really packed on the pounds. Why cook when I could buy a meatball sub or burger? It was easy and convenient—no muss, no fuss.

Now I've learned to pay attention to what I'm eating, and by cooking for myself, I don't have to rely on eating out. I can create my own healthy meals. And it's easy! If I want, I can even make my own healthy version of the meatball subs I used to buy.

When I was overweight, my primary veggie was the French fry and the occasional serving of broccoli. Today, I eat six to nine servings of fruits and veggies every day. I eat whole-grain breads, cereals, and pastas. I used to really love fried foods and buffalo wings. I ate them regularly. Today, I like grilled chicken or salmon. And I really do love my leafy green salads: I've learned to like bitter leafy greens like radicchio lettuce, chard, beet greens, mustard greens, kale, and spinach. Yes, I still eat pasta—eggs and butter, too. My motto is "all things in moderation." I do prefer lean, center-cut pork, turkey, and chicken to beef. I cook with extra-virgin olive oil and I eat plenty of nuts and seeds. I'd like to get more seafood into my diet, but I'm still working on that.

Since I made changes to my nutrition, I rarely get sick and if I do, it's only for a day or two and my symptoms aren't as severe. I have more energy and it's not just because of regular exercise. I am positive that the reason I was so sluggish when I was overweight was because I ate too much sugar. It weighed me down like an anchor. By cutting back on sugar, I feel absolutely amazing. And—bonus points—people tell me I have beautiful nails. I never heard that when I was overweight and eating poorly.

There's a quotation I read, perhaps from Confucius, that's really inspired me. It goes something like this: "When eating, leave a little space in your stomach." Seven years ago, I wouldn't think twice about eating until I was ready to burst. Today, I leave a little space in my stomach.

> **"When I was overweight, my primary veggie was the French fry and the occasional serving of broccoli. Today, I eat 6 to 9 servings of fruits and veggies every day."**

Success Story: A Family Gets Fit Together

by Stephanie Crane (IHEARTNOAHSDAD)
41 pounds lost

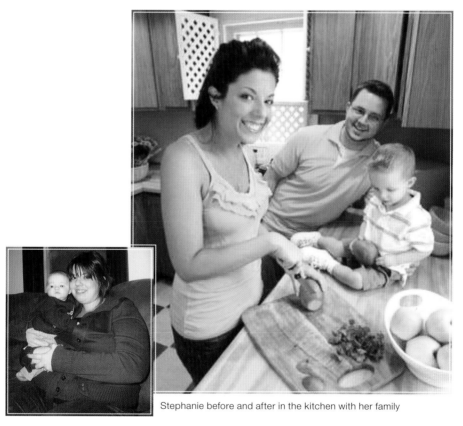

Stephanie before and after in the kitchen with her family

Stephanie can remember a time (not so long ago) when her family's refrigerator contained little more than a bottle of ketchup and a spoiled egg. She and her husband did not go grocery shopping (aside from a weekly soda run), and cooking was defined as reheating Chinese food or sprinkling extra cheese on day-old pizza.

But she can also pinpoint the moment when she decided to take back control of her family's nutrition—and their health. Stephanie had quit her intolerable job of six years and returned to college. She was reading a text on obesity and all the associated health risks, when it clicked.

My son was about seven months old and just beginning to eat solid foods. I realized he would grow up watching me eat McDonald's three (or more) times a week, probably eating the same, and he would likely be obese, too. And he could die. It was like something in me just snapped. That moment I began my journey back to fitness.

Now, we sit down together and plan out our week of meals, compiling a shopping list as we go. By preparing for meals ahead of time, we've been able to transform our lifestyle. We cook every single day, nearly every meal, and our definition of cooking has radically changed, as well. Yes, we still do eat out on occasion, but only after checking out a menu and pre-planning what we'll order. By knowing our calories ahead of time, it's much easier to say no to the hidden pitfalls (like predinner bread or appetizers). By making cooking a habit in our household, it no longer feels like a choice that we have to make every day; it's just something we do. With a plan in place, the time set aside, and the food already in the fridge, cooking meals at home has actually become easier than drive-thru!

> **"It's been vital to look at food in a new way—not as entertainment or happiness or therapy, but as fuel for my body."**

For me, a focus on nutrition and diet has been the single most important element to my weight-loss success. My zeal for exercise in any given week varies a great deal, but I've been able to eat well consistently for over a year thanks to my newly developed knowledge of cooking and nutrition. It's been vital to look at food in a new way—not as entertainment or happiness or therapy, but as fuel for my body. It's also been crucial to look at cooking in a new way—not as a hassle or a chore, but as a creative outlet.

And after a year of eating healthy, I think my taste buds had grown immune to fatty foods. In the past, the more sugary, salty, greasy food I ate, the more I craved. Pizza could never have enough cheese. Subs could never have enough mayo. Bread could never have enough garlic butter. It's incredible how you can reverse course by making small, consistent changes: the more good stuff I ate, the better it tasted (and the worse the cheese, mayo, and butter tasted). I never liked fish, but now salmon and haddock are staples in our diet. I used to be addicted to soda, but now it seems nauseatingly sweet. Green vegetables actually taste good on their own; they don't need to be drenched in butter and coated with salt. I think it's more than just getting used to "diet" food; it's allowing our bodies to appreciate the natural goodness of wholesome food without being overwhelmed and overshadowed by salt, sugar, and fat.

I do occasionally get that old, familiar fat craving, and we do allow ourselves splurge days now and then. It always seems exciting (exhilarating even!) to order that double-cheese pizza or turtle sundae, and it is always (*always*) followed by the same scenario: After the first few bites, I realize it doesn't taste as good as I had imagined it would. I continue, though, feeling almost obligated to realize the indulgence. Then comes the bloat, the stomachache, and the nausea. I feel physically bad, then I feel emotionally bad—I'm filled with guilt and disappointed in myself. I am forced to examine why I fell back into the old (bad) habit of covering up some psychological issue with food, and I realize that the psychological issue is still there, lurking. I still have to address the issue itself, and now I have to address the emotional eating on top of it. The next day is always the same, too. I find myself hungrier than usual, as if my body is aching for some nutrients that I deprived it of the previous day. Then comes the forgiveness, and, ultimately, the moving forward.

This lifestyle change was not a solitary choice, but a family decision, so I never really had to deal with any adverse reaction from my husband. We support each other in making choices that are good for ourselves and for our family. Ironically, it seems like we spend more time together than ever before! Instead of hitting separate drive-thrus on our way home from work, we plan meals together, collectively brainstorm new recipe ideas, grocery shop as a family, and cook as a team. We eat meals gathered around our dining-room table while chatting about our days, instead of silently in front of the television with brown bags in our laps and blank stares on our faces.

It has also created a new closeness between my husband and me. That's in part due to the intense levels of support that this journey has required and in part because we have had to form a united front against a world that shoves donuts and cheeseburgers in our faces and tells us that food is entertainment and happiness and love. It has forced us to really examine our parenting philosophies, our values, our hopes and dreams for our son; and it has required us to make a plan (as a team) as to how we can put that plan into motion.

My extended family has been shocked and amazed by our transformations but still more shocked and amazed by our dedication to this lifestyle. I think my greatest joy in this whole process has been to watch how our choices have influenced and motivated others around us to change. I couldn't be prouder of us, or them.

Success Story:
Using Food to Fuel
Fitness—and Faith

by Tara Behanan (HALLELUL)
38 pounds lost

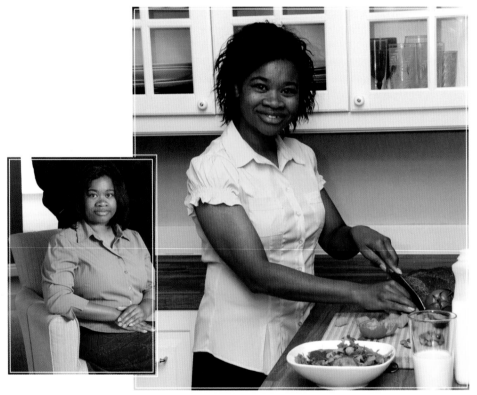

Tara before, and Tara now in her kitchen

Tara, a 38-year-old clerical worker for a Cincinnati-based nonprofit organization, has an infectious laugh and a smile that lights up her face. Single with no children, she was a member of our Ditch the Diet Taste Test. When Tara found she didn't have the energy to keep up with the rest of the congregation in church, she knew she needed to lose weight. Motivation came from a friendly competition in her church and SparkPeople helped her to meet her goals. Now, she's not only enthusiastically praising the Lord on Sundays, but she completed her first marathon in 2010.

I used to say I had "sweet teeth," not just one sweet tooth. My nickname was Froot Loop. I would literally bring an empty margarine tub of the sugary cereal to work with me and snack on it all day. Now I've replaced that with Kashi's GOLEAN cereal. Not only do I really like it, but it's also healthy for me so I don't have to feel guilty eating it. Of course I eat it in moderation—about a serving size (1 or 2) and not a tub.

It's taken me a little more than a year to lose the weight, but I've reached my goal since participating in the Ditch the Diet Taste Test! Cooking has been so important to my success. I've been hearing more and more about "superfoods" and knowing how to properly incorporate them into a meal each day makes me feel good. I now know that I'm doing what I can to ward off sickness and fuel my body for the all-important "playtime" (which is what I call exercise).

"Now I know that I don't have to cheat to have a mmm-good meal."

I cook about three to four times a week. I have to admit that I was apprehensive, thinking, once I got to my goal weight would I be able to keep it off?—thinking that since I lost so much, I could cheat. Now I know that I don't have to cheat to have an mmm-good meal.

Salt was a big no-no growing up because of my mom's high blood pressure issues, so I have a low tolerance for really salty things. But [at the Ditch the Diet Taste Test] when I bit into the sweet potato, carrot, and parsnip fries, they seemed spicy at first, but then just reminded me of regular French fries. What was even more interesting is that I didn't know I was eating carrot fries. I love to "drink" carrots in carrot juice, but I've never really enjoyed eating them. Well, I do now!

And though salt was never a problem for me, I have limited fat (especially bad fat). And I use a food scale to keep myself from overeating. Sugar is still a work in progress. I say progress because I do consume less of it but it still is a weakness. I'm used to things being sweet and I just don't like the taste of artificial sweeteners. Sometimes, when the meal is over and I still feel like eating or I'm not satisfied, adding my favorite fruit—cantaloupe—will help. It actually makes me feel full.

Before, I would buy a family-size roll of the 80/20 ground chuck, cut it into 2-inch slices, and eat two slices for dinner. I'd fry those up with slices of American cheese on top, alongside four potatoes—also fried in a skillet—and call it dinner. Dessert was cookies-and-cream ice cream—my favorite, but I don't crave it as much anymore—I'd eat two cups a few nights a week. That's four servings!

Now I use healthier condiments, and make substitutions, like Greek yogurt in place of butter and heavy cream. I bake more than I fry, too. Honestly, I haven't mastered all of this yet and I'm still working on planning meals ahead of time so that my kitchen is properly stocked. But I know I'll get there soon.

Success Story:
Healthy Eating Is
a Family Affair

by Greg Gaul (KSIGMA1222)
165 pounds lost

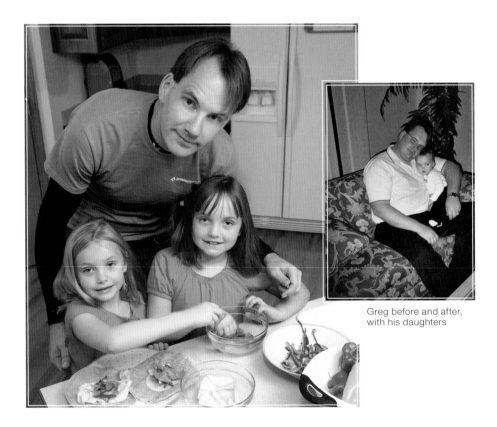

Greg before and after,
with his daughters

A former high-school athlete from Kansas, Greg has lost 165 pounds with SparkPeople, and this father of three says his family's lives will never be the same. His daughters are growing up healthy and happy, thanks in part to his family's commitment to the SparkPeople philosophy of small steps to reach larger goals. He has also grown closer with his father, who has always been active.

I lost the weight so I could be more the father I wanted to be—rather than the one I talked about being and thought about being. I want to see my daughters grow up and experience life. I went skiing with my dad for the first time last year, and it was amazing for me; I want to be able to do that with them. My dad is a very active man who was a runner when he was my age, and I have always aspired to be as much like him as I can. I want to give that to my kids as best I can and for as long as possible.

I am now more active and willing to go out and do things than I was before so they are as well. They come and cheer me on in races, and I get to play more with them and not be winded or all sweaty. Before, if it was hot outside—forget about me even thinking of going outside. Now I take them to the pool or playground and could care less about getting hot or sweaty. I can also show them that you can and should always remain active through-out life, as my father showed me.

Since I started losing weight and shaping up, much in our lives has changed. The changes are small, but they're significant. We started walking to school and church more since both are only about half a mile away. We take more walks as a family and go to the park more. We go swimming more in the summer and are outside more in general and do not sit nearly as much as we used to and watch TV.

We keep healthier foods around and encourage our children to try them. We are also teaching them about serving sizes and how to know when they are full. They've learned what a complete meal is—that they need to have a fruit, vegetable, and an entrée and to eat all three meals plus snacks. They prepare their fruit while we prepare dinner for them. We don't eat out as much as we did before; we sit down together at home and have dinner as a family. I've learned what my daughters like to eat and now we work new foods into our meals to get them to try things. Hopefully, they'll like them, but we don't force them to eat anything they don't want.

> "If you eat fast food and frozen dinners, well, then your family will spend just that much time preparing and eating it, which is not long and really mindless. Working together for our meals and then sitting down together to eat them is so HUGE to any family."

I cook at least 95 percent of my meals now, if not more, and it's been a huge part of my weight-loss success. I've learned that eating is all about balance and making sure your body has what it needs to keep you healthy mentally and physically. I appreciate, respect, and enjoy what I am eating now. Before, the comfort came from wolfing down whatever and not caring about what it was and what it did for or to me.

I reduced my salt intake without even trying—just by eating healthier and preparing my own fresh food. My taste buds are much more sensitive now and I use them to understand and appreciate what I am eating. Before, with such greasy, salty, and processed foods, my taste buds would get coated or overwhelmed with one taste; but now I use them more to truly determine if I will continue to eat something or decide it is not what I want and just not eat it.

I do not look at reducing my intake of sugar, salt, and fat as limiting but finally getting it right and understanding how these all work in my cooking. The family does not really notice because things taste better.

Healthy cooking slows us down and brings us together. If you eat fast food and frozen dinners, well, then your family will spend just that much time preparing and eating it, which is not long and really mindless. Working together for our meals and then sitting down together to eat them is so *huge* to any family. Growing the food, buying it at a farmers' market, buying at the grocery store or anywhere else—it all takes time and planning, but it is time spent with the family planning, thinking, and sharing. Doing so teaches you and your family so much: it shows that you have options and can be creative, and not just stuck with the way it comes.

Success Story: Confessions of a Reformed Country Cook

by Dawn Wilson (REVELATIONGIRL)
30 pounds lost: halfway to goal weight!

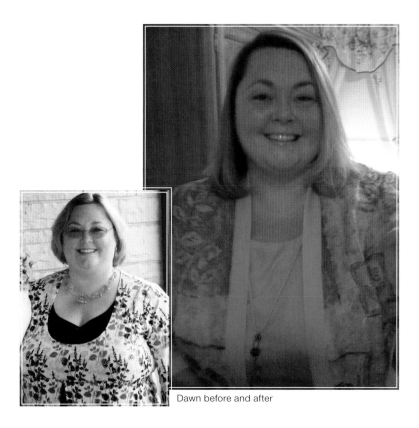
Dawn before and after

Married for 27 years and a mother of two grown sons, Dawn (REVELATIONGIRL)—the reformed "country cook" you met in Chapter 1—recently resigned her job in western Pennsylvania to get back "a little 'me' time." Having successfully made it through knee surgery this year, she finds that using SparkPeople.com's Nutrition Tracker feature helps her continue toward her weight-loss goals while improving her overall nutrition. One of our most popular features, the Nutrition Tracker allows members to enter food plans and receive a daily calorie count and nutritional analysis.

Once I realized how much my nutrition was off, it really helped me to be more conscious of the foods I was eating. I didn't feel well at all. I'm struggling with numerous health issues and I felt completely out of control of my quality of life, which was spiraling downward. I thought, *Okay, I can't do anything really to control, stop, or change arthritis. I can't control my body's fibro reactions. I can't fix my knees without replacing them. There is so much I have no control of, but I can control what I put in my mouth.* That was the beginning of my realization that I am responsible for that portion of my health; not God, not another person, not the doctor, just me.

I'm making it my goal to hit the proper nutrition and I also track some key elements like potassium, calcium, and iron, which are problem areas for me. I *love* it when the nutrition report gives me As! I have lost 4 inches from the bust, 3.5 inches from my waist, 3 inches from my hips, for a total of 10.5 inches! And I lost without exercising because I've had very serious knee problems. I have much more energy and desire to get up off the couch or tackle projects that before seemed too much to even start. My cholesterol has come down 20 points.

I am much more aware of the sodium content of things that I thought of as healthy before (like tomato juice—something I love!). I have really cut way back on canned goods and packaged side dishes, and I even started making homemade bread so I can control the ingredients, including the sodium.

> "My family is everything to me and feeding them well, instead of feeding them much, has become the goal."

I began to crave the steamed fresh or frozen veggies far more than the old canned stuff. The taste I thought was reserved for restaurant-style food—the crisp, fresh veggies that my family wasn't used to at home—became what I wanted on my own table. The taste of high-sodium, fatty gravy or rich cream sauces might still appeal to me initially, but after a couple bites I feel like I've ingested straight fat or straight cholesterol. I taste the sodium and it is so unappetizing. I feel like I've got to go grab some healthy fresh fruit and cleanse my palate.

My husband and adult children were very supportive of my efforts to lose weight and get healthy, but they were not sure that they wanted to eat like me. The SparkPeople recipes I've tried have won them over! They are my biggest supporters and my husband tells everyone about me making recipes off the site that are so good that even he is eating them!

My family is everything to me and feeding them well, instead of feeding them much, has become the goal. We have learned together about eating healthy. Instead of my husband judging if my food is "diet-approved" or not, he's learning about better choices and how to support me in them. We share our health successes, weight loss, goals met, and so on and it has made a really big impact. Now, instead of my husband egging my younger son to finish up something from the supper table, he's aware of his weight-loss efforts, his success, and my husband is learning not to push food on him. That was a big problem. My husband can eat a ton of calories and seemingly not gain weight. Something had to make him aware of my son's inability to do the same. SparkPeople has helped us to create an atmosphere in our home where directly, and indirectly, better choices, healthy foods, and support for each other's personal plans allow everyone the freedom to succeed.

I hope you begin to think of your journey as more than dieting to lose weight to get to a particular goal. Take it from me, your health is a very fragile thing. These are the times in your life to grab hold and start making really strong, good habits that will work for the rest of your life! If you're older and starting now, *good for you!* Get your health meter up and your nutrition in, and I bet you see a big difference in your mood, how you feel, and how you face the day.

Success Story:
Small Changes Lead
to Great Success

by Frances Kranik (CALIDREAMER76)
110 pounds lost

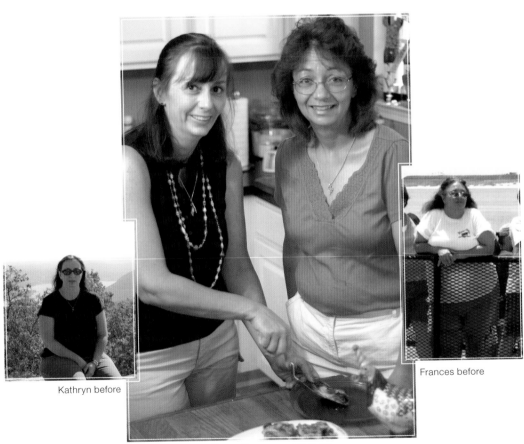

Kathryn before

Frances before

Sisters Frances and Kathryn

Sometimes a little sibling rivalry can be a good thing—especially when it provides a wake-up call to a healthier lifestyle. For Frances Kranik, the alarm clock rang when her sister Kathryn Garguilo revealed that she had been losing weight in her first two months as a SparkPeople member. (See Kathryn's story on page 69.) That was in 2007, and at this writing, Frances is only 15 pounds from her goal of being 125 pounds lighter. A 52-year-old teacher living in southwestern Pennsylvania, Frances uses the SparkPeople Nutrition Tracker daily and embraced our philosophy of small changes to keep her on track toward her goals.

I've never been happy with my appearance. In high-school gym I "majored" in what they called Slimnastics—a class I took every year, which included using a universal gym and running laps. I had tried Weight Watchers and lost about 20 pounds, but gained it back and then some when I got pregnant with my third child.

My sister was always smaller than me, but in 2007 she told me that she had joined a weight-loss study at work. We had gone to the beach a couple of times and I'd noticed she was thinner. Then she told me about SparkPeople. At that point I decided that she wasn't going to continue to get thinner while I still looked like a beached whale. I guess you could call that my "aha!" moment.

> **"I enjoy telling people to watch out on the road to my house, because there is 100 pounds of fat lying out there. That's where I walked and lost the weight."**

Over the course of two years, I have managed to keep the weight off and continue to lose, but I have hit plateaus and they are *very* frustrating and discouraging. But then I get mad at myself and refocus my efforts: I add some strength-training exercises and change up my routine.

I fight against the statistic that I won't keep it off. I refuse to be that kind of statistic! And I've had so many people tell me they are proud of me. They look at me a certain way and I couldn't stand the look they'd have if I gained weight. I'm sure most wouldn't say anything, but it would just hurt too deeply to feel as though they were disappointed in me.

I've been trying a few new recipes that I've found on SparkRecipes.com, but I also have a number of new healthy menu staples: frozen brown rice (half a bag is one serving, so it's good for two nights!); frozen vegetables when they're not in season; fresh root vegetables that I roast once a week for three or four days of roasted veggies; and oatmeal—I stock up when it's on sale. In addition to a variety of spices, I'm trying to incorporate more variety and use more fresh herbs in my cooking.

I use the Nutrition Tracker on SparkPeople.com every day. At midday I'll track my food to see what I need to do for dinnertime. I track my exercise daily, too. But it is the message boards—getting to know people and being able to get and give support—that takes it a step beyond other sites. SparkPeople is a community of loving, health-minded people.

As I've lost weight, my life continues to change. I've developed more confidence, and in September 2009 I drove by myself to Cincinnati to attend the SparkPeople convention. Although I didn't know anybody before I got there, I left with some dear friendships. No matter where we are now in regard to our health, we all have in common where we began and we can relate easily to everyone else's journey.

I would advise anyone who is just starting on this journey to make small changes that you can live with. If you don't like salads, then don't eat salads to lose weight, because that isn't something you'll stick with. Don't have forbidden foods. I didn't cut anything out—I just evaluated what I was eating. I have a goal to eat at least five fruits and veggies during the day. So if I'm doing that sometimes I don't have room in my daily meals for other things that may have empty calories or just aren't as helpful to my body. I used to be a big bread eater. I still have it, but not as much, and when I do I thoroughly enjoy every bite. I exercise in some form every day. Most of my weight was lost walking. I enjoy telling people to watch out on the road to my house, because there is 100 pounds of fat lying out there—that's where I walked and lost the weight. At the very least, get a good pedometer. I started out with the goal of 10,000 steps—now most days it's 12,000 to 15,000 steps. When I first started out, I'd check myself in the late afternoon and, if I was low, I'd take an extra walk.

My family is my biggest inspiration. My sister, who first inspired me and introduced me to SparkPeople, and my children; I continue on to be a good example to them and hopefully inspire them. And I would also say to my students: when they are down and say things like "I can't," I point to a picture of me by my desk when my oldest graduated college and say, "If I can do this, you can do whatever you put your mind to."

Success Story: Driving Away from the Drive-Thru

by Kathryn Garguilo (BIGDOGMOM3)
50 pounds lost

Kathryn Garguilo is the sister who inspired Frances Kranik to join SparkPeople. A nurse living in Nashville, Kathryn has learned to adapt both Italian and Southern cooking styles to her new healthy habits.

I truly enjoying cooking and use it as a means of relaxing. Cooking takes my mind off work and whatever else is going on in my life. I love trying new dishes. Most of the time I eat at home so learning to cook flavorful, healthy meals has really helped me in losing weight and feeling better.

I also really love cooking for people. Being Italian, I like to cook to please people. Nothing makes me happier than to cook for friends and family and make them feel good. I also enjoy sneaking healthy foods in and have people really like it without realizing they're eating healthy. Living in the south—where everything is cooked in butter, oil, or heavy cheese—that's a real triumph!

Today, my diet is much healthier and lighter—and I always try to make sure I have something quick to make for the days I work late. There have been many days when I get off work late and I think it would be so easy to stop and grab a hamburger somewhere. Then I tell myself by the time I get through the drive-thru I could warm some chicken up in the microwave and throw a salad together. In the past, the drive-thru would have won out. I also always bring my lunch to work. I used to bring the leftovers from my not-so-healthy dinner the night before. Now I eat Lean Cuisine, a light soup, or a turkey wrap with fresh veggies.

My favorite foods really haven't changed, I've just learned how to cook them healthier. I'm Italian and I love pasta. I stick with lighter pasta dishes, with a rare diversion of homemade Alfredo sauce. Homemade seafood Alfredo is a real weakness for me, but as long as it's only once or twice a year, I think I can treat myself.

Most people think of Italian food as heavy and very fattening, but I've managed to find lighter and healthier recipes or adapt old recipes to be healthier. I pretty much cook only with olive oil. I believe there's something to the Mediterranean way of eating: more fish, vegetables, and olive oil. I do a lot more baking, broiling, and braising. And I'm even getting my dad to eat healthier Italian foods. For example, when we make eggplant parmesan, we bake the slices of breaded eggplant instead of frying them.

People also think of Italian food as filled with lots of gooey cheese. But in the region that my dad's family comes from, the Amalfi Coast in southern Italy, they actually cook with lighter sauces and a lot of lemon. So I'm trying to adapt recipes we've always made with lighter sauces and healthier ways of cooking.

I do have to admit that I used to love fried foods, like fried chicken and French fries or onion rings. But I just can't handle greasy fried foods any more; if I try, my stomach gets upset. Foods I would have breaded and fried in the past, I now bake or grill. I love cooking on my grill year-round.

I eat a lot more fresh fruit and veggies and a lot more fish. I feel it's worth the expense of buying fresh fruit and veggies for the health and flavor benefits. I've learned to like a variety of fresh veggies—and a bigger variety of greens. I love putting baby spinach or arugula (or both) on a wrap. I have a fruit for a snack every morning and either fresh fruit or yogurt in the afternoon—I'm really hooked on Greek yogurt. Hummus is another of my favorite foods now—I never would have eaten that before.

When people bring tempting foods to work, like cookies and other goodies, I ask myself: *Is this really worth the calories?* Most of the time the answer is "no." It makes it easier to walk away from whatever temptation is put in my way.

> "I approach most foods with the question, 'Is this really worth the calories?' Most of the time, the answer is 'no.' It makes it easier to walk away from a cookie or whatever temptation is put in my way."

Part II

GET COOKING

BREAKFAST

In our house, we have three growing, active teen boys, a husband who is trying to lower his cholesterol, and a mom who has added strength training to her morning fitness routine—all trying to get out the door by 8 A.M. Despite our schedules, skipping breakfast is never acceptable in our house and everyone starts the day with a filling and nutritious meal.

It's not just a marketing ploy on the part of cereal companies: breakfast is the most important meal of the day. Think about it: your body has just spent (ideally) eight hours sleeping and your last meal was probably a few hours before bedtime. You've had no food or water in almost 12 hours. You're dehydrated, your blood sugar is low, and as a result, you have no energy. By skipping breakfast in favor of a snooze or getting the kids out the door in time for you to pick up coffee, you're sabotaging your healthy-eating efforts. By the time lunch rolls around, you're ravenous and more likely to reach for larger portions and unhealthy foods.

A 2002 study by the National Weight Control Registry of more than 3,000 people who had lost at least 30 pounds and kept it off for at least a year found that breakfast-eaters were more successful at maintaining their weight loss. SparkPeople members agree: when we surveyed members who had either lost 100 pounds or reached their weight-loss goals, we found that almost all of them either eat a substantial breakfast (66 percent of them) and or eat some breakfast (25.5 percent) every day. Less than 1 percent of successful members skip breakfast altogether.

WENDI_WA1 has lost 76 pounds in the past two years—and a good breakfast is part of her plan. "I went a few years with skipping a good breakfast," says the grandmother of five and retired nurse, "but am now back where I should be. I feel better and have more energy for the day when I do eat breakfast."

Even if, like my family, you're not trying to lose weight, breakfast should still be a part of your morning routine. It can improve your memory, brighten your mood, and even boost your performance at work and school. One study of college students found that those who ate breakfast scored 22 percent higher in word-recall tests than students who started the day with an empty belly.

Harvard researchers found that kids who skipped breakfast were twice as likely to be depressed, four times more prone to anxiety, and 30 percent more likely to be hyperactive. When those kids started eating breakfast regularly, their levels of depression, anxiety, and hyperactivity all decreased.

That same study showed that children who ate breakfast had 40 percent higher math grades and missed fewer days of school than non-breakfast-eaters. When children who "rarely" ate breakfast began eating breakfast "often," their math grades increased one full letter grade.

With all those benefits, why don't people eat breakfast? The No. 1 reason is time. Well, you don't need an hour to make breakfast. If you have five minutes, you have time for breakfast. You'll soon find it's worth it to make a good breakfast, like SparkPeople member ARTEMISIA47 did:

"I used to have a bowl of cereal and orange juice for breakfast, but found that I was ravenous by mid-morning. I have switched to having egg whites, a whole-wheat light English muffin, and O.J. I find that I have so much more energy—and breakfast stays with me a whole lot longer. It takes a bit longer but it's so worth it."

I remind my boys that I'm a chef—not a short-order cook—so breakfast during the week has to be quick and easy. As any mother knows, mornings require superhuman strength to keep everyone organized and on time. Just as *mise en place* (everything in its place and a place for everything) is the key to success in a restaurant, it is the guiding principle in my home kitchen as

well. Sunday is the day for organizing a week of filling healthy breakfasts. I take inventory of the pantry and fridge, making sure we have gallons of nonfat milk (my oldest son is growing like a weed and another chugs milk like it's going out of style), low-sugar cereal for our busiest days, and fresh fruit to round out our meals. We each have our favorite meals, but none takes more than a few minutes to prepare.

There's oatmeal for my husband, whose doctor recommended that he eat oats for high cholesterol. Oats contain soluble fiber, which can help reduce cholesterol absorption and lower blood cholesterol levels. (Learn more about the benefits of fiber on page 290.) He stopped at the store and picked up a box of instant oatmeal, a great first step—until I read the label and saw how much salt and sugar he was consuming. Instant oatmeal can contain up to 170 calories and a tablespoon of sugar in each 2-ounce packet. On my next trip to the store, I picked up a low-sugar version, but it still contained a lot of sugar and had more salt than the original.

Making oatmeal at home is cheaper and healthier, and each person can customize his or hers. I started with Stepfanie's recipe for a basic Oatmeal Mix (page 79) I found on SparkPeople's healthy living blog, the dailySpark. Each portion has fiber-rich nuts, dried fruit, and flaxseed, which can further help lower cholesterol. All the benefits of oats without all the sugar and salt, and it's still ready in just a couple of minutes.

One menu item all my boys can agree on is omelets. This is a perfect way to get your kids to eat right in the morning without having to get up at 4 A.M. Think ahead and always be on the lookout for omelet fillers and toppings as you prepare meals. If we have stir-fry for dinner, I put aside leftover vegetables for the morning.

If lasagna is on the menu, I save some of the sauce for an Italian cheese omelet.

We live just outside of Cincinnati, Ohio, where chili is king. The favorite omelet creation in this household is a chili-cheese omelet. Believe it or not, it can be done for a reasonable amount of fat and calories. (Try it with the Slow-Cooker White Bean Chicken Chili on page 172 or even Slimmer Sloppy Joes on page 221.) I always save some of my vegetarian chili for omelet fillings on cold mornings. The beauty of the omelet is that each of my boys can "have it his way" and head off to school with a healthy breakfast in his belly.

I could eat the same breakfast 365 days of the year: 1 cup high-protein cereal, 2 tablespoons ground flax seeds, and ½ cup skim milk; plus some fruit, so I try to plan for variety. To change things up, I eat granola (see recipe, page 87) with low-fat yogurt and berries as my go-to meal when I know I'll be tasting students' dishes all day at school. On days when I've had a harder workout, I have an egg-white omelet in a whole-wheat tortilla wrap with salsa.

SO WHAT SHOULD YOU BE EATING?

SparkPeople recommends a healthy breakfast of 300 to 400 calories, with a mix of quality carbohydrates, healthy protein, and healthy fat. Design a breakfast that includes something from at least three food groups, for example: Greek yogurt, fresh fruit, and granola.

If it's better to eat breakfast than to eat nothing, why should it matter what you're eating? Donuts, pastries, and other baked goods made from white flour are popular breakfast foods, but think about how you feel after eating them. Are you content after just one donut, or are you reaching for another? Does a croissant or sugary Danish sustain you until lunchtime?

Those meals are filling your belly with empty calories; along with fat, salt, and sugar. They're doing nothing to satisfy you. The donut will set you up for a sugar crash later on, and the simple carbs lack staying power. The same goes for that doughy bagel. Your belly will growl by mid-morning, and you'll count down the minutes until lunch arrives.

SparkPeople Cooking Challenge:
Swap your sweet and sugary breakfast for one that's higher in fiber and protein. Note any difference in your energy levels.

When we started our taste test, almost half the participants skipped breakfast. At the end of two weeks, everyone said they were eating breakfast. That was one change they could commit to with little effort!

The recipes in this chapter are meant to fuel you through a busy morning. They're well-balanced meals, not light bites. Savory or sweet, hot or cold, whatever you crave, we have a recipe for you. From Warm and Spicy Banana Waffles (page 98) for the weekend to Egg-White Omelets (page 89) for a busy morning, these recipes will quell your hunger.

Because breakfast is such an important meal, you should choose your food carefully. We start with high-fiber carbohydrates for staying power and energy, then add some protein—which takes longer to digest—to keep you satisfied and fill you up. Add a cup of nonfat milk or a serving of low-fat yogurt and a generous portion of fruit; such as berries, a pear, an orange, or a banana to any recipe for a well-balanced meal.

Though you might be tempted to skimp on breakfast and "save" calories for a splurge at dinner or dessert, don't do it! Studies have shown that that tactic usually backfires, and you'll end up eating more in the long run.

"I have breakfast every morning," says PFIFER80. "I find that as long as I eat a good breakfast, I am not searching the house for food the rest of the day mindlessly eating. Usually, since I go to the gym really early, I prepare everything the night before. When I get home it is just a matter of either microwaving something I have prepared, or pouring on some hot water or milk."

The trick is to find something that satisfies you. If your epitome-of-health best friend swears by oatmeal every morning, but you can't stand the texture, eat something else. Bake a batch of healthy muffins, make a smoothie, or whip up an egg-white omelet. Eat leftovers from last night. All of us have had those days where you say "I'll do better tomorrow." Eating a good breakfast is the No. 1 thing you can do to "do better tomorrow."

SparkPeople Cooking Challenge:

Tonight, set your alarm ten minutes earlier—or forgo the snooze button just one time. You'll have plenty of time to make a healthy breakfast, even if you need to eat it on the go. (Breakfast is the one meal we give you permission to eat away from a table!)

NO TIME TO COOK BREAKFAST? NO EXCUSES!

For those days when cooking breakfast just isn't an option, SparkPeople members share ten meals that are healthy and ready in no time, for 400 calories or less:

1. A cup of high-fiber cereal with a banana and a carton of plain or vanilla low-fat yogurt.

2. A hard-boiled egg, a handful of spinach, and some salsa in a whole-wheat tortilla. (Also good with low-sodium deli turkey, roasted chicken, low-fat Cheddar, or scrambled egg whites.)

3. A smoothie made with a banana, ½ cup of yogurt, and a handful of berries; plus a slice of whole-wheat toast on the side.

4. A peanut butter and banana sandwich on whole-wheat bread. (Try adding berries or sliced grapes, too!)

5. Handfuls of a few items for the car: grapes, almonds, and high-fiber cereal; plus a cup of low-fat milk in a to-go mug.

6. A toaster waffle sandwich with cashew butter and all-fruit spread.

7. One piece of string cheese, an apple, and a handful of whole-wheat crackers.

8. A serving of plain, low-fat yogurt topped with a spoonful of real maple syrup, a chopped pear, and a serving of cereal or granola.

9. A fruit cup and a mini whole-wheat bagel with almond butter.

10. Low-sodium turkey, a slice of low-fat Cheddar, and leftover stir-fry vegetables in a whole-wheat pita pocket.

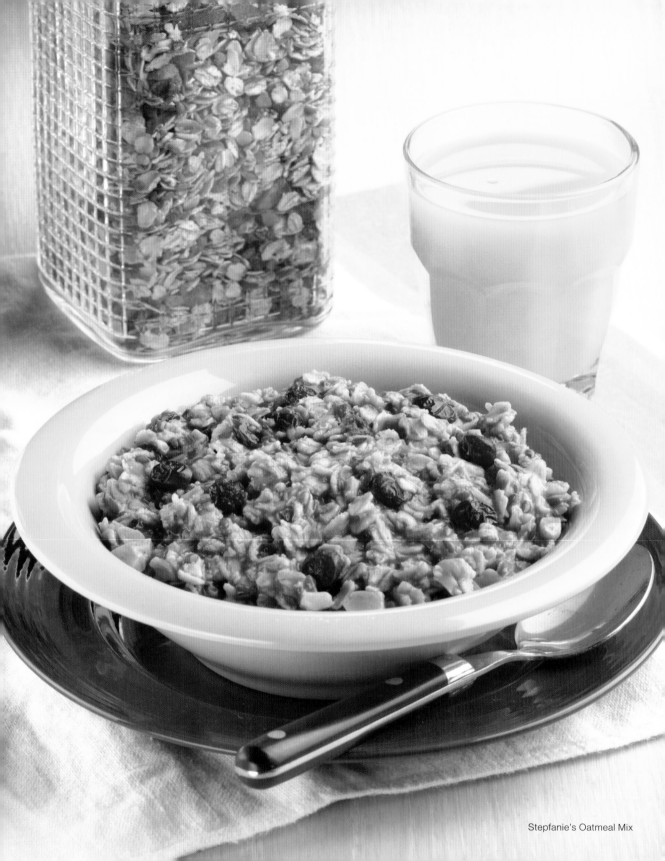

Stepfanie's Oatmeal Mix

Stepfanie's Oatmeal Mix

Who needs fancy oatmeal from the store? Stepfanie created this instant mix at members' request. Mix up a batch, and you'll have a gourmet breakfast each morning. This mix will keep in the refrigerator for up to a month. (Store it there because flax seeds and walnuts can go rancid quickly.) To cook the oatmeal, start with equal amounts water and oatmeal mix as we do here, then adjust the amount of water to achieve the texture you prefer. You can adjust the amount of cinnamon or swap in another spice, based on your preferences.

Makes 12 Servings:
¾ cup (1½ cups cooked) per serving

10 minutes or less to prep and cook

6 cups old-fashioned oats

¾ cup flaxseeds, ground

3 tbsp cinnamon

1½ cups chopped walnuts

1½ cups dried cranberries

1. Mix all the ingredients together and pour into a zip-top plastic bag or tightly covered container. Store in the refrigerator.

2. When ready to cook, bring ¾ cup water to boil on the stove or in the microwave. Place ¾ cup of the oatmeal mix in a bowl, pour the boiling water over, stir, and let stand for 5 minutes.

Note: Add more water if you prefer thinner oats, or use half milk and half water for richer oats and a boost of protein.

Per Serving: 329.2 calories, 15.3 g total fat, 0 mg cholesterol, 1.2 mg sodium, 44.9 g total carbs, 8.8 mg dietary fiber, 8.9 g protein

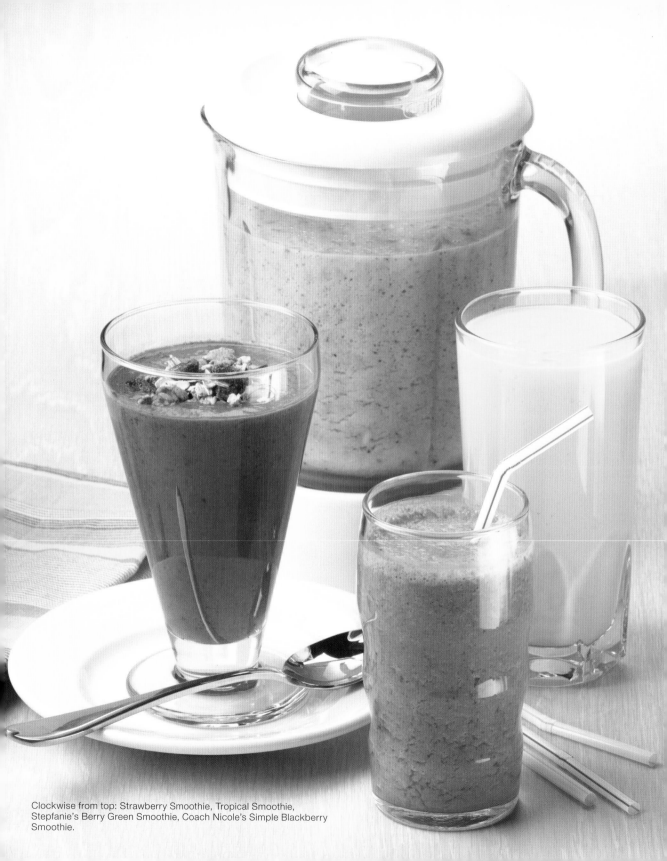

Clockwise from top: Strawberry Smoothie, Tropical Smoothie, Stepfanie's Berry Green Smoothie, Coach Nicole's Simple Blackberry Smoothie.

Superior Smoothies

Smoothies are a go-to breakfast at the SparkPeople offices. From SparkGuy's Spicy Vegetable Smoothie to Coach Nicole's Simple Blackberry Smoothie and Stepfanie's Berry Green Smoothies, it seems like the blender is always in use. Limited only by your imagination, smoothies are a great way to incorporate fruits and vegetables into your diet. You don't need a recipe to make a smoothie, but here are some tips to pack in the nutrition while keeping your portions under control.

Chef Meg's Tip: Add 1 cup of fresh spinach to your smoothies when you blend the liquids. You can see but not taste the spinach (I promise!), and you've just consumed one serving of vegetables without even trying.

For a sweet smoothie, choose one of the following base liquids:

½ to 1 cup skim milk

½ to 1 cup low-fat yogurt, plain or flavored

½ to 1 cup soy or other nondairy milk

½ cup 100% fruit juice

Choose from among the following to add texture and flavor:

1 tbsp nut butter (for added protein and satiety)

¼ cup oats (for added bulk and satiety)

1 scoop protein powder

1 tbsp flaxseed, ground

1 tbsp unsweetened cocoa powder

½ tsp cinnamon

1 tsp honey

Add your fruit (and even some vegetables). A serving is a ½ cup, but go ahead and pack in multiple servings.

1 small banana (to add thickness and creaminess)

½ cup each of the fruits and vegetables of your choice

1. If your fruit is fresh, add it when you blend the liquids. If it's frozen, add it at the end, and use the ice crushing setting on your blender and pulse until combined.

2. To ensure a perfect smoothie every time, blend your fresh fruit, nut butters, and liquids first. Pulse a few times to break up the chunks, then process until smooth. The time will vary based on your blender; it could take up to 2 minutes to reach the consistency you desire. Once the fruit and liquids are processed, add the ice or frozen fruit, pulse a few times, and process until thoroughly blended.

Note: Any fruit with a skin (pears, apples, grapes) doesn't blend well in a smoothie.

If you like, top your smoothie with something crunchy or creamy, for a nice contrast in texture:

½ graham cracker or 1 vanilla wafer cookie

¼ cup whole-grain cereal (add it a few tablespoons at a time as you eat the smoothie)

2 tbsp Nutty Fruity Granola (page 87)

1 tbsp chopped nuts

1 tbsp low-fat whipped cream topping

Pumpkin-Pie Smoothie

½ cup canned pumpkin

½ tsp pumpkin-pie spice

1 small banana

½ cup low-fat vanilla yogurt

½ graham cracker, crumbled

Per serving: 250 calories, 3 g fat, 6 g fiber, 7 g protein

Chocolate-Covered Cherry Smoothie

1 tbsp cocoa powder

1 cup frozen cherries

1 cup skim milk

1 small banana

Per serving: 265 calories, 2 g fat, 7 g fiber, 12 g protein

PB&J Smoothie

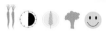

1 tbsp all-natural, no-salt-added peanut butter

1 tsp all-fruit strawberry preserves

½ cup strawberries

½ cup low-fat plain yogurt

1 small banana

Per serving: 318 calories, 11 g fat, 6 g fiber, 12 g protein

Coach Nicole's Simple Blackberry Smoothie

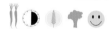

1 cup fresh blackberries

1 cup low-fat vanilla yogurt

Per serving: 276 calories, 3 g fat, 8 g fiber, 11 g protein

Stepfanie's Berry Green Smoothie

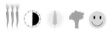

1 cup fresh spinach

½ cup soy milk

½ cup frozen blueberries

1 small frozen banana

1 tbsp almond butter

Per serving: 291 calories, 13 g fat, 6 g fiber, 8 g protein

Tropical Smoothie

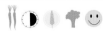

½ cup canned pineapple, with juice

½ cup frozen or fresh mango

½ cup low-fat vanilla yogurt

2 tbsp light coconut milk or 1 drop coconut extract

Per serving: 331 calories, 4 g fat, 5 g fiber, 7 g protein

SparkGuy's Spicy Vegetable Smoothie

1 cup low-sodium tomato juice

1 or 2 stalks celery, roughly chopped

1 carrot, roughly chopped

1 garlic clove, minced

½ tsp turmeric

½ tsp cayenne pepper

Salt and black pepper to taste

Note: Feel free to add any other vegetables you like to this smoothie. Spinach and broccoli are good choices.

Per serving: 106 calories, 0.5 g fat, 6 g fiber, 4 g protein

Muesli

Some people call it pottage, and other people call it overnight oats. I call it the good stuff. Muesli, a popular European breakfast cereal, was developed in 1900 by a Swiss physician. Recipes vary, but they always contain oats, which are mixed with other whole grains, and sometimes dried fruit and nuts. Once prepared, the mix is soaked overnight with milk, water, or yogurt for an easy, healthy breakfast. This is a basic recipe that can be changed to your liking with very little effort. It doubles well and makes a great hostess gift.

Chef Meg's Tip: Have you ever had a flip-flop dinner—breakfast for dinner? Muesli makes a great dinner when you add yogurt and fresh fruit.

Makes 8 Servings:
¼ cup per serving

7 Minutes to Prepare and Cook

For the dry mix:

2 cups old-fashioned rolled oats

¼ cup toasted wheat germ

¾ cup wheat or oat bran

½ cup flaxseeds, ground

½ tsp cinnamon

For serving:

¼ cup water

¼ cup skim milk or low-fat plain yogurt

½ cup strawberries, blueberries, bananas, mangoes, or apples (optional)

1 tbsp chopped pecans, walnuts, or almonds (optional)

1 tsp honey or maple syrup (optional)

1. To make the dry mix, combine the oats, wheat germ, bran, ground flaxseeds, and cinnamon in a large bowl. Store in an airtight container in the refrigerator for up to one month.

2. To make muesli for the next morning's breakfast, combine ¼ cup dry mix with the water and skim milk. Stir, cover, and place in the refrigerator overnight. Serve with fruit, nuts, and sweetener as desired.

Per serving of dry mix: 157.3 calories, 5.8 g total fat, 0 mg cholesterol, 4 mg sodium, 23.1 g total carbs, 8.7 g dietary fiber, 6.4 g protein

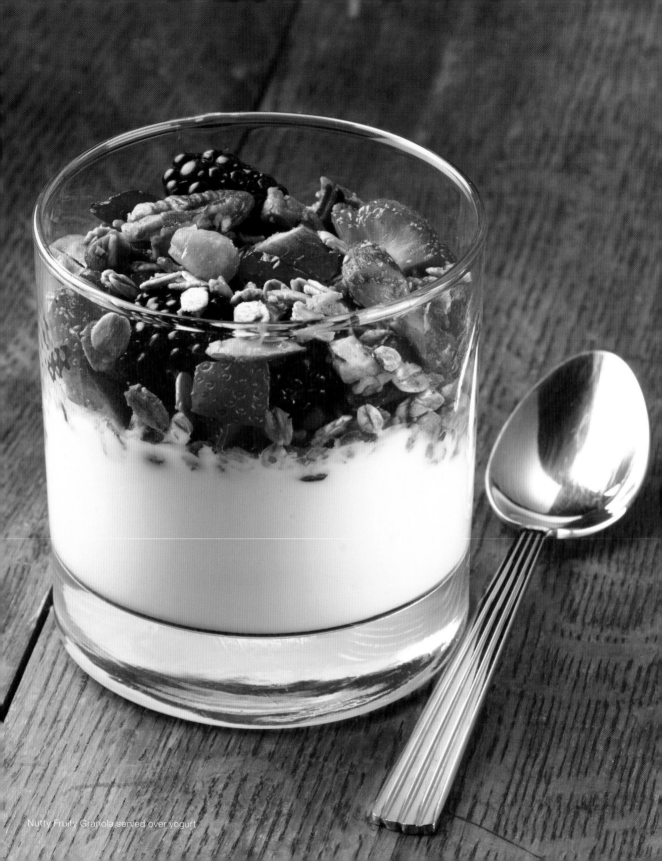

Nutty Fruity Granola served over yogurt

Nutty Fruity Granola

SLIM IT DOWN: Use half the nuts (save 33 calories) or omit them (save 66 calories).

While most people consider granola to be a cereal substitute—and want to eat it in larger servings—it is full of nutrient-dense ingredients like nuts and dried fruit. A serving of granola is considerably smaller than a serving of cold cereal—think of it as a topping for smoothies, yogurt, or fruit. It's also great as a snack in small amounts.

This recipe has a lot less fat than other recipes I've seen. It's very basic and easy to customize. You can use the seeds or nuts of your choice—try pistachios, walnuts, peanuts, sunflower seeds, or macadamia nuts instead of pecans and almonds. Swap dried blueberries, strawberries, or raisins for the cranberries, and use any dried fruit (dates, prunes, apricots, and figs) in place of the peaches.

This recipe makes a huge batch of granola, but it's much more cost-effective than store-bought versions. (It also makes a great gift!) If you're worried about controlling yourself around such a large amount, use a measuring cup to portion out the ¼-cup serving.

Makes 24 Servings:
¼ cup per serving

45 Minutes to Prepare and Cook

1 cup raw pecan halves

1 cup raw almonds

½ cup honey

3 cups old-fashioned rolled oats

1 tsp cinnamon

½ cup dried cranberries

½ cup dried peaches, chopped (see Note)

1. Preheat the oven to 375° F. Line a sheet pan with a silicone baking sheet or foil. Spread the pecans and almonds on the sheet pan and bake until toasted, about 10 minutes. (You'll notice the strong aroma of the toasted nuts.) Meanwhile, place the jar of honey in a bowl or saucepan filled with hot water for 5 minutes to thin its consistency.

2. Reduce the oven temperature to 300° F. Remove the nuts from the sheet pan and chop them using a knife or a food processor.

3. Return the nuts to the sheet pan. Add the oats, honey, and cinnamon; toss to combine. Bake for 25 to 30 minutes, stirring halfway through.

4. Line another sheet pan or a serving tray with paper towels (see Note). After the granola has baked, add the dried fruit and toss to combine. Transfer the mixture onto the paper towel–lined pan to cool. Store in an airtight container for up to one month.

Note: Kitchen shears make quick work of cutting up dried fruit. Also, cooling the granola on paper towels helps to keep the mixture crisp.

Per Serving: 156.2 calories, 7.5 g total fat, 0 mg cholesterol, 0.6 mg sodium, 20.3 g total carbs, 2.9 g dietary fiber, 3.7 g protein

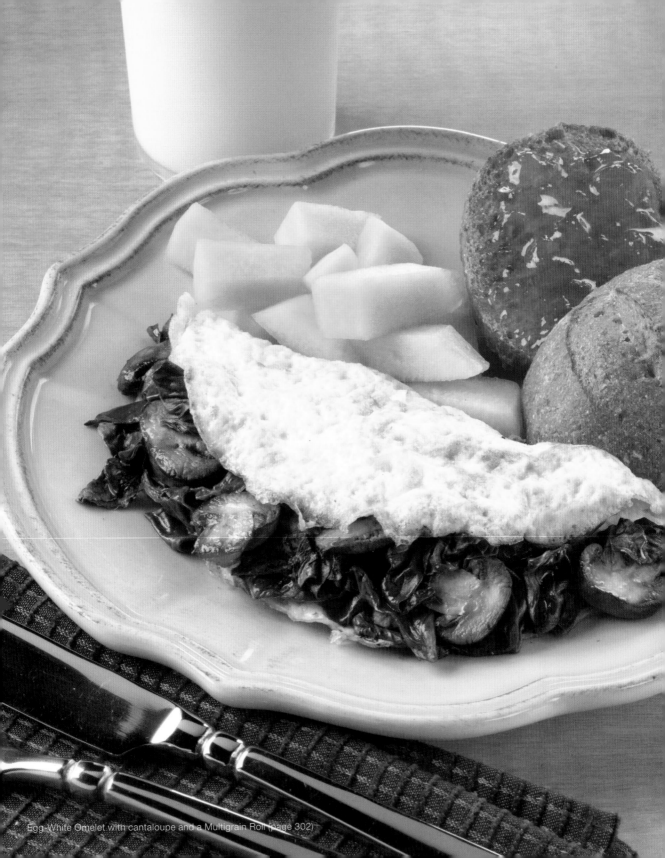

Egg-White Omelet with cantaloupe and a Multigrain Roll (page 302)

Egg-White Omelet with Spinach and Mushrooms

The egg-white omelet is a staple breakfast for many healthy eaters, but they're often rubbery and bland. After several trials, I've found that it's easy to make a flavorful omelet that's very low on fat: the secret is to add a tablespoon of Parmesan cheese to the eggs after beating them. You'll find it really improves the texture.

Adding cheese to the eggs leaves plenty of room to fill the omelet with vegetables. I recommend using baby bella or shiitake mushrooms because they have more flavor, but white button mushrooms would work as well—as would any combination of vegetables you prefer (see Awesome Omelets, page 90, for our suggestions). To make the weekday breakfast easy, sauté your vegetables ahead of time, then reheat them slightly in the microwave before adding them to the eggs.

Add two slices of whole-wheat toast, a cup of fat-free milk, and a cup of melon for a meal that has less than 400 calories, only 5 grams of fat, and four servings of fruits and vegetables!

Makes 1 Serving

15 Minutes to Prepare and Cook

Canola oil to coat the pan

½ cup sliced mushrooms, preferably baby bellas or shiitake

1 cup fresh spinach, washed and stems removed

Pinch black pepper

Pinch nutmeg (optional)

3 egg whites or ⅓ cup packaged egg whites

1 tbsp grated Parmesan cheese

1 tsp butter

1. Heat a nonstick sauté pan over moderate heat, and coat it with canola oil. Add the mushrooms to the pan and cook for 1 to 2 minutes. Add the spinach and cook just until wilted. Season with pepper and nutmeg, if using, then remove mixture from the sauté pan and set aside to cool slightly.

2. In a small mixing bowl, whisk the egg whites until fluffy, then whisk in the Parmesan.

3. Heat the sauté pan over moderate heat again. Add the butter to the pan, taking care to not let it brown. Add the eggs to the pan and swirl them around to coat the bottom. As the egg whites begin to set, lift the sides up with a rubber spatula so they don't overcook.

4. Once the omelet is partially set, add the vegetable mixture to half of the omelet. Cook the omelet until just set, 1 to 2 minutes more. Don't overcook: the egg whites should still be moist. Slide the omelet onto a plate, vegetable side first, folding the other half of the omelet on top.

Per Serving: 90.0 calories, 2.1 g total fat, 4.0 mg cholesterol, 283.3 mg sodium, 3.2 g total carbs, 1.2 g dietary fiber, 19.1 g protein

Awesome Omelets

You can fill an omelet with anything. Here are a few of our favorite combinations:

- Sautéed onions and bell peppers

- Sweet potato and black beans

- Red peppers and frozen artichoke hearts

- Asparagus and shallots

- Broccoli and yellow peppers

- Spinach and sun-dried tomatoes

Omelets vs. Frittatas

With three boys, we host our fair share of sleepovers. Teenage boys are always hungry, so the next morning I rely on two staples: omelets and frittatas. How do I decide which to make? The number of boys who stayed the night!

The two recipes contain the same ingredients. It's in the preparation where they differ.

Omelet	Both	Frittata
cooked in a sauté pan over high heat		cooked in a sauté pan over low heat, then baked in the oven until puffy
	filled with cheese, cooked meats, or vegetables	
	made from a base of eggs	
fillings cooked separately, added at the end		fillings mixed in and cooked with the eggs
served hot		served hot or at room temperature
folded over before serving		served open-faced

The next time you have a crowd of hungry people staring at you early in the morning, go the easy route and make a frittata.

Mushroom-Cheese Frittata

Though most people think of eggs as a breakfast meal (and we have placed this recipe in the breakfast chapter), in my house we like backwards breakfast—breakfast for dinner. On those nights that we get home late with grumbling bellies, I reach into the fridge, pull out eggs and whatever vegetables I find, and have dinner on the table in 20 minutes or less. See Awesome Omelets (opposite) for filling suggestions.

Frittatas are a staple of any Spanish tapas menu, cut into wedges and served hot or cold—and one of my family's favorite frittata ingredients is the traditionally Spanish twist of leftover roasted potatoes with smoked paprika.

Makes 2 Servings:
½ frittata per serving

15 Minutes to Prepare and Cook

½ cup chopped leeks, white and pale green parts only (about 1 large or 2 medium leeks)

½ cup finely chopped baby bella mushrooms

½ tsp black pepper

1 egg, beaten

2 egg whites, beaten

2 tbsp shredded Parmesan cheese

1. Preheat the oven to 375° F. Place a 6-inch, ovenproof omelet pan or small sauté pan over moderate heat. Spray the pan with nonstick cooking spray. Once pan is hot add the leeks, and mushrooms, and season with pepper. Sauté until leeks are tender, about 5 minutes.

2. In a small mixing bowl, whisk together the egg, egg whites, and Parmesan. Pour the egg mixture over the vegetables and stir just to combine.

3. Move the pan to the oven and bake until the frittata puffs and is just set in the center, about 5 minutes.

Per Serving: 104 calories, 4.7 g total fat, 112.5 mg cholesterol, 200.4 mg sodium, 5.7 g total carbs, 1 g dietary fiber, 11.5 g protein

Tomato-Cheese Frittata

Frittatas are a great brunch item. They're simple to prepare but look impressive. This particular frittata is a great dish for the summer months when your basil is flourishing and tomatoes are at their peak. Use one large or two plum (Roma) tomatoes instead of the cherry tomatoes if that's what you have on hand. The egg yolk creates a richer frittata, but you can use all egg whites if you prefer.

Makes 2 Servings:
½ frittata per serving

20 Minutes to Prepare and Cook

2 shallots, finely chopped

1 garlic clove, smashed and minced

1 egg, beaten

2 egg whites, beaten

1 tbsp crumbled feta cheese

1 cup cherry tomatoes, cut into quarters

4 large leaves of fresh basil, shredded

1. Preheat the oven to 375° F. Place a 6-inch, ovenproof omelet pan or small sauté pan over moderate heat. Coat the pan with nonstick cooking spray. Once the pan is hot, add the shallots and garlic, and sauté until the shallots are tender, about 5 minutes.

2. In a small mixing bowl, whisk together the egg, egg whites, and cheese. Add the tomatoes and basil and pour over the shallot mixture. Stir just to combine.

3. Move the pan to the oven and bake until the frittata puffs and is just set in the center, about 5 minutes.

Per serving: 88.5 calories, 3.7 g total fat, 110.3 mg cholesterol, 141.7 sodium, 5.8 g total carbs, 0.4 g dietary fiber, 9.6 g protein

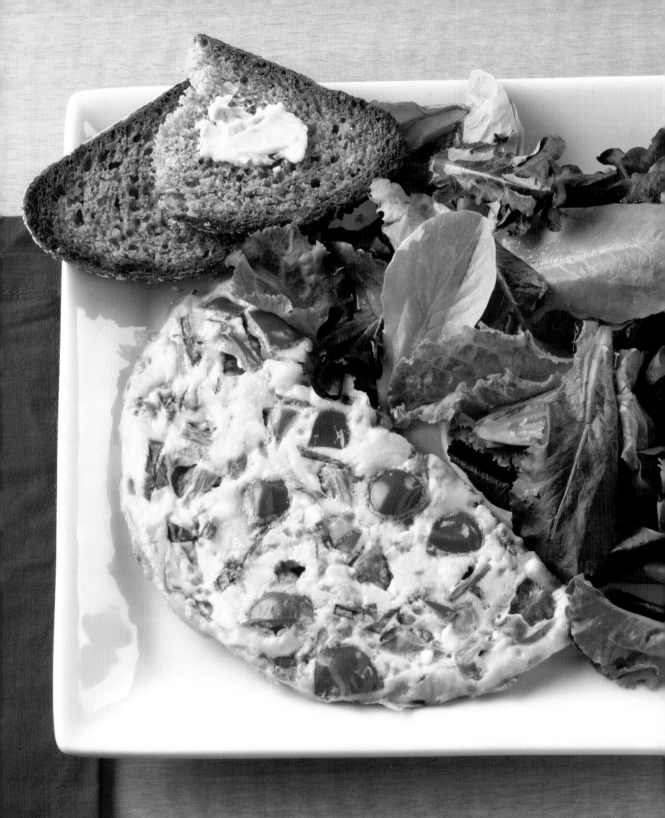

Tomato-Cheese Frittata with side salad and whole-grain toast

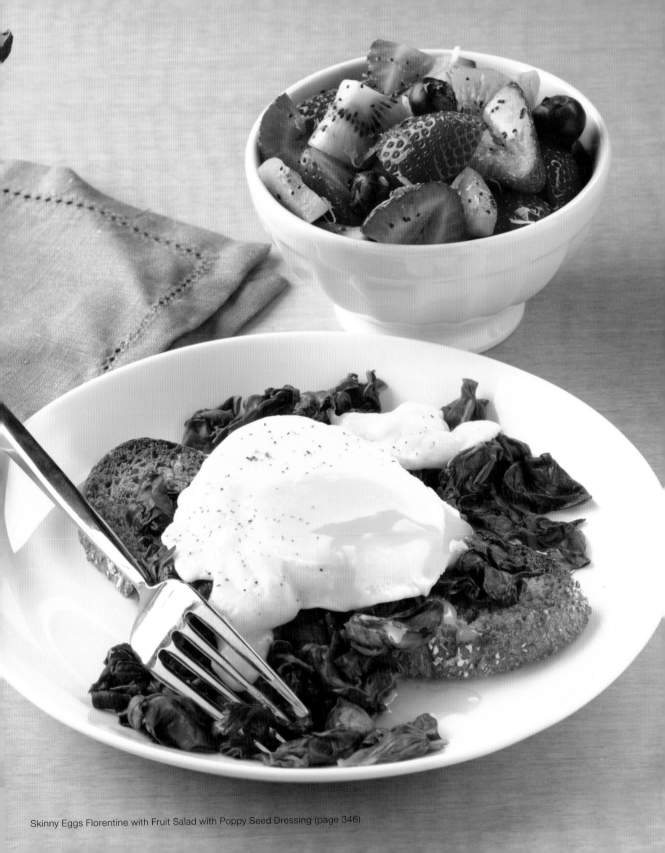

Skinny Eggs Florentine with Fruit Salad with Poppy Seed Dressing (page 346)

Skinny Eggs Florentine

Classic Eggs Florentine usually includes Hollandaise sauce, which is made with egg yolks, lemon juice, and butter. Our version has half the calories and a third of the fat of the traditional version, in part because I made a Mornay sauce using skim milk and a bit of Parmesan cheese for flavor. The recipe makes one cup of sauce, but you'll only need half. It's hard to make a small batch of this sauce, but it freezes beautifully for up to three months. Thaw it in the fridge and gently heat on the stove.

Poaching eggs is simple and, because there is no added fat, it's a very healthful cooking method. The trick to a perfectly poached egg is to use the freshest eggs possible.

Chef Meg's Tip: If you are making this recipe for a crowd, you can prepare the eggs ahead of time, hold them in cold water, then gently reheat by simmering them for 2 to 3 minutes.

Makes 4 Servings:
1 egg, 1 cup spinach, and 2 tbsp of prepared sauce per serving

30 Minutes to Prepare and Cook

For the Sauce:

1 tbsp light butter

1 tbsp flour

1 cup skim milk

2 tbsp Parmesan cheese

¼ tsp nutmeg, plus more for garnish

Pinch white pepper

For the Eggs:

4 cups spinach, washed and large stems removed (see Note)

2 tsp white vinegar

4 eggs

4 slices whole-wheat bread, toasted

1. Make the sauce. In a small saucepan, heat the butter until it begins to foam. Do not let it brown. Add the flour and cook for 1 minute, stirring constantly with a whisk. Slowly whisk in cold milk and simmer for 15 minutes, then add the Parmesan, nutmeg, and white pepper. Keep the sauce on very low heat.

2. Meanwhile, in a lidded steamer or sauté pan, steam the spinach just until wilted, then set aside.

3. Fill a saucepan with four cups of water, then add the vinegar. Stir to combine. Heat until just at a simmer. The water should not be boiling. Stir the water a couple of times to create a cyclone effect; this will keep the eggs from spreading out too far in the water.

4. One at a time, break the eggs into a ramekin or saucer, then slide them into the poaching water just above the surface. Poach for 3 to 5 minutes. Remove with a slotted spoon and place on a paper towel to remove any excess moisture.

5. To assemble the dish, place a slice of freshly toasted bread on a plate, then top with one quarter of the spinach, 1 egg, and 2 tablespoons of the sauce. Garnish with a pinch of nutmeg.

Note: You can use frozen spinach; just make sure that it's completely thawed and squeeze out all the moisture before using.

Per Serving: 254.2 calories, 9.9 g total fat, 216.6 mg cholesterol, 325.2 mg sodium, 29.0 g total carbs, 3.6 g dietary fiber, 13.3 g protein

Light Spinach and Mushroom Quiche

Quiches are another classic for brunch, but they make a great meal any time of day. This lighter version substitutes fat-free evaporated milk for cream. If you want to cut even more calories and fat, use nonstick cooking spray to sweat the vegetables, and choose light Swiss instead of regular. Once you learn how to make the custard filling, you can change up the ingredients according to your taste and what you have on hand. Try a variety of mushrooms (such as cremini, portobello, or shiitake) for extra flavor. Don't overcook your quiche: the filling should be just slightly firm and not too dry.

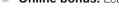 **Online bonus:** Learn how to make dough. Go to SparkRecipes.com for Chef Meg's videos.

Makes 8 Servings:
⅛ quiche per serving

1 Hour to Prepare and Cook (plus chilling of dough)

For the Crust:

1 cup all-purpose flour

½ cup whole-wheat flour

½ tsp salt

4 tbsp Smart Balance butter for baking, cold (see Note)

4 to 6 tbsp ice cold water

1 tbsp flour, for dusting work surface

For the Filling:

1 tbsp Smart Balance butter (see Note)

½ cup finely diced onion

½ cup sliced mushrooms

1 cup spinach, washed and stems removed

½ tsp black pepper

1 cup skim milk

1 cup fat-free evaporated milk

2 large eggs

1 egg white

¼ tsp salt

¼ tsp nutmeg

¼ cup shredded Swiss cheese

1. Make the Dough. Place the flours and salt in a food processor. Pulse 2 to 3 times to mix. Cut the butter into tablespoon-size pieces, drop them into the flour, then pulse until the butter is the size of peas. If you don't have a food processor the dough can be made by hand: use the backs of two butter knives to blend in the butter.

2. Add the water 1 tablespoon at a time, pulsing after each addition. Remove the dough from the processor and knead the dough lightly until smooth. Place the dough on a sheet of plastic wrap, cover, and press into a disc shape. Chill for an hour or overnight.

3. Prepare the Filling. Heat a sauté pan over moderate heat. Add the butter and melt until foaming; reduce heat and add the onions. Sauté the onions until tender, about 4 to 5 minutes. Add the mushrooms, spinach, and pepper; and continue to cook until the spinach is wilted.

4. Remove the pan from heat and allow the vegetables to cool slightly. This is important because if the vegetables are hot, they will start to cook the eggs when combined.

5. Prepare the Crust. Preheat oven to 350° F. Choose an 8" or 9" oven-proof pie plate. (If you are using a glass baking dish, reduce the oven temperature by 10 degrees.) Dust a work surface with the tablespoon of flour. Lightly roll out the dough to size, then place in the pie plate. Crimp the edges of the crust with a fork or your fingers.

6. In a mixing bowl, whisk together the skim milk, evaporated milk, eggs, egg white, salt, and nutmeg. Spread the vegetable mixture on top of the pastry crust then sprinkle the cheese over. Carefully pour the egg mixture over the vegetables. Place the pie plate on a sheet pan and bake for 45 minutes or until the center of the quiche is just jiggly (it will firm up as it cools). Let cool for 5 minutes before serving.

Note: The butter must be the stick variety; the tub butter is not suitable for baking because it has added water to make it fluffy.

Per Serving: 254.3 calories, 10.6 g total fat, 20.9 mg cholesterol, 282.6 mg sodium, 26.2 g total carbs, 1.8 g dietary fiber, 10.3 g protein

Warm and Spicy Banana Waffles

For most families, homemade waffles are a weekend or special-occasion meal, but with a little planning, you can have waffles in minutes, any day of the week, without having to resort to the pre-packaged toaster version. All you need to do is plan ahead. The next time you make waffles on the weekend, make a double batch. Freeze them in individual sandwich bags, and on a busy morning, just pull one from the freezer and pop it into the microwave or (even better) the toaster.

These banana waffles are so full of flavor that you won't even need syrup—though if you insist, opt for the real stuff instead of the imitation, maple-flavored corn syrup. You'll find that real maple syrup has such a strong flavor that you'll use far less and still be satisfied.

Try adding a dollop of Greek yogurt instead of butter on top. It provides a tangy contrast to the sweet waffles.

Makes 4 Servings:
1 waffle, plus banana and honey per serving

35 Minutes to Prepare and Cook

1 ripe banana

1 cup plain fat-free Greek yogurt

2 egg whites

⅓ cup skim milk

¾ cup whole-wheat flour

¼ cup oat flour (see Note)

2 tbsp brown sugar

¾ tsp baking powder

¼ tsp baking soda

¼ tsp salt

¾ tsp ground ginger

½ tsp cinnamon

½ tsp canola oil for the waffle iron

1 banana, sliced, for garnish

2 tbsp honey or maple syrup, for garnish

1. In a mixing bowl, mash together the banana and yogurt. Add egg whites and skim milk and mix until well combined. In a separate bowl, sift together whole-wheat flour, oat flour, brown sugar, baking powder, baking soda, salt, ginger, and cinnamon. Add the dry ingredients to the wet mixture, and mix until just combined. Allow to sit for 4 minutes to moisten flours.

2. Brush the surface of the waffle iron with the canola oil. Pour ½ cup batter onto the iron per waffle and cook according to waffle-iron instructions. Serve warm, topped with sliced banana and honey.

Note: Oat flour can be purchased, or you can grind your own by pulsing rolled or old-fashioned (not quick) oats in a food processor.

Per Serving: 259.8 calories, 1.7 g total fat, 0.4 mg cholesterol, 377.1 mg sodium, 56 g total carbs, 4.8 g dietary fiber, 12.6 g protein

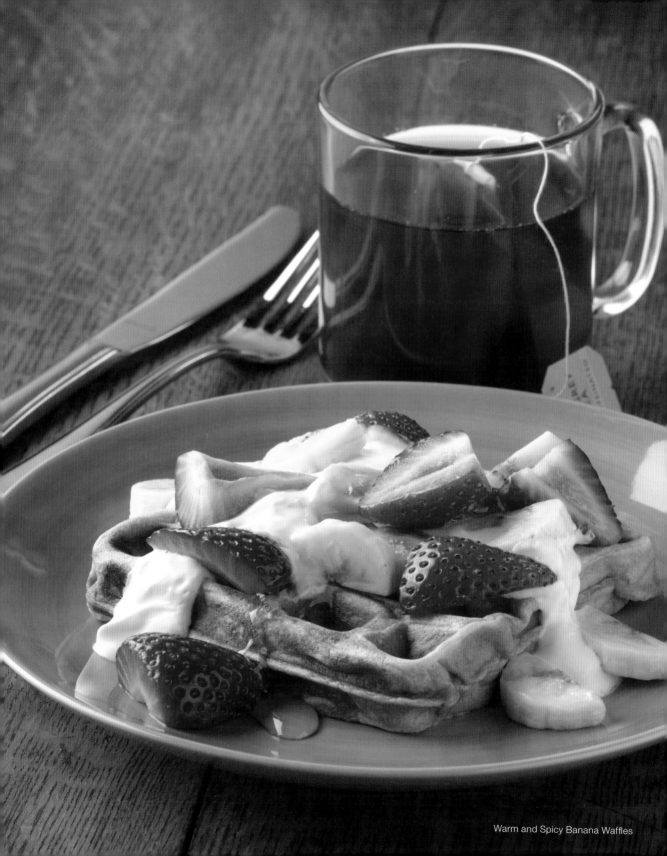

Warm and Spicy Banana Waffles

Blueberry Flaxseed Muffins

These healthful muffins freeze well, so make a batch over the weekend and then pop one in the microwave and serve it with a piece of fruit and a glass of low-fat milk for a quick and tasty weekday breakfast. Low-fat buttermilk and applesauce help lower the fat in this recipe, and the whole-wheat flour and flaxseed add fiber. Be sure to grind the flaxseed to get the full health benefits.

Makes 12 Servings:
1 muffin per serving

25 Minutes to Prepare and Cook

1 cup quick oats (do not use instant oatmeal)

1 cup low-fat buttermilk

1 cup whole-wheat flour

1 tsp baking powder

½ tsp baking soda

¼ tsp cinnamon

1 tsp salt

1 egg

¼ cup unsweetened applesauce

¾ cup brown sugar

1 cup blueberries, washed and dried

1 tbsp flaxseeds, roughly ground

1. Preheat the oven to 375° F. Spray the muffin pan with nonstick cooking spray or line the wells with paper liners.

2. In a small bowl, combine the oats and buttermilk and let the mixture stand at room temperature for 5 minutes. In a medium bowl, combine the flour, baking powder, baking soda, cinnamon, and salt; mix with a fork to blend and set aside.

3. In a large bowl and using a hand mixer, beat the egg, applesauce, and brown sugar at medium speed for 3 minutes.

4. Blend the oat-buttermilk mixture into the egg mixture, then stir in the flour mixture until just combined (try not to overwork the mixture). Fold in the blueberries. Fill muffin cups ¾ full and top with a sprinkle of ground flaxseed.

5. Bake 15 minutes or until a toothpick inserted into the center comes out clean.

Per Serving: 139.2 calories, 1.5 g total fat, 18.5 mg cholesterol, 320.5 mg sodium, 38.1 total carbs, 3.3 g dietary fiber, 3.7 g protein

- Blueberries are full of antioxidants and fiber. Buy organic when possible, and when they're in season, freeze them in large batches for use throughout the year.

- If using frozen blueberries, thaw them first and reserve the juice (use it in a smoothie or add to a glass of water for a treat).

- No blueberries? Substitute an equal amount of fresh strawberries or raspberries, or ½ cup dried cranberries or cherries. Dried fruit is concentrated in flavor and higher in calories so use half as much. (Rehydrate dried fruit by soaking it in water for about 10 minutes before adding to the batter.)

- Sprinkle in 1 teaspoon lemon or orange zest for an extra layer of flavor.

- Don't overmix the batter or the muffins will be tough. Mix just until the ingredients are blended.

- Fold in the blueberries using a spatula, not a mixer, to keep them whole.

Chew on This: Buttermilk

Too often you buy a quart of low-fat buttermilk, use a cup's worth, and then the rest of the container goes bad. Pour leftover buttermilk into the wells of a muffin pan and place the pan in the freezer. Pop the frozen buttermilk from the muffin pan into a plastic bag for up to 3 months, then thaw in the refrigerator when needed. (The wells of a standard muffin pan usually hold 3½ ounces.) Or make your own buttermilk by combining 1 cup nonfat milk with 1 tablespoon white vinegar or lemon juice.

SALADS & SANDWICHES

Easy to make and transport, customizable and affordable, salads and sandwiches are the cornerstone of a healthy lunch. Whether you're at work or at home, at school or on the road, this lunchtime duo is unbeatable—each can be loaded with flavor and healthy ingredients to create a meal that's low in calories with surprises for your taste buds in every bite.

SALADS

My boys love to buy their lunches from school, and I oblige a few days a week. They're fairly healthy eaters at home, so I trust them to make smart choices on the lunch line. When my son Noah was in third grade, I would ask him what he had for lunch. For the first two months of school, he would answer "salad bar." I was impressed!

Soon after, he was at the supermarket with me. While choosing lettuce, I asked him which varieties his school used. "Oh Mom, I don't eat lettuce off the salad bar," he said, making a confused face. "I eat the nacho chips and cheese." I almost died. That was my worst "mom" moment.

Lesson learned. To this day, I ask exactly what they eat each day, and I check up.

Just because it's on a salad bar—or atop a salad for that matter—doesn't make it healthy.

PCHEFLORA from Wisconsin told us:

"I work in a store that has a salad bar that's $4.99 a pound, and every day I see these people, usually women, whose bill is $10 or more! That's two pounds of 'salad,' but they pour on so much dressing it makes me nauseous, and [they think] that they're eating healthy. Also, they pile on ham cubes and cheese. You wouldn't believe how much they use! I had one lady say to me, 'I don't like lettuce so I don't use much of that, but I eat a salad because they're good for you.' Though I wanted to say something, I just smiled politely."

10 Ideas for Quick Salads

Use these ingredients as the basis for your next salad.

1. Mixed greens with grape tomatoes and cucumbers

2. Frisée with bean sprouts, spring peas, and herbs

3. Arugula with sweet onions, green beans, and nuts

4. Frisée with apples, nuts, and grapes

5. Leaf lettuce with artichoke hearts, hearts of palm, and asparagus

6. A BLT in a bowl: Romaine with turkey bacon, tomatoes, and whole-wheat toasted croutons

7. Mesclun greens with chicken breast, sliced apples, and walnuts

8. Spinach with mushrooms, red onion, and cranberries

9. Arugula with cannellini beans, roasted peppers, and capers

10. Bibb with carrots, leeks, celery, and peppers

To keep her salad light, PCHEFLORA brings homemade dressing and loads up on fruit. She's not tempted to pile on too much because she knows she's paying for every bite.

At restaurants, the salad comes early and can make or break your healthy meal. At home, most of us eat salad with our entrées. Either way, you can use it to set the tone for the rest of the meal. If you start the meal with a salad that's laden with ranch dressing, bacon bits, cheese, and croutons, that's what your taste buds will come to expect. You won't be satisfied by your healthy entrée, which will seem puny and bland. On the other hand, if you start the meal with a plateful of spinach or mixed spring greens, topped with bright vegetables, a sprinkle of flavorful cheese, and a bit of tangy vinaigrette, you won't feel weighed down. Your taste buds will be stimulated by all the tastes and textures, without being overwhelmed. You will feel better knowing you've started the meal with vitamins, antioxidants, and fiber rather than salt and fat.

You'll find plenty of nutritious and satisfying salad ideas on the pages that follow, but you don't really need a recipe. Learn the basics of building a better salad, and you'll be creating veggie-rich masterpieces in no time.

Start Strong

Just like a house is only as strong as its foundation, a salad is only as robust as its greens. Choose a mixture of greens, the greener the better! Not all lettuce tastes the same: they can be spicy (arugula and watercress), bitter (radicchio and endive), crisp (Romaine and iceberg), or soft and tender (Bibb or mesclun). Our recipes use varieties of lettuce you might have never tried, but be brave and branch out. If your market doesn't carry a specified lettuce, ask your greengrocer to recommend one with a similar taste and texture.

Always wash your greens right before eating, and only wash as much as you'll eat that day to prevent spoilage. After washing, dry the greens completely so the salad dressing will cling to the lettuce rather than pool in the bottom of the bowl. Whether you tear or chop your greens is up to you, but make the pieces small enough to fit on your fork.

A serving of greens is one cup (about one overflowing handful), but don't stop there. Use at least two! The only time I use a large bowl is when I'm building a salad. I want to be able to pack in all the veggies I can.

SparkPeople Cooking Challenge:
Buy a different kind of lettuce at the market this week. If you shop at a farmers' market, ask to sample the greens before you buy them. If you're wary of bitter lettuces, choose baby varieties, which are sweeter and more tender.

Keep Building

Once you've selected your greens, move on to the toppings—vegetables in particular. Use a ratio of 2 parts greens to 1 part vegetables. So, if you're starting with 2 cups of greens, add a cup of vegetables. It doesn't matter what kind of vegetables you use, as long as you like them. Raw or cooked (salads are a great way to use up leftovers), all are welcome.

When you return from the store, wash and prep a couple of days' worth of salad veggies. It's much easier to pull together a healthy salad for lunch or dinner if all you need to do is wash and dry greens, toss them in dressing, add your toppings, and sit down to eat.

- *Be creative with your chopping.* If you're learning to like vegetables, start with smaller, more manageable pieces. Shred carrots, cabbage, and zucchini. Dice celery, onions, and peppers. Chop tomatoes, mushrooms, and cucumbers.

- *Consistency is key.* Try to make all of your ingredients the same size, or at least small enough to fit on your fork.

- *Don't forget the fruit.* Halved grapes, chopped apples and pears, berries, and even melon can be tasty additions to a salad.

- *Choose seasonal toppings.* Strawberries in summer are among my favorite salad ingredients, but in wintertime, no thanks. Leftover roasted root vegetables are tasty salad toppers in cold weather. Eating what's in season tastes better and can help you save money.

SparkPeople Cooking Challenge:
Start your meal with a new salad once this week. Use at least three different kinds of fruits and vegetables.

Call in Reinforcements

One of the chief complaints we hear about salads is that they don't satisfy. An hour after lunch, members say they're starving, and by mid-afternoon, they're racing to the vending machines for a snack. It's usually a quick diagnosis. The salad contains little more than vegetables, often topped with a fat-free dressing. Vegetables, while a crucial part of a healthy meal, are low in protein, and it's protein that takes longer to digest and keeps us feeling satisfied.

While vegetables are high-volume foods that are high in fiber, they are relatively low in calories and need some help when it comes to satisfaction. Lean protein sources and whole grains are the support your salad needs.

Lean protein Beans, reduced-fat cheese, nuts, meat, eggs, and seafood are all good lean proteins to include in salads. One serving is enough to turn your salad from a side dish into a meal. That equals:

- ½ cup beans

- 1 ounce reduced-fat cheese

- 3 ounces meat or seafood

- 1 ounce nuts or seeds

- 1 hard-boiled egg

To minimize the effort of lunchtime prep, maximize your cooking. Grill an extra chicken breast or an extra skewer of shrimp. Eat half of your steak at a restaurant and save the other half for the next day. Measure out servings of beans or nuts ahead of time.

Whole grains The only grains that are present at most salad bars are croutons and greasy crackers, and any healthy eater knows to avoid those. But to maximize your satisfaction and keep your belly happy until dinner or your afternoon snack, add some complex carbs to your salad in the form of whole grains.

Unrefined or "whole grain" carbohydrates found in products like brown rice, whole-wheat pasta, and bran cereals are digested slowly. They contain vitamins, minerals, and fiber, all of which promote health.

Whether your whole grains are on the side or in your salad is up to you. Just be sure to include them.

- Sprinkle leftover grains like quinoa, brown rice, or bulgur over your salad.

- Chop up a piece of whole-wheat toast or crumble on a serving of whole-grain crackers or baked tortilla chips to replace croutons.

- Serve a Multigrain Roll (page 302) or a piece of whole-wheat toast with a bit of heart-healthy margarine on the side.

SparkPeople Cooking Challenge:
Make a salad into a meal at least once this week. Choose a salad from this chapter or use what you've learned to create your own. Be sure to include a serving of protein and whole grains. Notice how much fuller and more satisfied you feel.

DRESS IT UP

I love vegetables, but even I can't chow down on a bowl of dry greens. It's a matter of preference, but I always dress my greens before I serve a salad. Each bite is well coated and flavorful, and I'm not tempted to overload on dressing at the table. Some people prefer to have dressing on the side, which is a good idea in theory. The next time you ask for dressing on the side at a restaurant, notice the amount they give you. While I use less than a tablespoon of dressing per salad, restaurants deliver up to four times that much. Even if you daintily dip the tines of your fork into the salad before each bite, you'll still likely use more.

At home, when you're in charge, try tossing your greens in a measured amount of dressing. You'll find flavor in every bite.

If you're opting for fat-free dressings because you think it's better for you, think again. Small amounts of healthy fats are an important part of the satisfaction of a salad. A little fat will do, but you'll find that a vinaigrette with a balance of rich oil and tangy vinegar is more enjoyable than vinegar alone.

Still not convinced? Your body can't make use of certain vitamins and antioxidants (beta-carotene, vitamin D, and vitamin E in particular) without a bit of fat to help process them. In addition, fat helps transport vitamins A, D, E, and K.

In 2004, a study in the *American Journal of Clinical Nutrition* found that people who consumed salads with fat-free dressing absorbed fewer phytonutrients (the organic components of plants) and vitamins than those who ate the same salad of spinach, lettuce, tomatoes, and carrots with a dressing containing fat.

13 Unconventional Salad Toppers

1. Hummus (especially good with chopped cucumbers, shredded cabbage, and carrots)

2. Better-than-Pesto Puree (page 377) (try it with a Mediterranean salad)

3. Poached egg (the yolk serves as your dressing—very European and great on bitter greens)

4. Low-fat Greek yogurt (mix in some herbs)

5. Salsa (fat-free and full of veggies)

6. Guacamole (puree it for a thinner consistency)

7. Low-fat cottage cheese (adds protein and flavor)

8. A bound salad (egg, chicken, or tuna)

9. Pasta salad or other dressed grains (like the Herbed Bulgur and Lentil Salad, page 301)

10. Lemon juice (or lime, orange, or grapefruit juice)

11. Honey (thinned with a little water)

12. Flavored oils, like Spicy Garlic Oil (page 384), a nut oil, or an herb-infused oil

13. Grilled vegetables, chicken, or fish (the "juices" will flavor the salad more than you think)

Our taste testers agreed. Remember when we looked at the taste test results in Chapter 2? Those who ate the iceberg lettuce with a fat-free dressing rated it lower than our mixed greens salad with Tomato-Basil Vinaigrette (page 387).

SparkPeople Cooking Challenge:
Add some fat to your dressing. Whether you make your own (see any of the recipes in this chapter or check out Chapter 12) or buy one with a short ingredient list is up to you. Your salad will be so much more flavorful and satisfying.

FINISHING TOUCHES

What draws you to a salad on a restaurant menu? Is it the bed of baby spring greens or the heirloom carrots? Most likely, it's the candied pecans, crumbled maple-smoked bacon, or the sprinkle of local goat cheese. While many restaurants (especially chains) can go overboard with the accoutrements—fried tortilla strips, crispy battered onions, and even French fries—a few bites of something decadent can transform a salad from basic to brilliant. The trick is to keep your portions in check.

Cheese and nuts tend to be higher in calories and fat than other salad ingredients, so consider using them as a flavoring rather than a protein source. Some suggestions:

- Half a slice of bacon (turkey or pork)

- ½ ounce of a flavorful cheese (feta, blue, Gruyère, goat)

- ½ ounce of chopped, toasted, or candied nuts

- 1 or 2 tablespoons of dried fruit

- A quarter of an avocado

- 1 tablespoon of seeds (sunflower, pumpkin)

- 1–3 olives or 1 tablespoon of capers

To stretch these calorie-dense ingredients, chop, crumble, or slice them. Would you rather enjoy 4 bites of olives or 12? By stretching those flavor-boosting ingredients, there's more flavor in every bite.

SparkPeople Cooking Challenge:
Make one of the salads in this chapter and try to identify the "flavor booster" ingredient. Take a bite of the salad with it and without it. Which version do you like better?

SELL IT

Presentation is key when it comes to foods, and salads are no exception. Since most salads are vibrant in color, I prefer to serve them on a white plate with a rim or in a white bowl. The plate is your canvas, so splash it with color. Chefs tend to aim high when plating food, so to make your dishes more interesting, go vertical. Toss the salad in a separate bowl with the dressing, then lift your greens with a pair of tongs or two forks and place them on the plate, twisting as you release the greens. Your salad should have contrasting elements of texture, flavor, and color.

SparkPeople Cooking Challenge:
Instead of throwing your ingredients in a bowl and digging in, take a few seconds to creatively plate your salad. Did you notice anything different? Does your salad seem more exciting? Taste better? Feel more decadent?

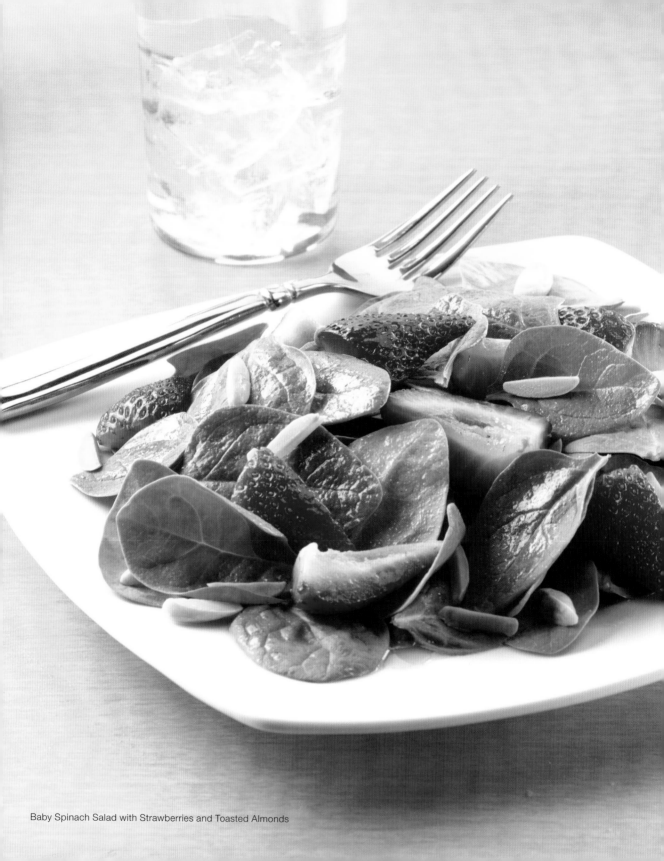

Baby Spinach Salad with Strawberries and Toasted Almonds

Baby Spinach Salad with Strawberries and Toasted Almonds

SLIM IT DOWN: Skip the almonds (50 calories).

Strawberries move from the dessert course to the salad course. Fresh and juicy during spring and summer months, strawberries are delicious when combined with tender spinach and crunchy toasted almonds. This dish was inspired by a member-submitted recipe. We reduced the amount of sweetener used and then increased the vegetables.

Makes 4 Servings:
2 cups spinach with ½ cup berries per serving

15 Minutes to Prepare and Cook

⅓ cup almonds, slivered

8 cups baby spinach, stems trimmed

1 tbsp balsamic vinegar

1 tsp Dijon mustard

1 tsp honey

3 tbsp extra-virgin olive oil

2 cups strawberries, quartered (see Note)

Salt and pepper, to taste

1. Place the almonds in a dry skillet or sauté pan. Cook over low heat, shaking the pan the entire time until the almonds are toasted (watch carefully—they burn quickly!). The almonds are done when they turn brown and you start to smell their aroma. Remove almonds from the pan to cool. (Do not cool in the skillet because they will burn from the heat that remains in the pan.)

2. Wash and dry the spinach.

3. Prepare the dressing by placing the vinegar, mustard, and honey in a mixing bowl. Slowly whisk in the oil until all is incorporated. Place the spinach in a large bowl; add the strawberries and almonds, and pour the dressing over. Toss to coat. If desired, season with a pinch of salt and pepper. Divide evenly onto 4 plates and serve.

Note: Instead of slicing strawberries for the salad, quarter them. Quartered strawberries are easier to pick up with a fork.

Per Serving: 180.9 calories, 15.1 g total fat, 0 mg cholesterol, 79.4 mg sodium, 9.9 g total carbs, 3.7 g dietary fiber, 4 g protein

Lunch Box Carrot Slaw with Apples

My kids really like this—it's crunchy and sweet. Feel free to add another apple—and if you don't have pineapple on hand, consider raisins, nuts, or grapes. I sometimes sprinkle celery seed or poppy seeds on top for a more adult flavor.

Makes 4 Servings:
    1 cup per serving

5 Minutes to Prepare and Cook

3½ cups shredded carrots

½ cup plain, low-fat yogurt, drained of any
    excess liquid

½ cup crushed pineapple, no sugar added

1 Granny Smith apple, not peeled, diced
    into ½-inch pieces

1. In a mixing bowl, combine the carrots, yogurt, pineapple, and chopped apple.

2. Cover and chill for at least 10 minutes before serving.

Per Serving: 89.9 calories, 0.8 g total fat, 1.8 mg cholesterol, 87.1 mg sodium, 18.7 g total carbs, 3.5 g dietary fiber, 2.5 g protein

Spinach Salad with Cherries and Pomegranate Vinaigrette

If ever there was proof that salads don't have to be boring to be healthy, this is it. A luxurious combination of bright, bitter spinach is paired with sweet dried cherries and tangy goat cheese for maximum flavor satisfaction—and topped with a bit of almond crunch. Our pomegranate vinaigrette is loaded with flavor *and* antioxidants.

Online bonus: Learn how to toast almonds, wash spinach, and slice onions without tears. Visit SparkRecipes for Chef Meg's videos.

Makes 4 Servings:
1 cup per serving

20 Minutes to Prepare and Cook, with optional, additional 10 Minutes to soak onions

For the Dressing:

2 tbsp bottled or fresh pomegranate juice

1 tbsp balsamic vinegar

1 tsp honey

2 tbsp olive oil

¼ tsp black pepper

For the Salad:

8 cups fresh spinach, cleaned and stems removed

½ cup red onion, thinly sliced (see Note)

⅓ cup dried cherries

¼ cup slivered almonds, toasted

2 ounces goat cheese, crumbled

1. Make the Dressing. Prepare the vinaigrette by placing the pomegranate juice, vinegar, and honey in a blender. Slowly drizzle in the oil while the blender is running to emulsify. Add the pepper.

2. Make the Salad. In a large bowl, toss together the spinach, onion, and dried cherries. Add the dressing and toss to coat. Divide the salad evenly onto 4 plates and garnish with the toasted almonds and goat cheese.

Note: To tame the bite of the red onions, soak them in ice water for 10 minutes.

Per serving: 198.8 calories, 13 g total fat, 6.5 mg cholesterol, 105.1 mg sodium, 16.5 g total carbs, 2.8 g dietary fiber, 6 g protein

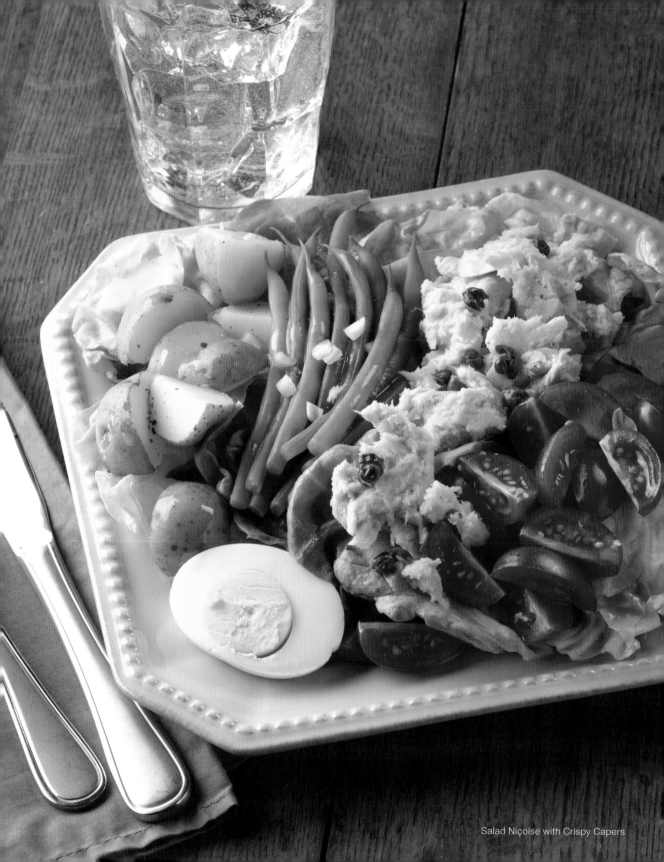

Salad Niçoise with Crispy Capers

Salad Niçoise with Crispy Capers

SLIM IT DOWN: Omit the potatoes (131 calories).

A salad from the South of France, Salad Niçoise is found on menus up and down the Mediterranean coast, and every chef has a slightly different recipe. One constant: this salad fills you up.

In our version, we added extra flavor and texture by frying the capers in the oil we use to dress the salad. Tuna from a can or a pouch is great in this salad, but you can also use grilled tuna or salmon. Perfect for a summer lunch or a light supper, Salad Niçoise is as hearty as it is simple to prepare.

Makes 4 Servings:
2 cups dressed greens with ½ egg, ½ cup each potatoes and beans, ¼ cup tomatoes, and 2 ounces tuna per serving

20 Minutes to Prepare and Cook

4 small red-skinned potatoes, quartered

2 cups green beans

3 tbsp olive oil

1 tbsp capers, drained, rinsed, and patted dry (see Notes)

2 tbsp rice-wine vinegar

1 tsp Dijon mustard

2 heads Bibb lettuce (see Note)

1 cup cherry tomatoes, cut into fourths

One 8-ounce pouch of tuna, packed in water, drained

2 eggs, hard-boiled

2 tsp finely diced shallots

Pinch black pepper

1. Bring a medium saucepan of water to a boil. Place the potatoes in boiling water and simmer until just tender, about 10 minutes. Using a slotted spoon, remove the potatoes from the water and set aside to cool. Reserve the water.

2. Prepare a large bowl of ice water. Add the green beans to the pot of potato water and simmer for 5 minutes. Drain the beans, then immediately place them in the ice water to stop the cooking process and keep the beans bright green and crisp.

3. Place the oil in a small saucepan. Have a slotted spoon and paper towels nearby. Heat the oil until hot over moderate heat, then add the capers and fry for 1 minute. Caution: they can pop. Remove the capers from the oil with the slotted spoon and place on paper towels to drain and cool. Place the oil in a small bowl and set it aside to cool.

4. Make the dressing. Put the vinegar and mustard in a blender. Pulse to combine. Slowly add the oil from the capers while the motor is running.

5. Tear the lettuce into bite-size pieces, then place in a large bowl and toss with 2 tablespoons of the dressing.

6. Divide the lettuce among 4 plates. Top each salad with one fourth of the tomatoes, beans, and potatoes; 2 ounces of tuna; and half an egg. Drizzle the remaining dressing atop the vegetables, and garnish with shallots, black pepper, and the crispy capers.

Note: Make sure the capers are very dry before frying, or they will spatter when added to the hot oil. Bibb lettuce is also called Boston or butter lettuce. You could also substitute Romaine.

Per Serving: 344 calories, 14.1 g total fat, 131.3 mg cholesterol, 163.4 mg sodium, 38.8 g total carbs, 7.7 g dietary fiber, 19.7 g protein

Roasted Beet and Apple Salad

Is there another vegetable that's been more maligned than our friend the beet? Survey ten people about beets, and nine of them will likely wrinkle their noses at those ruby orbs. They don't know what they're missing. If you think you don't like beets, try roasting them, then serving them in a salad. Beets are naturally sweet, and roasting only enhances their natural flavor.

. . . .

Chef Meg's Tip: Every piece of citrus is going to yield a slightly different amount of juice and zest. Don't sweat it. This is one time you don't need to measure.

. . . .

Makes 4 Servings:
   1 overflowing cup per serving

1 Hour, 15 Minutes to Prepare and Cook

2 small red beets, fresh, washed and
     scrubbed (see Note)

2 tbsp pecans

2 Granny Smith apples, thinly sliced

2 heads Belgian endive, pulled apart and
     tough stem removed

2 tbsp olive oil

1 lemon, juiced

½ tsp black pepper

2 tbsp crumbled feta cheese

1. Preheat oven to 375° F. Wrap the beets in aluminum foil and roast until they are just tender to the touch, about 1 hour. Remove from the oven and unwrap to cool.

2. While the beets are roasting, spread the pecans on a baking sheet and toast them in the same oven until fragrant, about 3 minutes. Allow them to cool and then chop and set aside.

3. In a large mixing bowl, combine the apples and endive leaves. Peel and slice the cooled beets and toss them into the mixture.

4. Prepare the vinaigrette by slowly whisking the oil into the lemon juice. Season the dressing with pepper, then pour over the salad and mix. Divide the salad among 4 plates and top with the nuts and cheese.

Notes: Pick beets that still have the greens attached. You get two vegetables for the price of one: Remove the greens and use them in place of your favorite greens in a sautéed dish.

Roast and chop the beets ahead of time for a quick meal.

Per Serving: 195.4 calories, 11.2 g total fat, 4 mg cholesterol, 123.6 mg sodium, 24.8 g total carbs, 12.1 g dietary fiber, 5 g protein

Watercress Tomato Salad

Watercress is a nutritional powerhouse that's often overlooked for more common greens like spinach and Romaine. With just four calories a cup, as much vitamin C as an orange, and more iron than spinach, consider giving it a try. Peppery and tangy, watercress pairs well with tomatoes and a strong dressing, such as my Tomato-Basil Vinaigrette (page 387). If you can't find watercress in your supermarket, substitute arugula or your favorite greens.

Makes 4 Servings:
1 cup watercress, 4 tomatoes, with 1 tablespoon vinaigrette per serving

10 Minutes to Prepare and Cook

4 cups watercress, large stems trimmed

16 cherry tomatoes, quartered

¼ cup crumbled feta cheese

¼ cup Tomato-Basil Vinaigrette

1. In a large bowl, combine the watercress, tomatoes, and cheese. Add the dressing and toss to coat well.

2. Divide the salad onto 4 chilled plates and serve.

Per Serving: 79.5 calories, 6.3 g total fat, 8.3 mg cholesterol, 136.3 mg sodium, 4.1 g total carbs, 0.9 g dietary fiber, 2.7 g protein

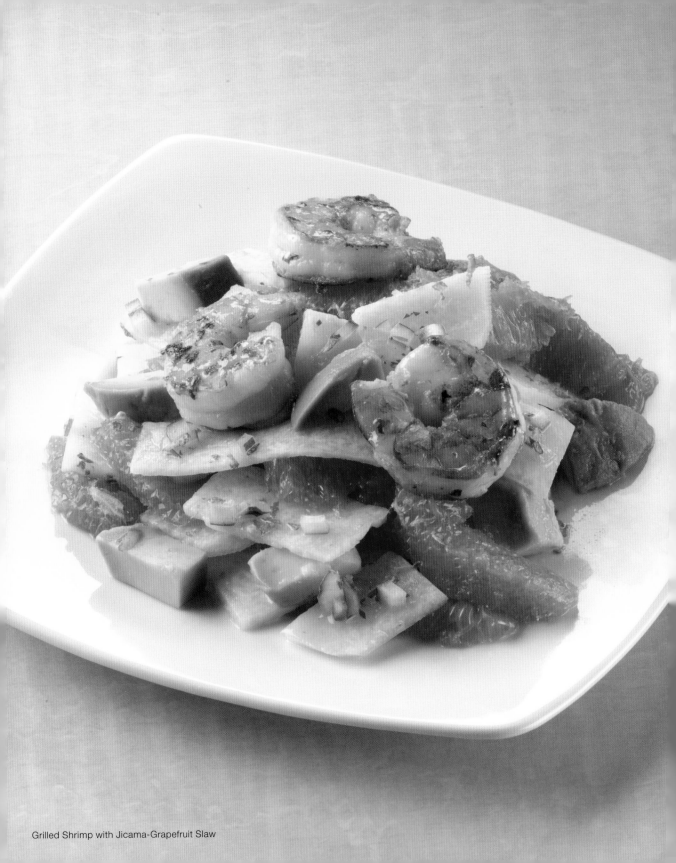

Grilled Shrimp with Jicama-Grapefruit Slaw

Grilled Shrimp with Jicama-Grapefruit Slaw

Grapefruits are the Rodney Dangerfield of the citrus family—no respect! They're either eaten for breakfast as part of a crash diet or ignored entirely. And that's a shame, because they can add a bright, tart flavor to all kinds of salads. I prefer the pink variety for their great color and less-sour taste.

This dish is a great balance of flavors and textures. Creamy avocado, tart grapefruits, tangy red onions, firm shrimp, and crunchy jicama (see Chew on This on page 120 for more info) have a party in your mouth. It's great for a light supper or a brunch with friends—and it's perfect summertime fare, as you don't have to turn on an oven. The slaw is just so refreshing—try serving it on a bed of lettuce to bulk it up or leaving out the shrimp for a vegetarian version.

Online bonus: Learn how to peel and cut an avocado and segment citrus. Visit SparkRecipes.com for Chef Meg's videos.

Makes 4 Servings:
    1 heaping cup slaw and
    6 shrimp per serving

45 Minutes to Prepare and Cook

3 tbsp red onion, finely diced

2 grapefruits

2 limes

2 tbsp grapeseed oil or canola oil

1 tbsp cilantro leaves

1 pound medium (21–25 per pound) shrimp, peeled and deveined

1 small jicama, peeled, sliced (see Note)

½ avocado, peeled and cubed (see Note)

1. Soak the raw onion in cold water for 10 minutes to temper its bite, then drain well. Meanwhile, peel the grapefruits and, with a sharp knife and holding the fruit over a bowl to catch the juice, peel away the remaining pith. Segment the grapefruits and remove the tough membrane so you only have the sweet inner fruit remaining. Set the fruit segments aside and reserve 2 tablespoons of the juice for the marinade. Zest and juice the limes.

2. Make the marinade. Place the grapefruit and lime juices and half of the lime zest in a blender and drizzle in the oil while the blender is running. Add the cilantro and pulse to combine, then pour into a bowl. Stir in the onion.

3. Preheat the grill to medium-high heat. Pour 2 tablespoons of the marinade over the shrimp;

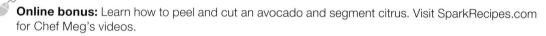

Chew on This: Cilantro vs. Coriander

Cilantro is a leafy herb that looks somewhat like parsley but packs a fresh, almost soapy flavor that people either love or hate if too much is used. Cilantro and coriander come from the same plant: cilantro is the leaves; coriander seeds are the fruit and have an entirely different spicy, sometimes citrusy taste. Cilantro goes to seed in 21 days, so it does have a short life if you don't harvest on a regular basis. It is really a two-for-one plant.

reserve the remaining marinade to dress the slaw. Marinate for 10 minutes. (Do not marinate the shrimp for longer than 10 minutes, as the citric acids will begin to "cook" the shrimp, as in ceviche.)

4. Make the slaw. Combine the grapefruit sections and jicama, toss with the reserved marinade and the reserved lime zest.

5. Remove the shrimp from the marinade and grill for 2 minutes per side, or until the flesh is firm. Discard the marinade you used for the shrimp.

6. To assemble the dish, divide the slaw onto 4 plates, top each with 5 to 6 shrimp, and garnish with the avocado.

Note: Use a vegetable peeler to remove the skin of the jicama, thinly slice it, and cut into 1-inch strips. (You can also use a box grater or a slicing attachment on a food processor.) The jicama should be about the size of a small stick of gum.

We only used half an avocado in this dish. To store the rest, keep the pit attached, sprinkle with a bit of juice from the grapefruit or lime, and wrap tightly in plastic wrap. Use within a day. Or, if you have room in your meal plan for more heart-healthy fat, go ahead and use the other half of the avocado in the dish.

Per Serving: 318.9 calories, 12.2 g total fat, 172.3 mg cholesterol, 173.7 mg sodium, 29.4 g total carbs, 12.5 g dietary fiber, 25.3 g protein

Chew on This: Jicama

Jicama (pronounced HICK-uh-muh) is a large legume with brown skin and white flesh that's native to Mexico. Crunchy in texture, with a sweet nutty flavor, jicama is a great addition to any salad. Often served raw with just a sprinkle of chili powder, jicama is very high in fiber. When purchasing jicama, always look at the spot where the root was attached. If you see any mold, don't buy it. The flesh should be very firm and the skin fairly dry and not slimy, although the high starch content can make the thick flesh a bit sticky and slippery.

Black Bean and Corn Salad

This salad is super easy to make, and it's ready in no time. Like most salads, it's even better the next day. Consider taking this to your next potluck or summer barbecue.

Together with the acid in the lime, the Anaheim pepper really makes the salad. Anaheim peppers are red when ripe and often seen dried. They're spicier than a banana pepper but still quite mild. Use a banana or poblano pepper if you can't find an Anaheim.

Makes 8 Servings:
½ cup per serving

20 Minutes to Prepare and Cook

2 tsp canola oil

½ cup diced red onion

2 cloves garlic, smashed and minced

1 Anaheim pepper, seeded and diced

¼ tsp black pepper

½ tsp chili powder

1 tsp cumin

2 cups corn, cut from 3 ears (or 1 can, drained and rinsed)

1 cup diced tomato

1 can (15 ounces) black beans, drained and rinsed (1½ cups)

2 limes, zested and juiced (see Note)

2 tbsp chopped cilantro

1. Place the oil into a sauté pan over moderate heat. Once hot, add the onion, garlic, and diced pepper. Sauté until the vegetables have softened, 3 to 4 minutes.

2. Add the black pepper, chili powder, cumin, and corn to the pan. Toss to combine, and cook until the corn just begins to brown, 3 to 4 minutes. Add tomatoes and beans to the mixture and cook for 3 minutes more. Add the lime zest and juice.

4. Remove from heat, pour into serving bowl, and sprinkle the chopped cilantro on top. Serve warm or cold.

Note: To extract more juice from your limes (or lemons), roll them on the counter a few times or pop them in the microwave for 10 seconds to warm, then slice and juice.

Per Serving: 80.2 calories, 1.9 g total fat, 0 mg cholesterol, 10.7 mg sodium, 14.8 g total carbs, 3.3 g dietary fiber, 3.2 g protein

CHEF MEG'S TIPS:

- If you make this salad in the summertime when fresh corn is abundant, grill your corn before adding it to the salad.

- Add one large roasted sweet potato to the salad or even a cup of cooked brown rice to turn it into a light meal.

- Leave out the corn and tomatoes and turn this into a three-bean salad by adding chickpeas, kidney beans, black-eyed peas, or your favorite beans.

- Swap pinto or red beans for the black beans, bell peppers for the tomatoes, parsley instead of cilantro—you're only limited by your imagination.

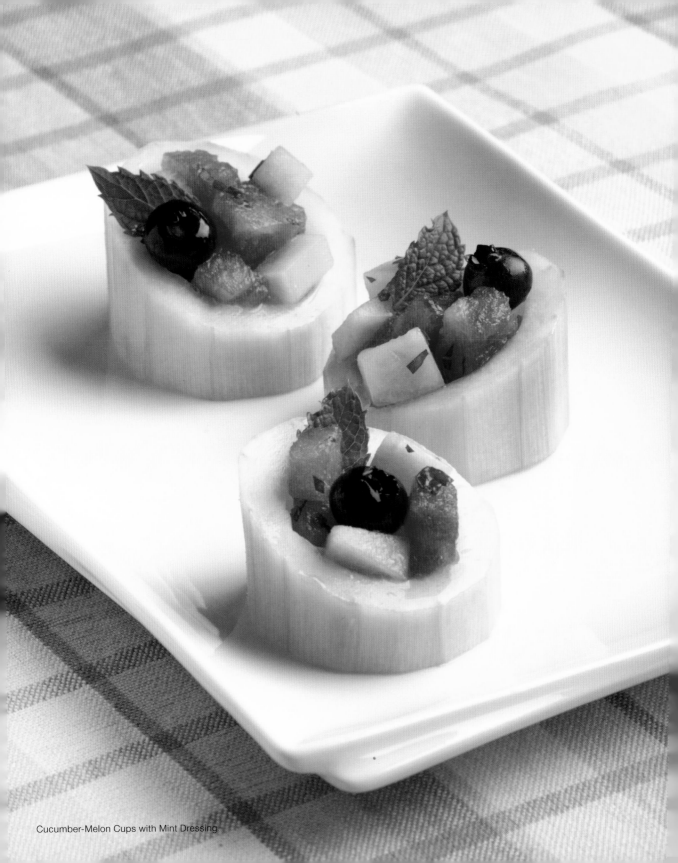

Cucumber-Melon Cups with Mint Dressing

Cucumber-Melon Cups with Mint Dressing

The cool-sweet, fruit-vegetable combination of melon and cucumber is so refreshing, it's no wonder we see it used in everything from lip-gloss to shower cleaner. Any fruit that's in season and affordable will work well here: try honeydew, raspberries, strawberries, papaya, or guava. This is a great appetizer for a summer party—a melon baller makes the work easy and you can cut the cucumber slices on an angle for a fancier presentation.

Makes 4 Servings:
    3 filled cucumbers per serving

10 Minutes to Prepare and Cook

1 cup cantaloupe, cubed

1 cup watermelon, cubed

½ cup blueberries

2 tbsp watermelon

1 tbsp rice-wine vinegar

1 tbsp salad oil

2 tsp chopped fresh mint, plus 12 small leaves for garnish

1 English cucumber, peeled and cut into 1-inch slices

1. Combine the cantaloupe, watermelon, and blueberries in a large bowl and set aside.

2. Prepare the dressing by crushing 2 tablespoons of watermelon in a small bowl. Add the vinegar, oil, and chopped mint; stir well and pour the mixture over the cut fruit.

3. Scoop out 1 tablespoon of inner flesh from each cucumber slice. Fill each cucumber with fruit mixture and garnish with mint sprig.

Per Serving: 67.8 calories, 1.4 g total fat, 0 mg cholesterol, 6.9 mg sodium, 13.2 g total carbs, 2.1 g dietary fiber, 1.4 g protein

Grapefruit-Pear Salad with Fennel

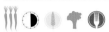

Could you pick fennel out of a lineup of vegetables? It's the white or pale green bulb with celery-like stalks and lacy green fronds that look like dill. The bulb, fronds, and seeds are edible and have diverse uses (see Chew on This for more on fennel). Here, we've combined fennel with grapefruit and pears and served it over arugula for an unconventional salad that will have your taste buds on edge as they wait for each bite.

Makes 4 Servings:
  1 cup arugula and 1 cup grapefruit, pear, and fennel slaw per serving

10 Minutes to Prepare and Cook

2 Ruby Red grapefruits

1 bulb fennel

1 tbsp white-wine vinegar

2 tbsp grapefruit juice

1 tsp Dijon mustard

2 tbsp canola oil

2 tbsp fennel fronds, chopped

2 red pears, sliced (do not peel)

4 cups arugula, torn into bite-size pieces

1. Peel the grapefruits and, with a sharp knife and holding the fruit over a bowl to catch the juice, peel away the remaining pith. Segment the grapefruits by cutting away the sections in a V, leaving behind the membrane. Set the fruit segments aside and reserve 2 tablespoons of the juice.

2. Thinly slice the fennel bulb using the slicing side of a box grater, a mandoline, or a slicing attachment on a food processor.

3. Make the Dressing. Place the vinegar, grapefruit juice, and mustard in a blender. While the blender is running, add the oil in a thin stream. Turn off the blender and stir in the chopped fennel fronds.

4. In a large bowl, combine the grapefruit sections, sliced fennel, and pears; toss with the dressing. Arrange the arugula on 4 plates and divide the fruit and fennel mixture on top.

Per Serving: 170.8 calories, 7.7 g total fat, 0 mg cholesterol, 65.9 mg sodium, 27 g total carbs, 5.5 g dietary fiber, 2.2 g protein

Chew on This: Fennel

Fennel has a subtle licorice flavor and a crunchy texture, and is a refreshing addition to any salad. The bulb, which is prevalent in Mediterranean cuisines, is what most cooks recognize and use, and sometimes you'll see it sold without the stalks and fronds. Those fronds are great garnish, and I like to add chopped fennel fronds to any recipe that uses the fennel bulb. Fennel seeds, often used in Italian and Indian cooking, are also edible. In India, fennel seeds are also used to freshen breath and aid digestion. (In fact, sliced fennel bulb can also aid digestion, and it is served as a palate cleanser in Italy.) The seeds are commonly found in tomato sauce and Italian sausage. Fennel can also be cooked, which mellows its flavor. Usually served braised, it is a nice accompaniment to fish and pork. When buying fennel, select a firm round plant with bright green stalks and fronds that look fresh.

Edamame Confetti Salad

I love the crunch of this salad and it makes a terrific light lunch when served over a cup of raw spinach or a half cup of whole-wheat pasta or brown rice. Think of this as more of a technique than a strict recipe: chop a variety of vegetables into equal sizes—try cucumbers, zucchini, lightly steamed broccoli, cauliflower, carrots, or celery—then toss with a vinaigrette. Edamame, which are young soybeans, add protein to the salad. (See Chew on This for more on Edamame.) You could substitute any kind of legume in its place—try chickpeas, kidney beans, or even lentils. Instead of parsley, try fresh dill, cilantro, or basil.

Makes 4 Servings:
1 cup per serving

10 Minutes to Prepare and Cook

2 cups edamame, shelled and thawed if frozen

1 red pepper, diced

1 yellow pepper, diced

2 plum (Roma) tomatoes, seeds removed and diced

4 green onions, white and green sections, sliced

2 tbsp rice wine vinegar

1 tbsp brown or Dijon mustard

¼ tsp salt

¼ tsp black pepper

2 tbsp olive oil

1 tbsp parsley, chopped

1. In a large mixing bowl, combine the edamame, peppers, tomatoes, and green onions.

2. Make the Dressing. Place vinegar, mustard, salt, and pepper in a blender. With the motor running, remove the cap from the lid and add the olive oil in a steady stream. Turn off the blender and stir in the parsley.

3. Toss the dressing with the vegetables. For the best flavor, refrigerate the salad for an hour before serving.

Per Serving: 209.5 calories, 12.1 g total fat, 0 mg cholesterol, 250.9 mg sodium, 14.1 g total carbs, 6.8 g dietary fiber, 11 g protein

Chew on This: Edamame

Edamame is actually the Japanese word for the preparation of young soybeans that are still in the pod. The pods are boiled in salted or seasoned water and served whole as a snack. Instead of sprinkling the warm pods with sea salt, consider herbs or spices, or simply coarsely cracked pepper. Simply pop the beans out of the tough pod to eat them. Shelled, edamame can be added to salads and soups as you would other beans. Soybeans are rich in carbohydrates, protein, dietary fiber, and omega-3 fatty acids; and are a good source of folic acid, manganese, and vitamin K.

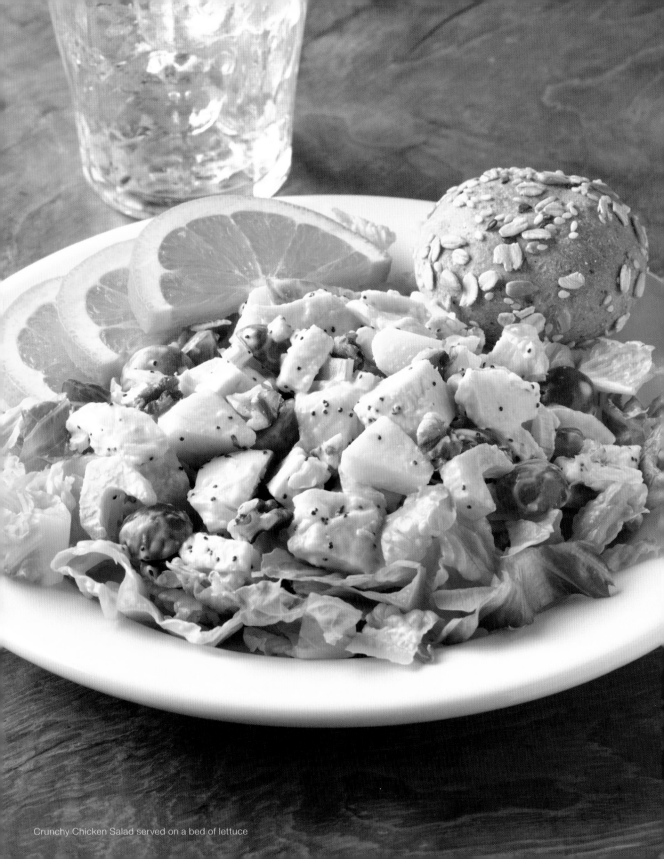

Crunchy Chicken Salad served on a bed of lettuce

Crunchy Chicken Salad

Salads that are held together by a dressing (usually mayonnaise), like tuna, chicken, or egg salad, are called bound salads, but more often than not, all that gloppy mayo yields a bound-and-*gagged* salad! Bound chicken salad is a great way to use up leftovers, and by adding fruit and vegetables, this is a salad you can feel good about eating.

For the dressing, I used equal amounts of reduced-fat mayo and nonfat Greek yogurt to keep that satisfying creaminess. Lemon and poppy seeds round out the dressing, but you could swap dried tarragon, dill, or thyme for the poppy seeds, depending on your preferences. I make a double batch of chicken for dinner, then put this in the fridge for the next day's lunches. This salad is even better the next day!

Makes 4 Servings:
1¼ cups per serving

25 Minutes to Prepare and Cook

1 pound boneless, skinless
    chicken breast

2 tbsp chopped walnut halves

1 cup red grapes, seedless, sliced in
    half lengthwise

1 cup celery, finely sliced

1 Granny Smith apple, cored and diced
    into cubes

For the Dressing:

2 tbsp reduced-fat mayonnaise

2 tbsp plain nonfat Greek yogurt

1 tbsp lemon juice

1 tsp poppy seeds

1. Preheat the oven to 325° F. Spray a casserole dish with nonstick cooking spray. Place the chicken in the dish and cover with warm water. Poach the chicken in the oven until no longer pink in the center, about 20 minutes. If you have a convection oven, turn the fan off or to low.

2. Spread the walnuts in a single layer on a baking sheet and toast in the oven while the chicken is poaching. Toast until the nuts are fragrant, about 5 minutes (watch carefully, as they can quickly burn). Remove from the oven and set aside to cool.

3. Cool the cooked chicken in the refrigerator. Once cool, dice into ½-inch cubes.

4. In a large mixing bowl, combine the mayonnaise, yogurt, lemon juice, and poppy seeds. Add the diced chicken, walnuts, grapes, celery, and apple. Toss to combine. Chill 30 minutes before serving.

Per Serving: 202.1 calories, 5.1 g total fat, 65.7 mg cholesterol, 168.3 mg sodium, 14.8 g total carbs, 2.1 g dietary fiber, 27.8 g protein

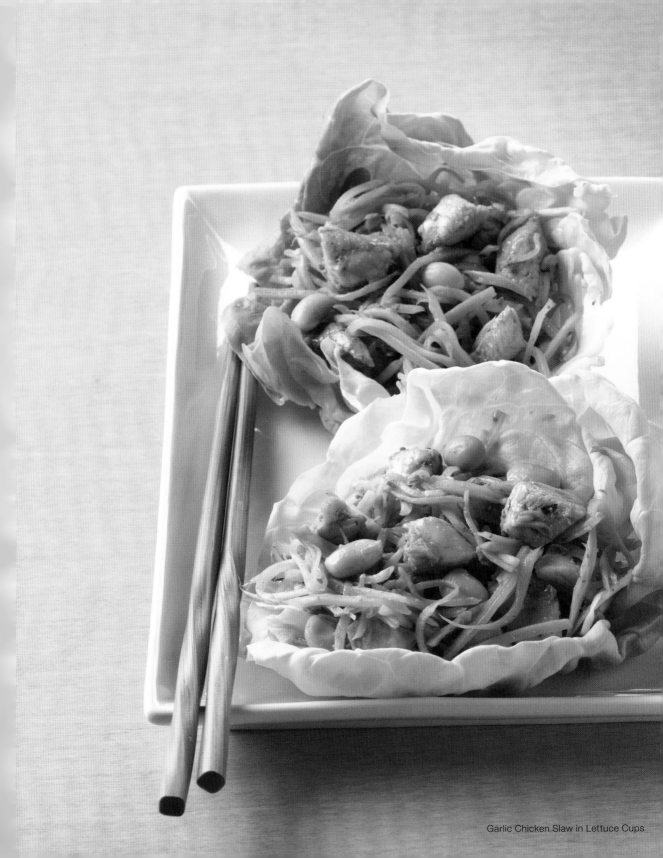

Garlic Chicken Slaw in Lettuce Cups

Garlic Chicken Slaw in Lettuce Cups

Has your dinner become monotonous and predictable? Then your family will love this dish. We transformed stir-fry and a salad into an exciting main dish that contains many ingredients you already know and love. Broccoli slaw is made from the often-discarded stalks, and grated carrots are sometimes added. Find it near the bagged lettuce at the supermarket, or make your own by peeling the tough outer layer from broccoli stalks and shredding them in the food processor. Bonus: kids who won't touch a broccoli floret will gobble up this slaw version, and the lettuce cups make this a fun meal to eat.

Serve two lettuce leaves each filled with a half cup of the slaw or, if you want more greens, serve a cup of the chicken and slaw alongside a plate of lettuce leaves and allow everyone to make their own wraps at the table.

Makes 8 Servings:
2 lettuce leaves with
½ cup chicken salad in each leaf

30 Minutes to Prepare and Cook

1 pound boneless, skinless chicken breasts

1 tbsp black bean garlic sauce (see Note)

2 cloves garlic, chopped

1 tbsp canola oil

One 10-ounce bag broccoli slaw, or 4 cups shredded broccoli stems and carrots

1 cup edamame, shelled and thawed if frozen

4 green onions, sliced, white and green sections

2 tsp Sriracha sauce (see Note)

8 Bibb lettuce leaves

1. Dice the chicken into ½-inch cubes (see Note), then place in a bowl. Combine the black bean sauce with 3 tablespoons of warm water, then stir in the garlic. Pour the entire mixture over the chicken. Cover and refrigerate for 15 minutes.

2. Heat a flat-bottomed saucepan or wok to moderate-high heat, then add the oil. Once the oil is hot, add half the chicken and stir fry until fully cooked. Remove the cooked meat and set aside, then repeat with the remaining chicken.

3. Once all the chicken is cooked, return it to the pan, add the broccoli slaw and sauté for 2 minutes. Add the edamame and cook for 2 minutes more. Stir in the green onions and Sriracha sauce. To serve, place 2 lettuce leaves each on 4 plates and divide the mixture among them, about a ½ cup per lettuce leaf.

Note: Black bean garlic sauce is made from fermented black soybeans. It has a rich, salty taste and can be found in the Asian food aisle of most supermarkets.

Sriracha is a Thai-style hot sauce with a sweet and spicy flavor. Sometimes called "rooster sauce" because of the rooster on the bottle, it works great on everything from eggs to chicken wings. Omit the Sriracha if you're cooking for kids or watching your sodium intake.

To dice or slice raw meat more easily, freeze it for 10 or 15 minutes.

Per Serving: 235.6 calories, 6.6 g total fat, 65.7 mg cholesterol, 243.6 mg sodium, 10.1 g total carbs, 4 g dietary fiber, 32.3 protein

SANDWICHES

Sandwiches have come a long way. Just a short time ago, bologna, peanut butter and jelly, ham and cheese, or maybe some leftover meatloaf were the only thing found slapped between two slices of (usually white) bread in most cafeterias. No vegetables, no whole-wheat bread, and no fun!

These days, sandwiches bear little resemblance to those from lunch boxes past. The trouble is, they're usually not much healthier—just bigger. Jared and his beloved subs are a safe bet if you're on the road, but most deli meats are packed with salt. A 6-inch ham and cheese sub can have half a day's worth of sodium—about a half teaspoon! Check out these stats:

- *Fast-Food Double Cheeseburger:* 440 calories, 23 grams fat, 1,150 milligrams sodium

- *6-inch Turkey Sub with Provolone:* 530 calories, 14 grams fat, 1,490 milligrams sodium

Skip the processed deli meat and you'll be off to a better start. Pile on the veggies, add some low-fat cheese, and choose whole-wheat bread, and you're doing well. Building a better, satisfying sandwich is simple. It comes down to one word: balance.

lost; too little and those precious fillings will end up in your lap. See Chapter 9 for more details on choosing a bread, but I prefer bread from a bakery rather than a supermarket. Good bread becomes an ingredient of the sandwich, rather than just a wrapper. I ask the baker to slice my whole-wheat sandwich bread for me, saving me a step at home and preventing me from being too generous with my slices.

When I want to branch out from sliced bread, I choose one of these whole-grain sandwich wrappers:

- 1 English muffin

- 1 6-inch pita

- 1 tortilla

- 1 bun or roll

- 1 mini or thin bagel

- 3-inch baguette

SparkPeople Cooking Challenge: Swap your usual bread for a higher-fiber one. How much longer does the whole-grain bread sustain you? If you already eat whole-wheat or whole-grain bread, choose a different type of sandwich wrapper.

The Bread

Bread is the most important structural element of a sandwich. It holds all the good stuff in. Too much bread and your toppings will be

The Fillings

A good sandwich is neither too dry nor too wet, neither too big nor too small. It's a study in contrasts, a perfect mix of tastes and textures. If your usual sandwich (turkey and Swiss) no longer appeals to you, make it more satisfying with a few simple changes. Add a burst of flavor with Dijon mustard, crunch with pickles or lettuce, or tang with apricot preserves. Keep your taste buds guessing, and that mundane sandwich suddenly satisfies.

The Chicken Kebob Pitas with Creamy Cucumber Sauce (page 140) are a lesson in building a superior sandwich. The chicken is juicy and tangy thanks to the lemon-pepper rub; the sprouts offer freshness and crunch; creamy cucumber sauce adds mouth feel; and the pita is slightly sour, with just enough bread to soak up the flavors of the chicken without bulking it up too much. Nothing falls out, no bite lacks flavor.

In our house, we usually cook extra meat for sandwiches instead of spending money on deli meat. Leftover grilled or poached chicken, roasted turkey, pork tenderloin, and roast beef all work just fine on a sandwich. The meat contains less salt and more flavor than processed deli meats, which means it doesn't overwhelm the rest of the sandwich. Fancy as it might seem to use leftover pork tenderloin or pot roast on a sandwich, the math is in your favor.

Look at this example:

	Deli Chicken	Chicken Breast
Cost/lb.	$5.99	$1.99
Calories/ serving	68	94
Sodium/ serving	630 mg	56 mg

The deli meat chicken has fewer calories than real chicken because it contains fillers, along with more than ten times the sodium. Read the

Ditch the fat, not the flavor

You can enjoy your lunch and feel good about eating it, too, with these tips:

- Make your own mayo substitute. Mix low-fat or fat-free yogurt (try Greek-style) with your favorite herb or spice blend. Be creative—try curry powder, your favorite salt-free grill rub, dried herbs like dill or tarragon, spicy mustard, or even your favorite jam. Spread this on your bread.

- Shrink your sandwich. Make it with a couple of mini-pitas or mini-bagels instead of full-size bread.

- Go halvsies. Split a sandwich with a friend and add a side salad or a piece of fruit.

- Go topless. Use only one slice of bread, then pile on the toppings.

- If you're toasting your bread, don't butter or oil it first. Use a quick spritz of nonstick cooking spray.

- Think of the vegetables as a main ingredient, not an afterthought. Add an extra serving!

- Berries, grilled onions, spinach, tomatoes, or roasted peppers are great on grilled cheese. Pile extra lettuce or spinach on any sandwich.

- Use mustard, vinegar, or chutneys instead of creamy condiments.

ingredient list on your deli meat sometime. You're getting far more than meat in every bite.

I could eat my weight in cheese, but I restrain myself. When I do eat cheese, I really want to taste it. In a sandwich, where there are so many other textures and flavors competing for my attention, the cheese doesn't stand out. Try leaving the cheese off your sandwich next time. Chances are, you won't miss it. Or, if you're a fromage fanatic like me, base your sandwich around cheese. Try sharp Cheddar, spinach, and raspberry preserves; Brie, green apple, and red onion; or Havarti and spicy mustard with tomatoes.

If you can't wrap your mouth around your sandwich, it's probably better to split it with a friend or save half for another meal. Tempting as it might be to pile on the toppings, standard serving sizes apply:

- 3 ounces meat

- 1 ounce cheese

- ½ cup bound salad (egg, chicken, or tuna)

- ½ cup vegetables

- 1 to 2 tbsp nut butter

SparkPeople Cooking Challenge:
Ditch the deli meat on your
next sandwich. Use leftovers from
last night's dinner, or cook meat
especially for your sandwiches.
What taste differences
do you notice?

The Extras

Condiments should not be the focus of the sandwich. The real reason we all like mayonnaise so much is that it adds desperately needed fat and moisture to a sandwich. By now, with better bread, flavorful fillings, and juicy home-cooked meats, your sandwich won't even need the mayo. Reach for something that will bring more than fat to the party. Mustards and ketchup are fat-free, and offer tang and contrast—and Chapter 12 offers other great condiment suggestions.

This is the time to be creative. Try some of these ideas and you could eat that same turkey sandwich every day of the week without getting bored.

- *Avocado:* tastes buttery and creamy like mayo, but with heart-healthy fats

- *Mustard:* choose Dijon, brown, yellow, or honey

- *All-fruit spread:* great with turkey or cheese

- *Ketchup:* classic and easy (choose low-sodium, low-sugar varieties)

- *Salsa:* drain most of the liquid

- *Barbecue sauce:* see our recipe on page 383

- *Tomato sauce:* add an Italian flair

- *Vinaigrette:* just a drizzle will do

- *Roasted garlic:* mild and sweet, it adds great flavor

SparkPeople Cooking Challenge:
Say no to mayo on your sandwich. Whether you choose one of the condiments above or skip it altogether, you won't miss it.

Tips to reduce the sodium in your condiments

Even if you've lowered the fat, many condiments get much of their flavor from salt or sugar. Here are some ideas to keep the flavor without the harmful additives.

- Choose low-sodium, low-sugar ketchup.

- Use mustard sparingly or blend your own using dried mustard seeds and vinegar if you're watching your salt intake.

- Rinse olives and capers before using. If they're still too salty, soak them in water for a few minutes.

- Make your own marinades and salad dressings.

- Use chili powder or red pepper flakes instead of hot sauce.

- Let a salty ingredient like capers or Worcestershire sauce provide the salt in a dish. You'll impart flavor and a salty taste at the same time.

Lower Count of Monte Cristo Sandwich

SLIM IT DOWN: Serve as an open-faced sandwich (you'll save 60 to 80 calories).

My son Ian loves Monte Cristo sandwiches. With ham, turkey, Swiss, and a crispy egg-coated exterior, who wouldn't? A traditional Monte Cristo sandwich has 600 calories, 30 grams of fat and 1,500 mg sodium! Yeeks! Needless to say, that's not on the menu at our house. One slimmed-down makeover later, my son was none the wiser. He cleaned his plate when I served this version.

Just a few quick swaps were all it took. I used low-sodium bread to counteract the ham. I added tomato slices, which are not in the traditional version, because I love a grilled tomato sandwich. I used just one ounce of reduced-sodium deli ham. Like bacon, ham is a meat that is packed full of flavor but also salt. That small bit of ham stretched its flavor. I used leftover roasted turkey breast instead of salty deli meat. And I used egg whites instead of a whole egg for the coating.

The boys had this with a cup of Minestrone Soup with Parmesan Crisps (page 154), to add more vegetables to their meal and balance the heaviness of the sandwich.

Makes 4 Servings:
1 sandwich per serving

15 Minutes to Prepare and Cook

2 egg whites, beaten

2 tbsp skim milk

2 ounces reduced-sodium deli ham, thinly sliced or shaved

6 ounces roasted turkey breast, thinly sliced or shaved

4 slices reduced-fat Swiss cheese

8 slices low-sodium, whole-wheat bread

2 plum (Roma) tomatoes, sliced

1. In a flat-bottomed bowl or pie plate, whisk together the egg whites and milk.

2. Warm a nonstick skillet over moderate heat. Divide the turkey and ham into four portions. Place the ham on top of the turkey and transfer to the warmed skillet. Cook for 1 to 2 minutes, then top with the cheese.

3. While meat is warming, dip each slice of bread into the egg mixture. Remove the meat and cheese from the skillet, set aside and keep warm. Spray the same skillet with nonstick cooking spray and add the bread.

4. When the bread is nicely browned on one side, flip, and add one portion of meat and cheese to the top of one slice of bread, then top each with one-fourth of the tomato slices. Cover with a second slice of bread and remove the sandwiches from the pan. Slice the sandwiches in half and serve.

Per Serving: 261.3 calories, 6.2 g total fat, 16.4 mg cholesterol, 225.7 mg sodium, 51.5 g total carbs, 2.3 g dietary fiber, 28.3 g protein

Chicken Vegetable Quesadillas with Ranch Yogurt Sauce

This is a great kids' meal, or cut each quesadilla into eight pieces for an appetizer. If you are unsure you can flip the quesadilla as described below, make individual servings with one wrap each, folded in half like an omelet.

Makes 4 Servings:
½ quesadilla with 1 tsp of sauce each

45 Minutes to Prepare and Cook

¼ cup low-fat plain yogurt

2 tsp Ranch Seasoning Blend (page 367)

12 ounces boneless and skinless chicken breast

1 tsp canola oil

2 red or orange bell peppers, top and bottom removed, cored and seeded

4 whole-wheat tortillas

2 tomatoes, diced

½ cup shredded Monterey or pepper Jack cheese

1. In a small bowl, make the sauce by combining the yogurt and ½ teaspoon of the seasoning blend. Cover and chill in the refrigerator.

2. Place the chicken into a plastic bag. Using a meat mallet or rolling pin, pound out the meat to ¼-inch thickness. Add oil and remaining seasoning blend to the bag. Marinate meat 10 minutes or up to 8 hours.

3. Place a cast-iron skillet or nonstick skillet over moderate heat. Once warmed, add the peppers. Sear the peppers by pressing down on them, 2 to 3 minutes. Remove from heat, let cool slightly, and dice.

4. Place the chicken in the skillet, and cook over moderate-high heat for 4 to 5 minutes. Turn, and continue to cook until internal temperature reaches 165° F, about 5 minutes more. Remove the meat from the skillet, let cool slightly, and dice. Wipe out the skillet with paper towels.

5. Reheat the skillet to moderate heat. Build the quesadillas one at a time by placing a tortilla in the pan, then layering on half of the chicken, peppers, tomatoes, and cheese. Top with a second tortilla and cook for 2 minutes on each side until the cheese melts. Remove the cooked quesadilla to a cutting board. To serve, cut each quesadilla in half, with a pizza wheel if you have one

Per Serving: 235.2 calories, 6.5 g total fat, 57.7 mg cholesterol, 436.1 mg sodium, 20.9 g total carbs, 10.7 g dietary fiber, 29.2 g protein

Chef Meg's Beef and Blue Sandwich

Forget grabbing deli sandwiches on the way home from work. You can feed a family of four healthy, gourmet-quality roast beef sandwiches, complete with sweet caramelized onions and creamy blue-cheese dressing, for about $8. That's $2 a sandwich—just try to spend that little at a deli! Use leftovers from our Beef Roast (page 211) or any other lean beef roast, serve the sandwiches with a piece of fruit and a cup of skim milk, and you've got a healthy dinner in no time flat.

Makes 4 Servings:
1 sandwich per serving

5 Minutes to Prepare and Cook

2 tbsp crumbled blue cheese

¼ cup low-fat plain Greek yogurt

4 Multigrain Rolls (page 302)

2 cups shredded Romaine or leaf lettuce

12 ounces thinly sliced lean roast beef

½ cup Caramelized Onions (page 310)

1. Make the blue-cheese sauce. In a small bowl, gently combine the crumbled blue cheese and the yogurt.

2. Cut open the rolls and layer the lettuce, beef, onions, and dressing between the bread.

Per Serving: 356 calories, 10.8 g total fat, 79.6 mg cholesterol, 283.7 mg sodium, 31.5 g total carbs, 5.3 g dietary fiber, 33.2 g protein

Easy Ways to Cut Calories

You know those days when you're craving a food and nothing else will do? This sandwich was created on one of those days. When you have a taste for something that you know isn't a food you should be eating regularly, go ahead and indulge. To keep yourself on track, here are a few helpful hints that allow you to enjoy your food and still eat a balanced meal.

- Share the dish with someone. Half of a rich dish is usually more than enough to satisfy.

- Serve a small portion with a high-volume, low-calorie food. If you're eating a creamy pasta, pair a modest amount with a large green salad. I always serve macaroni and cheese with a heaping pile of steamed or roasted vegetables, and you'll find a large salad on the table any time I serve steaks.

- Use the rich dish as a condiment. Three ounces of steak goes farther when sliced and served atop a salad. Chicken salad and other mayo-based salads are also good salad toppings.

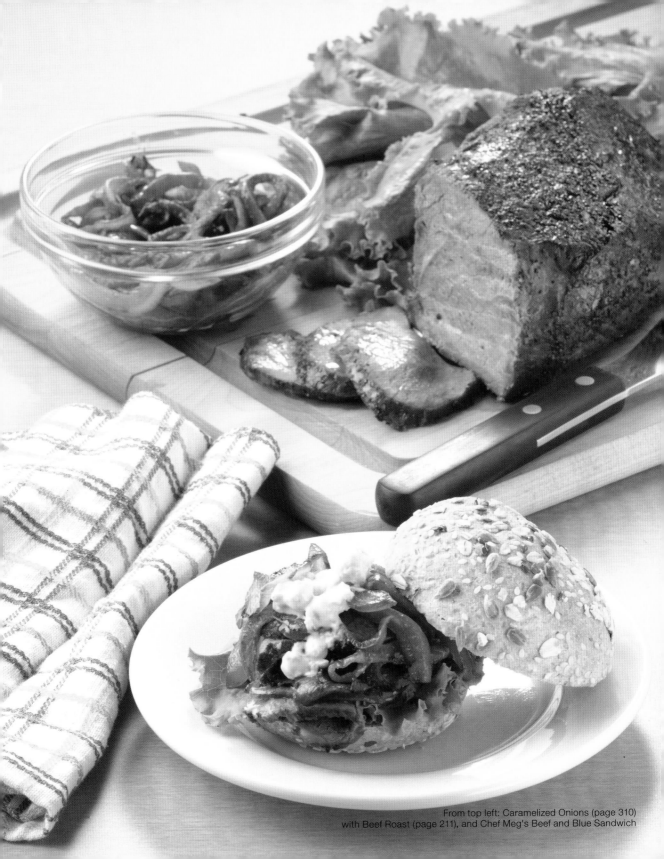

From top left: Caramelized Onions (page 310)
with Beef Roast (page 211), and Chef Meg's Beef and Blue Sandwich

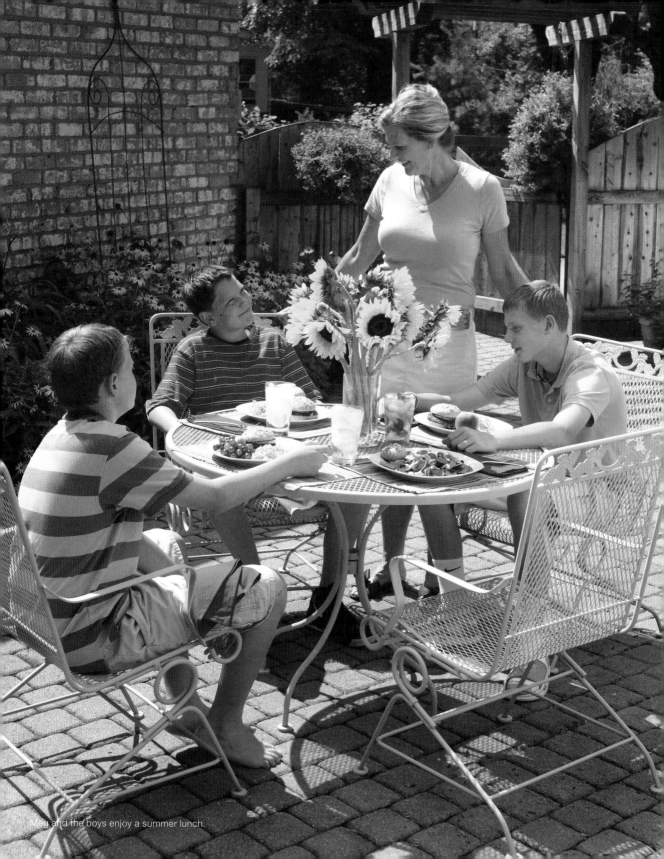

Meg and the boys enjoy a summer lunch.

Black-Bean Burgers with Lime Cream

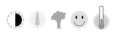

SLIM IT DOWN: Serve without a bun (137 calories).

Who says meat eaters get the best burgers? These black-bean burgers are full of fiber and flavor. For this member makeover, we added more vegetables and some cheese to help them stick together and upped the flavor profile with our Taco Seasoning (page 371). I've placed the cheese in the middle of the burger for a gooey surprise, but you can place it on top, if you prefer. A couple of slices of avocado are a good swap for the lime cream, too.

If you're trying to eat more meatless meals, add this recipe to the lineup. It's a real crowd-pleaser. If you do have leftovers, these burgers are great atop a taco salad or in any Mexican dish where you would use taco meat. Crumble one up and wrap it in a whole-wheat tortilla with your favorite burrito toppings—or use it to top baked tortilla chips for nachos.

Makes 8 Servings:
One 3-ounce burger per serving

30 Minutes to Prepare and Cook

¼ cup fat-free Greek yogurt

1 lime, juiced and zested

Two 15.5-ounce cans black beans, drained and rinsed

¼ cup whole-wheat breadcrumbs

2 tbsp chopped cilantro

1 tbsp diced jalapeño pepper

½ cup grated carrot

2 egg whites, beaten

1 tbsp Taco Seasoning

½ cup shredded reduced-fat Monterey Jack or pepper Jack cheese

4 whole-wheat sandwich thins or Multigrain Rolls (page 302)

2 cups shredded Romaine lettuce

1 large tomato, sliced

1. Combine the yogurt, lime juice, and zest in a small bowl; stir and set aside.

2. In a large mixing bowl, mash the beans slightly with a fork or potato masher. Add the breadcrumbs, cilantro, jalapeño, carrot, egg whites, and Taco Seasoning and combine. Divide into 8 patties. Place the bean mixture in the palm of your hand, place 2 tablespoons of cheese into the center, then fold over into a patty.

3. Preheat a flat nonstick skillet over moderate heat. Once warm, add the burgers and cook 3 minutes per side. You can also cook the burgers on a baking sheet in a 350° F oven for 20 minutes.

4. Serve on a sandwich thin with lettuce and tomato, then divide the lime cream among the sandwiches or serve on the side.

Per Serving: 326.6 calories, 6.0 g total fat, 10.4 mg cholesterol, 274.5 mg sodium, 52.4 total carbs, 13.7 g dietary fiber, 19.2 g protein

Chicken Kebob Pitas with Creamy Cucumber Sauce

This is a great recipe for a busy summer night. If, like mine, your family is out late at baseball games, this meal is for you. Marinate the chicken in the morning or before you leave for the game, and dinner will be on the table in no time flat. Lemon pepper is a versatile spice combination. You'll find endless uses for this juicy and flavorful chicken.

If you think you don't like sprouts, look for broccoli or sunflower sprouts, which are less bitter than bean or alfalfa sprouts. Still don't like sprouts? Use a cup of shredded Romaine or baby spinach in each pita. Want more veggies? Add chopped onions or tomatoes to the pockets. You can also serve the chicken over a green salad, and serve the sauce on the side, if you prefer.

Makes 4 Servings:
½ stuffed pita per serving

50 Minutes to Prepare and Cook

For the Sauce:

½ cucumber, peeled, seeded, and chopped

6 ounces low-fat plain yogurt

1 tsp dried dill or 1 tbsp fresh, chopped

1 tbsp lemon juice

¼ tsp salt

2 tbsp Lemon-Pepper Rub (page 375)

2 tsp canola oil

1 tbsp lemon juice

1 pound boneless, skinless chicken breasts, cut into ½-inch cubes

4 ounces alfalfa sprouts (about 2 cups, tightly packed)

2 whole-wheat pita pockets, cut in half

1. Make the Sauce. Drain the chopped cucumber on a paper towel for 5 minutes; then combine with the yogurt, dill, lemon juice, and salt in a small mixing bowl. Refrigerate the sauce until you're ready to eat.

2. Combine the rub, oil, and lemon juice in a small bowl. Place the chicken in a shallow container with a lid, pour the marinade on top, and refrigerate for 20 minutes.

3. Preheat a grill to moderate high heat. Soak four wooden skewers in water for at least 10 minutes (see Note).

4. Thread the chicken onto the wooden skewers, then place on the preheated grill. Grill until the chicken is cooked through, about 15 minutes. Remove meat from skewers.

5. Divide the chicken, sprouts, and sauce evenly among the four pita halves and serve immediately.

Note: Soaking wooden skewers prevents them from burning on the grill. No skewers? Cut the chicken into strips instead.

Per Serving: 257.7 calories, 4.8 g total fat, 70 mg cholesterol, 354.9 mg sodium, 138.8 total carbs, 4 g dietary fiber, 34.3 protein

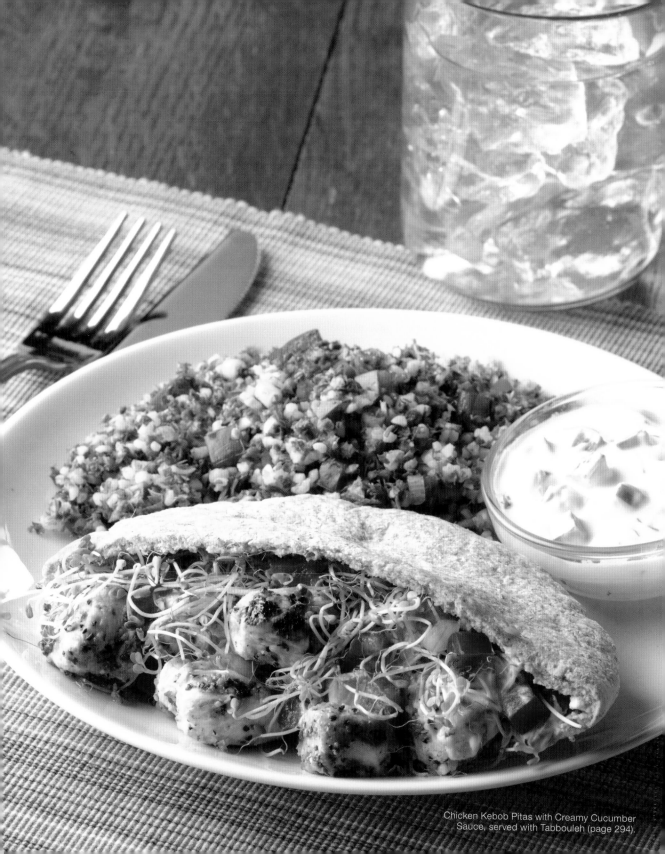

Chicken Kebob Pitas with Creamy Cucumber
Sauce, served with Tabbouleh (page 294).

Crunchy Cod Sandwich with Tartar Sauce

SLIM IT DOWN:
Eliminate the Tartar Sauce (45 calories).

In my hometown, eating fish sandwiches during Lent is a long-standing tradition. Every spring, greasy, bland fish fillets on soggy white-bread buns become a menu staple.

Not only are they rather tasteless, fish sandwiches also render a lean protein unhealthy as well. A popular fast-food fish sandwich has 640 calories, 32 grams of fat, and 1,370 milligrams sodium. Though our version has more sodium than we would usually recommend, you can cut that down by rinsing the pickles and capers before chopping them.

We keep the crispy coating, but inject some flavor with a salt-free lemon-pepper rub, use a whole-wheat sandwich thin or homemade roll, and create our own reduced-fat tartar sauce. If you're really watching your sodium, omit the tartar sauce and use the Spicy Yogurt Sauce (page 380) or Light Lemon Sauce (page 379) instead. By topping it with plenty of tomatoes and lettuce, we add texture and a serving of vegetables—and, of course, our sandwich is baked, not fried.

Makes 4 Servings:
1 sandwich per serving

30 Minutes to Prepare and Cook

For the Tartar Sauce:

¼ cup reduced-fat mayonnaise

4 slices sweet pickles, about 1 tbsp, drained and finely chopped

1 shallot, finely chopped

1 tbsp capers, drained, rinsed, and chopped

1 tbsp lemon juice

2 egg whites, slightly beaten

1 cup panko or whole-wheat breadcrumbs

2 tbsp Lemon-Pepper Rub (page 375)

1 pound cod fillets, cut into four equal portions, patted dry (see Note)

4 whole-wheat sandwich thins or Multigrain Rolls (page 302)

2 plum (Roma) tomatoes, sliced

2 cups Romaine lettuce, torn

1. Preheat the oven to 400° F. Grease a baking sheet with nonstick cooking spray.

2. Make the Tartar Sauce. In a mixing bowl, combine the mayonnaise, pickles, shallot, capers, and lemon juice. Cover and place in the refrigerator to chill.

3. Set out two pie plates or other flat-bottomed bowls. Place the egg whites in the first plate, then place the breadcrumbs and 1 tablespoon of the rub in the second. Sprinkle the remaining rub over the cod. Dip the fish into the egg whites one piece at a time, then transfer to the breadcrumb mixture, coating evenly.

4. Place the breaded fish on the baking sheet and bake for 20 minutes. If the fillets aren't as brown as you would like, change the oven set-

ting to broil. Leave the oven door ajar while broiling and watch until browning occurs.

5. To assemble each sandwich, spread 1 tablespoon of sauce on the top half of each sandwich thin. Place cooked fish on the bottom half of each sandwich thin. Divide tomatoes and lettuce evenly on top of fish before adding the top half of the sandwich thin.

Note: You can swap any white-fleshed fish for the cod in this recipe.

Per Serving: 265.8 calories, 5.7 g total fat, 0 mg cholesterol, 509 mg sodium, 44.2 total carbs, 5.5 g dietary fiber, 9.8 g protein

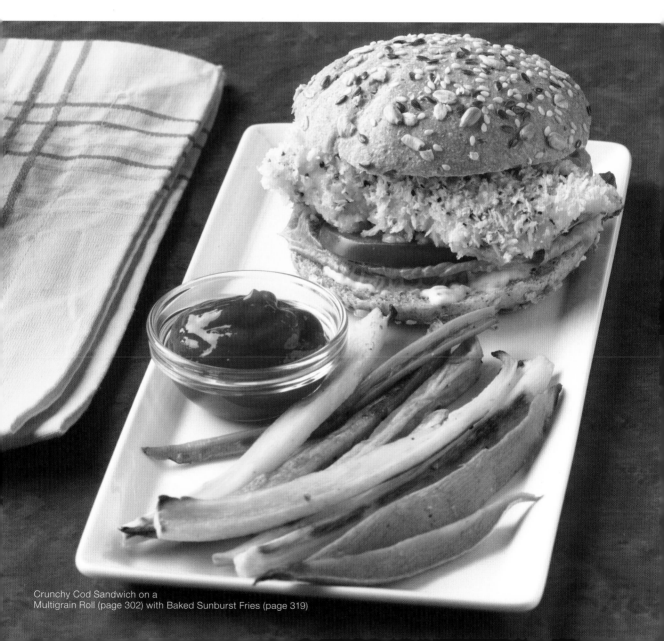

Crunchy Cod Sandwich on a
Multigrain Roll (page 302) with Baked Sunburst Fries (page 319)

Cheesy Pesto Bella Burgers

SLIM IT DOWN: Nix the provolone (50 calories) or the bun (137 calories).

Portobello mushrooms have a distinctly beefy taste and a thick, chewy texture when cooked, making them an ideal vegetarian "burger." Meat eaters and vegetarians alike will love these burgers. Think of your favorite burger toppings: mustard and pickles, grilled onions and peppers, blue cheese and bacon. They'll all be just as delicious atop a mushroom burger!

To turn your 'shrooms into burgers, start by removing the stem and use a spoon to scoop away the gills, which are the dark brown areas on the underside. Doing so allows more room for stuffing, and the gills impart a dark gray color to anything they touch. (You can skip this step if you're less concerned about aesthetics.) For a variation on this burger, try drizzling the mushrooms with balsamic vinegar or your favorite vinaigrette before grilling them. These also make a great appetizer when cut into quarters.

Makes 4 Servings:
    1 burger per serving

15 Minutes to Prepare and Cook

4 portobello mushroom caps, stems removed, gills removed, and discarded

2 tbsp Better-than-Pesto Puree (page 377)

2 slices provolone cheese, cut in half

4 Multigrain Rolls (page 302)

1 large tomato, sliced

1. Preheat the grill to medium heat. Spray the mushrooms on both sides with nonstick cooking spray. Place the mushrooms on the grill, gill side down. Cook for 2 minutes.

2. Flip the mushrooms, top each with 1½ tsp of pesto and ½ slice of cheese.

3. Close the grill lid and cook for 3 minutes more.

4. Serve each mushroom burger on a roll with tomato slices.

Per Serving: 238.6 calories, 7.8 g total fat, 9.8 mg cholesterol, 296.9 mg sodium, 33.5 g total carbs, 6.9 g dietary fiber, 11.5 g protein

Grilled Veggie Sandwiches with Fresh Mozzarella

This vegetable sandwich is one of my favorite recipes in this collection. I love the contrast of textures and tastes: the acid of the vinaigrette, the creaminess of the cheese, and the crunch of the veggies. It's a truly satisfying sandwich that will please meat eaters and vegetarians alike, and it embodies the SparkPeople philosophy of packing every bite full of flavor and nutrition.

If you haven't tried fresh mozzarella, you're in for a treat. It's slightly salty, creamy, and velvety—and it melts really well. It is a little bit more expensive, but a little goes a long way. Look for small *bocconcini* ("little mouthfuls" in Italian); they're about the size of cherry tomatoes (in fact, they're sometimes called *ciliegine,* which is Italian for cherries), that come packed in a tub of water. In smaller supermarkets, you might only find fresh mozzarella in large balls, which you'll need to slice. If you can't find fresh mozzarella, you can use goat cheese or regular mozzarella.

Makes 4 Servings:
1 sandwich per serving

45 Minutes to Prepare and Cook

12 thin asparagus spears

½ red onion, sliced

2 bell peppers, cored and seeded, quartered

1 small eggplant, sliced lengthwise with skin on

2 zucchini, sliced lengthwise with skin on

8 cherry tomatoes

⅔ loaf (about 8 ounces) whole-wheat baguette

¼ cup Tomato-Basil Vinaigrette (page 387)

4 ounces fresh mozzarella, or 8 cherry-sized balls (see Note)

Dash black pepper

1. Preheat grill to moderate heat.

2. Blanch the asparagus. Bring a saucepan of water to boil and prepare a large bowl of ice water. Drop the asparagus in the boiling water for 2 minutes then, using a slotted spoon or kitchen tongs, remove immediately to the ice-water bath to stop the cooking process.

3. Place the onion on a sheet of foil, then wrap to form a packet. Place the packet on the grill and cook for 15 minutes. Place the peppers directly on the grill to char.

4. Place the asparagus, eggplant, zucchini, and tomatoes on the grill, and cook until they are just tender, then set aside on a platter. The tomatoes and asparagus should be removed after 5 minutes, the eggplant and zucchini after 6 minutes, and the peppers after about 12 minutes. The tomatoes' skin will split when they are ready to be removed.

5. Place the peppers in a bowl, cover with plastic wrap, and set aside for 5 minutes. This will help release the charred skin. Meanwhile, use a serrated knife to cut the bread horizontally.

Slice almost all the way through, but keep the bread attached on one side.

6. Remove the peppers from the bowl, and peel off the charred skin. Rinse the peppers to remove any blackened bits, then pat dry. Spread the bread with half of the vinaigrette, then layer on the vegetables, ending with the tomatoes. Sprinkle with black pepper. Place the cheese on top and close the "hinge" on your sandwich.

7. Place the sandwich on the grill for 5 minutes to melt the cheese. Use a serrated knife to cut the sandwich into four servings, then serve with the remaining vinaigrette.

Note: When you buy fresh mozzarella, don't drain the liquid. Use a slotted spoon to remove the balls as you need them. The liquid keeps the refrigerated cheese flavorful and fresh.

Per Serving: 297.6 calories, 10.5 g total fat, 20 mg cholesterol, 335.3 mg sodium, 38.5 total carbs, 8.3 g dietary fiber, 14.3 g protein

SOUPS & STEWS

Here's a cooking riddle for you: It's one of the easiest dishes to make, but it can also take hours in the kitchen. It can contain 1 ingredient or 17, be chunky or smooth. It can be light and cool or hot and heavy. It fills the belly and warms the soul. What is it? It's soup, of course!

Our humble friend soup can be served as an appetizer, main course, or even dessert. Add a few more ingredients or let it cook awhile longer, and you have its cousin, the stew. Research has shown that eating a small bowl of broth-based soup as a first course will reduce the amount of food you consume throughout the entire meal. Slowing down and sipping a bowl of soup or stew, waiting for it cool enough to enjoy it, and savoring one taste at a time is a great way to let your brain and your stomach sync up. Soup is meant to be savored, which is why it's the perfect food for healthy eaters.

Soups deserve a medal of honor; they truly are multitaskers. When a member of the family or a friend is sick, we serve them chicken soup. When a friend moves in to a new home, when I donate a meal to a food pantry, when I take food to a new neighbor, or when I want to console someone from church, I make them soup or stew. Emotions aside, soups and stews are workhorses. They will hold for several days in the refrigerator and freeze well. And you can often get your slow cooker to do the heavy lifting, one more reason soups and stews are so crucial to the busy, healthy cook.

SparkPeople Cooking Challenge:
Start your meal with a cup of soup. Notice that you feel more full and satisfied at the end of your meal.

TAKING STOCK

Stock and broth are both flavorful liquids that we use as the foundation of soups and stews. Meat stocks contain bones, vegetables, herbs and seasonings; vegetable stocks contain only the latter three. Broth is made with the same ingredients, plus meat left on the bones.

The cardinal rule in soup making: taste thy broth or stock before adding it to your soup. If your broth tastes salty or bland, your soup will too. I've tasted many a soup ruined by salty stock or overly seasoned broth. I recommend homemade stocks and broths because you can control the sodium content, but if you are strapped for time, purchase a low-sodium variety. Once you taste the stock you will have an idea of how much seasoning to add to your soup or stew. Though you're always striving to make foods as delicious as possible, broths and stocks are the exception. I tell my students that you shouldn't take a sip of stock and say "that's the best thing I've ever tasted!" Stocks and broths are supporting ingredients.

Making your own stock is so important for the healthy cook. Stocks can form the basis of healthy sauces; be used instead of oil for sautéing; be a base for steaming; and even flavor whole grains, vegetables, and dried legumes.

I make stock once a month or so, saving up bones in the freezer each time I cook. Homemade stock has roughly the same nutritional value as store-bought stock, but it has a fraction of the sodium—13 milligrams compared with 960 milligrams. Those little cubes—which are mostly salt and artificial ingredients—have more than 700 milligrams each! Homemade chicken stock costs about $2.50 a gallon, but a small can at the store will cost about $1. You're really saving money with this recipe.

Store your homemade stock in the freezer—pour cooled 1-cup servings into freezer bags or plastic containers, or freeze in ice tube trays for smaller portions. I put the frozen cubes in a bag and pull them out as needed. One cube plus ½ cup water equals a cup of stock. These stocks are so simple and the final products so crucial to healthy cooking, that they're included here, separate from the rest of the recipes.

SparkPeople Cooking Challenge:
Make a batch of chicken stock
and store it in the freezer. The next
time you want to reach for a pat
of butter to flavor your rice, use
homemade stock instead.

Chicken Stock

Makes 16 servings;
   1 cup per serving

3 Hours, 30 Minutes to Prepare and Cook

3 pounds chicken bones

2 stalks celery, diced

3 carrots, peeled and diced

1 onion, diced

6 parsley stems

8 whole peppercorns or ½ tsp ground
   black pepper

1. Place a large stock pot over moderate heat. Add the chicken bones and cover with 5 quarts of cold water. Bring to a boil, then reduce to a simmer. Remove any impurities or "scum" that may float to the surface.

2. Add the celery, carrots, onion, parsley, and peppercorns and simmer for 3 hours. Line a strainer with cheesecloth, strain, and cool before storing in freezer or refrigerator.

Vegetable Stock

Makes 16 servings;
   1 cup per serving

45 Minutes to Prepare and Cook

2 tbsp olive oil

2 leeks, white and light green parts only,
   sliced

3 carrots, peeled and diced

3 ribs celery, diced

2 cups mushrooms, sliced or quartered
   (see Note)

1 onion, diced

½ tsp black peppercorns

½ tsp thyme, dried, or 2 sprigs fresh

6 parsley stems

1. Place a stock pot over medium heat. Add the oil and heat to warm.

2. Add the leeks, carrots, celery, mushrooms, and onion and cook them slowly until the onions are transparent and the vegetables are softened. Do not let them brown.

3. Slowly add 5 quarts of cold water to the mixture along with the peppercorns, thyme, and parsley stems. Bring to a boil, then reduce to a simmer. Simmer for 30 minutes. Strain and cool before storing.

Note: When cleaning mushrooms for other dishes, save the stems for use in vegetable stock.

SOUP vs. STEW

Before the soup's on, we need to understand the difference between soups and stews.

They start out the same: meats and or vegetables are sautéed, then liquid is added and the mixture is simmered. Stews are heartier, usually with larger pieces of food and less liquid. Soups are thinner, with smaller, uniform ingredients, and can be pureed or served chunky.

For the healthy eater, soups and stews are a must. In addition to slowing down your appetite, they are a great way to pack in multiple servings of vegetables. Pureed soups are a sneaky way to get your five a day. I know plenty of people who won't touch a broccoli spear but will happily slurp down broccoli-cheese soup. (We have a light recipe on page 161!) While sneaking in vegetables isn't a long-term solution for healthy eaters, it is a quick fix for picky palates.

A pound of protein goes much farther when mixed into a pot rather than served on its own. That 3-ounce cooked serving is interspersed with other ingredients, maximizing the flavor of the meat while minimizing the portion.

Roasted Squash Soup

Try a two-for-one: The next time you are turning on the oven to 375° F, cut up a butternut squash and roast it along with whatever else you're cooking. Let it cool slightly, peel, and package to freeze. You'll have cooked butternut squash on hand whenever you need it, and you can have dinner on the table pronto! You'll find very little fat in this soup—it gets a boost of flavor from cilantro pesto.

Makes 8 Servings:
   1 cup per serving

1 Hour to Prepare and Cook

1 large butternut squash (about 3 pounds)

1 tbsp olive oil

1 medium onion, finely chopped (1 cup)

4 cups homemade or low-sodium
   chicken stock

1 orange, zested and juiced

For the Pesto:

½ bunch cilantro, stems removed

¼ cup unsweetened flaked coconut

1 orange, peeled

1 serrano chile pepper, seeded

1. Preheat oven to 375° F. Peel, halve, and remove the seeds from the squash. Cut into ¾-inch cubes. Add the cubed squash to a roasting pan and cook until tender, about 20 to 25 minutes.

2. In a Dutch oven or medium, heavy-bottomed saucepan, heat the oil over medium heat. Add the onion and sauté over medium-low heat until softened. Add the squash and stock and cook, covered, for 10 minutes. Add the orange zest and the juice, and continue to simmer, uncovered, for 10 minutes more.

3. Puree the soup using an immersion blender, or transfer in batches to a blender or food processor (taking care not to be splashed with hot soup). For a smoother texture, strain the soup through a sieve, though you'll remove some of the fiber.

4. Make the Pesto. In a blender or food processor, blend the cilantro, coconut, orange, and hot pepper until the mixture forms a puree. If the consistency is too thick, add warm water to thin it.

5. Ladle the soup into cups and garnish each serving with about a teaspoon of the pesto.

Per Serving: 128.6 calories, 2.8 g total fat, 0 mg cholesterol, 304.5 mg sodium, 25.6 g total carbs, 6.2 grams dietary fiber, 3.7 g protein

Watercress and Spring Pea Soup

I love starting a summer meal with chilled soup or even making one into a light meal. After a long day of working in the garden, the last thing I want is to eat a heavy meal. In springtime, when the season's first peas are popping up in the farmers' markets, this soup is a familiar addition to our dinner table.

The best way to clean watercress—and spinach, too—is to fill a sink a third of the way full with cold water. Drop the greens into the water, swish them around, then remove them from the water. You will find all the dirt that you did not want to eat in the bottom of the sink, not in your soup or salad.

Online bonus: Learn how to chop an onion and make vegetable stock. Visit SparkRecipes.com for Chef Meg's videos.

Makes 4 Servings:
1 cup per serving

30 Minutes to Prepare and Cook

1 tbsp canola oil

1½ cups finely diced onion

1 cup thinly sliced leeks, white and pale green parts only

4 cups homemade, low-sodium, or no-salt-added vegetable stock

2 small russet potatoes, peeled and diced (about 1½ cups)

1 cup spring peas, 10-ounce bag found in the produce section, or shelled from pods

¼ tsp salt

½ tsp black pepper

1 large bunch watercress, washed, stems removed (about 2 cups) 1 lemon, juiced

4 tbsp reduced-fat sour cream

1. In a large saucepan, heat the oil over moderate heat. Once hot, add the onion and leeks and sweat until softened, 3 to 4 minutes. Add the stock and the potatoes and simmer until the potatoes are well cooked, 8 to 10 minutes. Add the peas and salt and pepper, simmer for 2 minutes, then remove from the heat.

2. Place watercress in a food processor or blender. Process or blend until reduced to a puree. Carefully add the soup to the watercress and process to blend. You may need to do this in batches. Add lemon juice to taste.

3. The soup can be served warm or chilled. Garnish each serving with 1 tablespoon of the sour cream.

Per Serving: 190.8 calories, 5.7 g total fat, 5.9 mg cholesterol, 182.6 mg sodium, 27.5 g total carbs, 5.3 g dietary fiber, 5.2 g protein

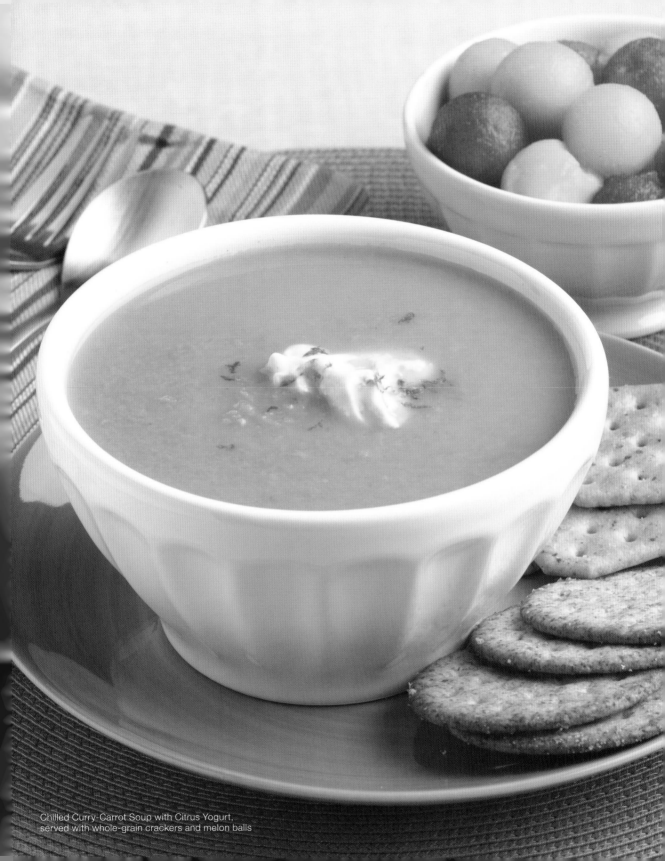

Chilled Curry-Carrot Soup with Citrus Yogurt,
served with whole-grain crackers and melon balls

Chilled Curry-Carrot Soup with Citrus Yogurt

Cold soups are great when you are watching your waistline because traditionally they contain very little fat. When fat melts, it gives you that great mouth feel. When it's cold, it just coats your mouth and feels greasy. To achieve a refreshing chilled soup that's light in texture, go easy on the fat. This particular soup can also be served barely warm. Notice the difference in flavors as the soup cools.

Makes 4 Servings:
1 cup soup and 1 tbsp of citrus yogurt

45 Minutes to Prepare and Cook

1 tbsp unsalted butter

1 cup chopped onions

6 cups shredded carrots

2 tsp grated ginger, either fresh or jarred

1 tsp curry powder

¼ tsp table salt or fine sea salt

3 cups homemade or low-sodium vegetable stock

1 orange, zested and juiced

2 limes, zested and juiced

4 ounces low-fat plain yogurt

1. Heat the butter over moderate heat in a large saucepan. Once the butter is melted, add the onions, stir frequently, and cook until tender, about 2 minutes. Add the carrots, ginger, curry powder, and salt to pan; stir; and cook for 2 minutes more.

2. Pour the stock over the vegetables and stir to combine. Bring the mixture to a boil and reduce heat to a simmer. Cook until carrots are tender, 15 to 18 minutes.

3. Remove the pan from the heat, then puree the soup using an immersion blender, or transfer to a food processor or blend. Add the orange and lime juices, then transfer the soup to a large bowl. Stir half of the orange and lime zest into the soup. Refrigerate until completely chilled.

4. In a small bowl, combine the remaining orange and lime zest with the yogurt, and chill.

5. When ready to serve, top each cup of soup with 1 tablespoon of citrus yogurt.

Per Serving: 159.6 calories, 4.1 g total fat, 9.6 mg cholesterol, 296.5 mg sodium, 28.8 g total carbs, 6.3 g dietary fiber, 4.5 g protein

CHEF MEG'S TIPS:

- Kosher salt is too coarse to dissolve in cold soups. Use table salt or a fine sea salt.

- When zesting citrus, always rotate the fruit after each run on the grater. You are zesting the skin not the white pith.

- If your citrus is room temperature it will yield more juice. Pop your fruit in the microwave for 10 seconds and watch the juices flow.

- To save time, look for bags of preshredded carrots. In a pinch, you could use diced frozen carrots.

Minestrone Soup with Parmesan Crisps

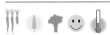

Minestrone is a classic Italian soup that's packed full of flavor and nutrition. You can use any vegetables you have in the kitchen, but always keep the onion, carrot, and celery, which are the "holy trinity" of flavorful vegetables.

I make this soup year-round, but the ingredients change based on the season. I might add spinach in springtime, tomatoes from my garden in summer, and some root vegetables in fall and winter.

Makes 6 Servings:
2 cups of soup and 1 crisp per serving

50 Minutes to Prepare and Cook

1 tbsp canola oil

1 cup diced onion

1 cup diced celery

1 cup diced carrots

2 cups chopped cabbage

¼ cup tomato paste

One 4.5-ounce can diced tomatoes

1 tbsp dried basil

½ tsp salt (optional)

½ tsp pepper

One 5.5-ounce can cannellini (white kidney) beans, drained and rinsed

6 cups homemade, low-salt, or no-salt-added vegetable or chicken stock

½ cup lentils, yellow or pink, rinsed (see Note)

1½ cups diced zucchini

½ tsp red pepper flakes

1 tbsp basil pesto, or Better-than-Pesto Puree (page 377)

2 tbsp shredded Parmesan cheese

1. Heat the oil in a large saucepan, then add the onion, celery, carrots, and cabbage. Cook over moderately low heat until the vegetables are translucent, about 5 to 7 minutes. Add the tomato paste, tomatoes, dried basil, salt (if using), pepper, and cannellini beans. Cook for 1 minute, then slowly add stock, stirring to combine. Simmer for 20 minutes.

2. Add the zucchini and lentils and simmer 10 minutes more. Add the red pepper flakes, crushing with your hands to release the heat (see Note). Stir in the pesto.

3. To make the Parmesan crisps, preheat the oven to 400° F. Line a sheet pan with parchment paper or a silicone pan liner. Place teaspoon-sized mounds of Parmesan on the pan, then spread the cheese into a single layer. Bake until just browned, 3 to 4 minutes. The crisps will appear slightly melted, but they'll firm up after you remove them from the oven.

Note: I prefer pink or yellow lentils, which take less time to cook but become mushy when overcooked. For a firmer lentil, use the green variety, but they need to go in with the cannellini beans and cook for 20 minutes.

Always wash your hands after handling hot peppers or red pepper flakes, and avoid touching your eyes, which could cause irritation.

Per Serving: 197 calories, 4.8 g total fat, 2.1 mg cholesterol, 222.5 mg sodium, 29.2 g total carbs, 9.4 g dietary fiber, 10.4 g protein

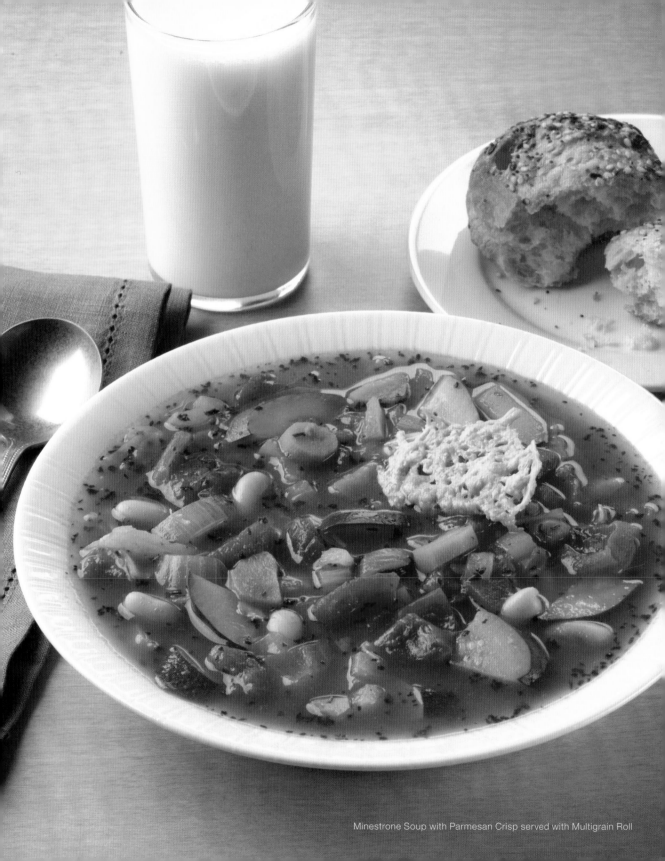

Minestrone Soup with Parmesan Crisp served with Multigrain Roll

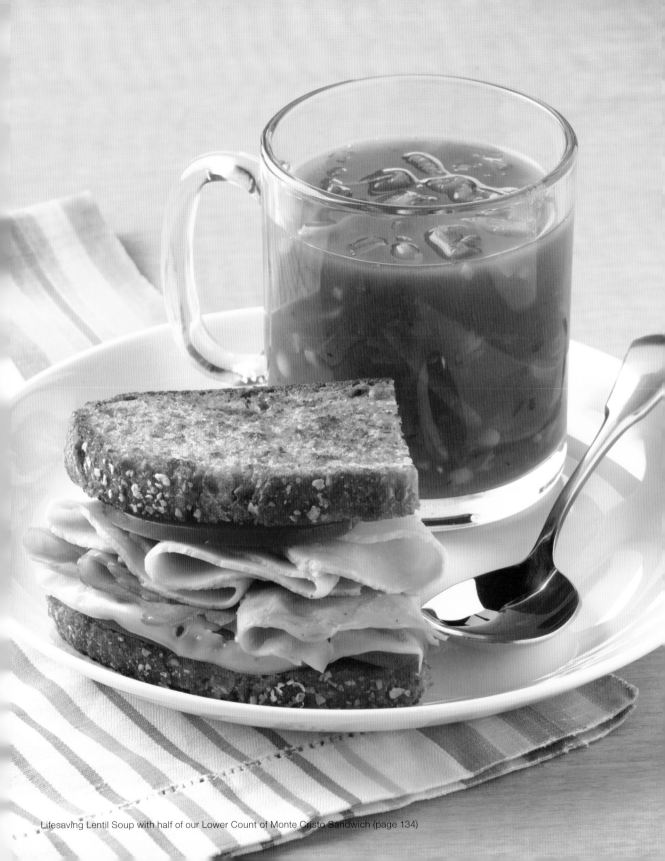

Lifesaving Lentil Soup with half of our Lower Count of Monte Cristo Sandwich (page 134)

Lifesaving Lentil Soup

This soup truly is a lifesaver for busy families! On days that we are occupied with homework and sports until dinnertime, I can mix this together in a flash and put everything in the slow cooker before picking the boys up from school. When we arrive home at dinner time, there's a warm meal waiting for us to enjoy.

If I am making this soup in the spring or summer, lemon is a great way to finish the soup; when it is cold outside I reach for the hot sauce!

Makes 6 Servings:
  1 cup per serving

20 Minutes to Prepare, 4 Hours to Cook

1 onion, finely diced

One 14.5-ounce can diced tomatoes, juice
    included

One 6-ounce can tomato paste

½ cup diced celery

2 cups shredded carrots

1 cup brown lentils

1 tbsp Italian Herb Seasoning (page 369)

½ lemon, juiced, or 3 drops hot sauce

1. Place the onion, tomatoes, tomato paste, celery, carrots, lentils, and herb seasoning in the slow cooker. Add 5 cups water.

2. Set the cooker on low and slow cook for 4 hours. Just before serving add a squeeze of lemon juice or a few drops of hot sauce to the soup.

Per Serving: 110.8 calories, 0.4 g total fat, 0 mg cholesterol, 58.5 mg sodium, 22.5 g total carbs, 8.1 g dietary fiber, 5.4 g protein

CHEF MEG'S TIPS:
HOW TO COOK LENTILS

Lentils need no presoaking and cook much more quickly than other dried legumes. Just place them in a strainer (use a mesh strainer rather than your pasta colander so they don't fall through the holes) and give them a rinse. Pick out any debris or shriveled or discolored lentils.

Cook lentils with a 2:1 ratio of water or broth to lentils and simmer until soft. Depending on the variety, this can take 10 minutes up to an hour. Most varieties will take about 15 to 20 minutes.

Do not add salt to the lentils, as that will make them tough. Add salt to taste after the lentils are cooked.

LEAN ON LENTILS

Lentils are a cheap and versatile protein source—I buy lentils for about a dollar a pound in the bulk bins at my local supermarket. Most people limit lentils to lentil soup, but these legumes have a lengthy list of uses.

- Add a cup of cooked lentils to ground beef or turkey to mix into meatballs, meatloaf, or burgers.

- Add pureed lentils to chili, soups, or stews to thicken.

- Toss cooled French or green lentils with vinaigrette and some chopped vegetables for a quick salad. Or add lentils to your favorite pasta salad. Try the Herbed Bulgur and Lentil Salad on page 301.

- Substitute lentils for half or all the ground beef in your favorite pasta dish. In meat sauce, lasagna, or stuffed shells, the texture is indistinguishable.

A half cup of lentils has 115 calories, less than half a gram of fat, and 366 mg potassium. It contains 9 grams each of protein and fiber (about a third of your recommended amount of fiber), and 45 percent of your Daily Recommended Value of folic acid. Lentils are frequently included on lists of the world's healthiest foods.

French lentils are dark green and peppery in flavor. They hold their shape well after cooking but can take longer to cook than brown or orange lentils. These are the lentils to use in salads or dishes where you want the lentils to retain their shape.

Red or pink lentils are a bright shade of salmon when they're dry, but they become mushy and yellow when cooked. They're quite tasty and cook in less than 10 minutes. They are milder and sweeter than other lentils, and because they lose their shape when cooked, they are easier to mix into soups, burgers, and stews.

Brown lentils (also called green lentils, German lentils, or Egyptian lentils) are the most common lentil seen in grocery stores. Khaki in color and mild in flavor, they also hold their shape after cooking—as long as they're not overcooked. Add a bit of oil to the cooking water and cook until just tender, about 15 minutes at a simmer.

Black lentils are sometimes called beluga lentils because they shimmer after cooking and look like caviar.

Slim Down Your Soup

Creamy, rich soups feel great on the tongue but not in the belly. To reduce the amount of fat—in the form of cream, butter, and meat drippings—but still retain flavor, try one of these tips:

- Pack in flavor with herbs, spices, and citrus instead of salt or meat drippings.

- Use legumes as a filler to boost fiber in your soups.

- Sweat or roast vegetables in minimal fat to extract the most flavor.

- Thicken soups with legumes, whole-wheat bread, and vegetable purees instead of commercial thickeners (cornstarch) or a roux (flour and fat mixed together).

- Finish soups with low-fat Greek yogurt, salsa, or pesto instead of heavy cream. Even a dollop of hummus can add low-fat richness.

CHEF MEG'S TIPS: THE RULES OF CREAMY SOUPS

In classical cooking, there are rules for everything, even creamy soups. While I use lower-fat alternatives in my creamy soups, those rules still apply.

- If the cream (or milk) is warm, it will blend into the soup better. (Since the evaporated milk that we often use is shelf-stable and at room temperature, there's no need to heat it.)

- Cream should always be added at the end of the cooking process. I prefer adding it after I puree the vegetables.

- Once the cream (or evaporated milk) is in the soup, do not allow the mixture to boil—it will curdle.

- One more to grow on: When you reheat the soup, heat it slowly and do not allow it to boil or you'll have a lumpy, curdled soup.

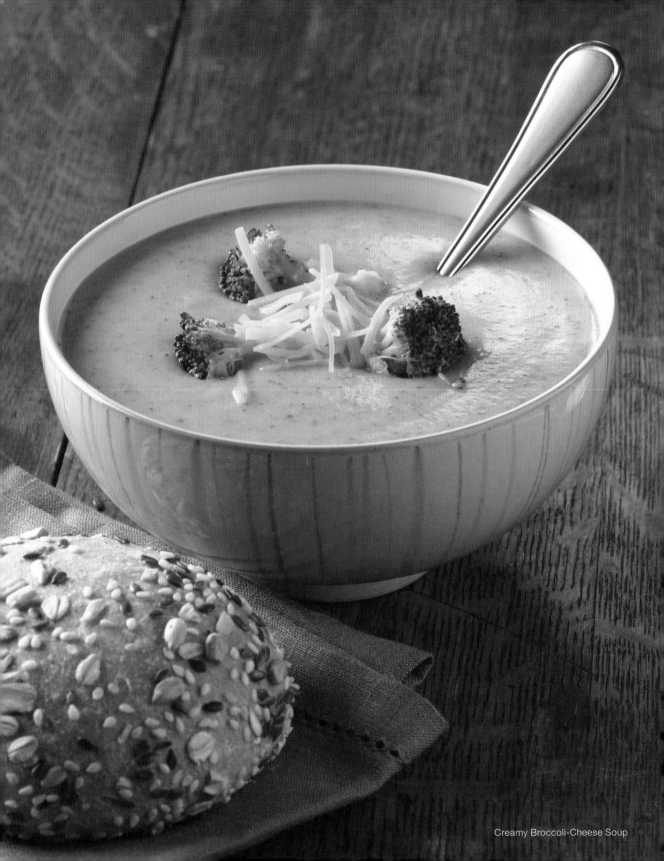

Creamy Broccoli-Cheese Soup

Creamy Broccoli-Cheese Soup

Everything's better with cheese, isn't it? So if you think you don't like broccoli, start here! Fat-free evaporated milk is substituted for heavy cream, which gives this soup richness without the fat. This is a basic cream-soup recipe that can be used with almost any vegetable: try asparagus, cauliflower, celery, mixed vegetables, or mushrooms.

I prefer to use fresh broccoli because it is simple to prepare, but feel free to use a 10-ounce bag of frozen florets as a substitute. Just don't throw away the broccoli stalks, peel them and shred them to use in broccoli slaw (make Garlic Chicken Slaw in Lettuce Cups on page 129 for dinner the next night with the leftover broccoli).

Makes 4 Servings:
  1 cup per serving

45 Minutes to Prepare and Cook

2 tsp unsalted butter

1 cup chopped onion

1 large head of broccoli, florets separated from the stalks (about 4 cups)

1 large or 2 small russet potatoes, peeled and diced (1 cup)

2 cups homemade, low-sodium, or no-salt-added chicken or vegetable stock

1 cup fat-free evaporated milk

½ tsp white pepper

¼ cup shredded sharp Cheddar cheese

1. Place a large saucepan over moderate heat. Add butter and cook until melted. Add the onions, reduce heat to low, and cook until onions are tender, about 3 minutes, stirring occasionally.

2. Add the broccoli, potato, and stock; stir, and bring to a boil. Reduce to a simmer, cover, and cook for 20 minutes.

3. Uncover the soup and remove from heat. Puree with an immersion blender, or carefully transfer the soup to a blender or food processor to puree, then return the soup to the saucepan.

4. Stir in the evaporated milk, season with pepper, and add 2 tablespoons of the cheese to the soup. Simmer for 1 minute. Serve hot, garnished with the remaining cheese.

Per Serving: 178.1 calories, 4.6 g total fat, 13.9 mg cholesterol, 156.3 mg sodium, 23.5 g total carbs, 4.6 g dietary fiber, 10.2 g protein

French Onion Soup with Whole-Wheat Croutons

SLIM IT DOWN: Lose the cheese (70 calories).

The predominant flavor in most versions of this classic French soup is salt. Commercial versions can have almost an entire day's worth of sodium in one serving—about eight times the amount in our recipe. We created rich, deep flavors by slowly caramelizing the onions and using homemade stock. And, of course, no onion soup would be complete without the signature crouton and cheese. This soup freezes well. Use leftovers as a sauce in braised meat dishes. (You can also make this recipe with the Caramelized Onions on page 310. Just start the recipe with Step 2.)

Makes 4 Servings:
1 cup per serving

45 Minutes to Prepare and Cook

2 large onions

1 tsp butter

2 tbsp sherry or white wine

1 tsp dried thyme

½ tsp black pepper

¼ tsp salt

1 quart beef or vegetable stock, homemade or low sodium

Four ½-inch slices whole-wheat baguette

4 slices reduced-fat Swiss cheese

1. Peel the skin from the onions, cut them in half from root to tip, and then thinly slice them into half-moons.

2. Heat a large saucepan over moderate heat. Add the butter, heat until foaming, then add the onions. Reduce heat to medium. Once the onions are light brown, add two tablespoons of water to deglaze and scrape the brown bits from the bottom of the pan with a wooden spoon (see Note). Continue to cook the onions, and when the pan starts to turn brown again within a few minutes, deglaze it a second time by adding the sherry or wine and scraping the browned bits from the bottom of the pan. The onions will take about 20 minutes to turn dark golden in color.

2. Add the thyme, pepper, and salt to the onions, then slowly pour in the stock and simmer for 15 minutes.

3. Preheat the broiler and toast the bread.

4. Ladle a cup of soup into an ovenproof bowl, then top with the toasted bread and a slice of cheese. Repeat for all four servings. Place the soup dishes on a sheet pan, then place under the broiler, leaving the door slightly ajar. Keep a close eye on the soup, and broil until cheese is bubbly and toasted.

Note: As the onions cook, you will notice the bottom of the pan developing a *fond* (French for "base" or "foundation"), or starting to turn brown. To get great caramelization, deglaze the pan by adding a liquid and stirring with a wooden spoon to pull the *fond* back into the food.

Per Serving: 194.5 calories, 6.4 g total fat, 17.8 mg cholesterol, 320.4 mg sodium, 22.5 total carbs, 4.1 g dietary fiber, 7.9 g protein

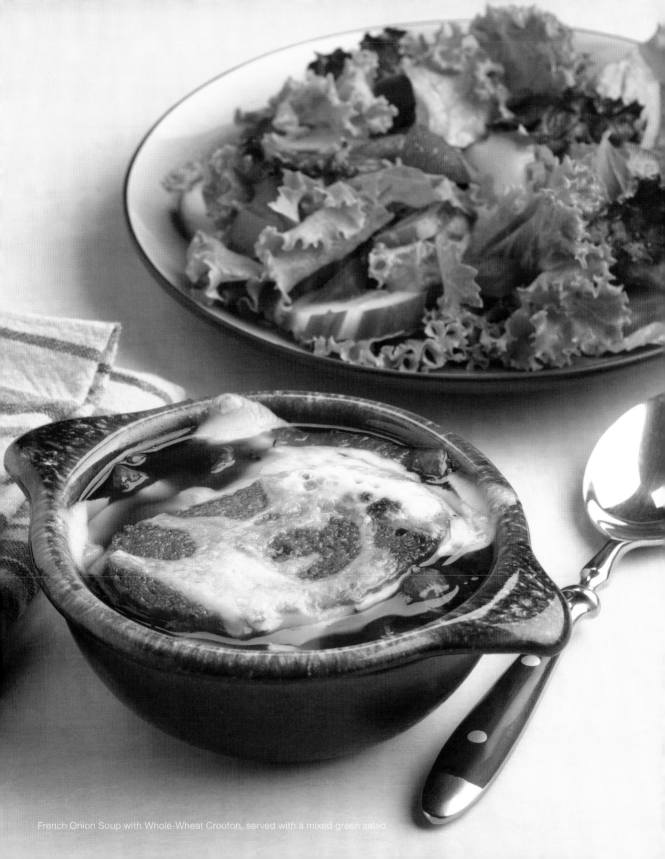

French Onion Soup with Whole-Wheat Crouton, served with a mixed green salad

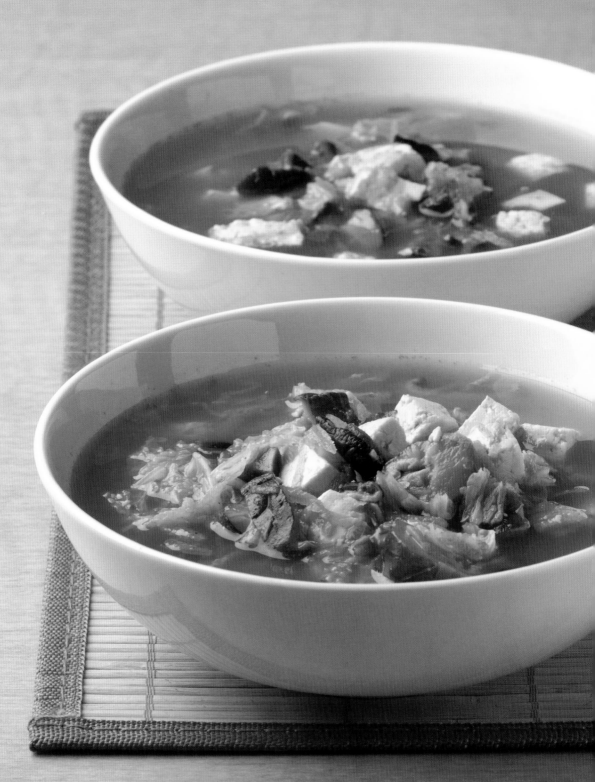

Miso Vegetable Soup for two

Miso Vegetable Soup

Have you ever had miso soup, the rich, salty soup made from a paste of fermented soybeans and rice that's a staple of Japanese restaurants? The traditional soup is quite high in sodium, and contains many ingredients not commonly found in home pantries.

After much thought and testing I came up with a version that's not only easy to make at home, but contains a fraction of the sodium. This recipe goes down in our family history—I got my husband to eat tofu! Miso is Japan's version of chicken noodle soup, and I think you'll find it just as comforting.

Makes 4 Servings:
    1 cup per serving

20 Minutes to Prepare and Cook

1 ounce dried shiitake mushrooms (about 14)

3 tbsp miso paste

8 ounces firm tofu, drained, cut into ½-inch cubes

2 cups shredded Napa cabbage

½ cup grated carrots

1 tsp Sriracha (see Note)

4 green onions, white and green parts, sliced (about ½ cup)

1. Soak the mushrooms in 1 cup of hot water for 5 minutes.

2. Drain mushrooms, reserving the liquid. Add additional water to the liquid to equal 5 cups. Slice mushrooms, underside up, into ¼-inch slices. Place a saucepan over moderate heat and add the mushrooms and liquid. Bring to a simmer, add the miso paste, tofu, cabbage, carrots, and Sriracha. Simmer for 5 minutes more.

3. Ladle the soup into individual bowls and garnish with the green onions. Serve warm.

Note: Sriracha is an Asian hot chili pepper sauce. It is widely available and most commonly found in plastic bottles bearing a rooster logo. Look for it in the Asian foods aisle.

Per Serving: 87.4 calories, 5.4 g total fat, 0 mg cholesterol, 220 mg sodium, 8.8 g total carbs, 1.9 g dietary fiber, 12.9 g protein

Light and Creamy Crab Chowder

Chowders are thick and creamy soups that are usually loaded with fat. With this recipe, fat-free evaporated milk replaces the cream, and the potatoes cook down and help thicken the soup, too. A small amount of butter lends richness.

The basis of this chowder is a *mirepoix* of celery, onion, and mushrooms replacing the traditional carrots. In this case, leeks bring a more delicate flavor. Don't sauté the vegetables, just sweat them over low heat. Canned crabmeat is already fully cooked, and it's easy to overcook the meat by adding it to the chowder too early. Add it at the end just to heat through.

Drain the crab well and give it a quick rinse to further reduce the sodium in this soup. If you have access to fresh-cooked crabmeat, you could use that as well. No crab? Substitute canned clams. Basil eliminates the need for any added salt.

Makes 4 Servings:
1 heaping cup per serving

45 Minutes to Prepare and Cook

1 tsp unsalted butter

1 cup sliced leeks, white and pale green parts only

1 cup thinly sliced celery

½ cup finely diced mushrooms

½ pound russet or Yukon gold potatoes, peeled and cut into ¼-inch cubes (2 cups)

½ tsp white pepper

2 cups homemade, low-sodium, or no-salt-added chicken stock

1 cup crabmeat (about 8 ounces), drained and rinsed

1 cup fat-free evaporated milk

2 tbsp shredded fresh basil leaves

1. Place a medium saucepan over moderate heat and add butter to melt. Once the butter is foaming, add the leeks, celery, and mushrooms. Reduce the heat to low and sweat the vegetables until soft, 5 to 6 minutes.

2. Add the potatoes and season the mixture with pepper. Slowly pour in the stock and stir to combine. Bring to a boil, then reduce the heat and simmer until the potatoes are tender, about 15 minutes.

3. Add the crabmeat and evaporated milk to the mixture. Simmer without boiling until heated through, 2 to 3 minutes. Stir in the basil and remove from heat. Serve warm.

Per serving: 181.8 calories, 1.3 g total fat, 40.1 mg cholesterol, 385.5 mg sodium, 27.6 g total carbs, 3.2 g dietary fiber, 14.4 g protein

Vegetable Chicken Soup

If roasted chicken is a blank canvas, then chicken soup is a canvas that has been primed and given a rough coat of paint. How you fill in the details is up to you, but the possibilities are endless. Add beans for more fiber, whole-wheat orzo pasta for a change in texture, or green beans for crunch and color. Change up the vegetables, the herbs, and the starches. You really can't mess up this soup. Even better, it's ready in less than 30 minutes!

Soup is a great way to make a second meal from roasted chicken, like our Lemon Herb-Roasted Chicken (page 184). This is the perfect soup for cold winter nights or days when you're fighting off a cold.

Makes 8 Servings:
  1 cup per serving

30 Minutes to Prepare and Cook

1 tbsp canola oil

1 cup sliced onion

1 cup carrots, sliced into strips

½ cup celery, sliced into an angle

One 14.5-ounce can diced tomatoes, no salt

1 tbsp Italian Herb Seasoning (page 369)

2 cups homemade, low-sodium, or no-salt-added chicken stock

1½ cups whole-wheat penne pasta

1. Place a large saucepan over moderate heat; once warm, add the oil. When the oil is hot, add the onions and carrots, and sauté for 2 to 3 minutes. Add the celery and cook for 2 minutes more.

2. Add the tomatoes, herb seasoning, stock, and pasta; simmer for 15 minutes stirring occasionally. Serve hot.

Per Serving: 99.3 calories, 2.1 g total fat, 0 mg cholesterol, 39.6 mg sodium, 17.3 g total carbs, 3.2 g dietary fiber, 3.1 g protein

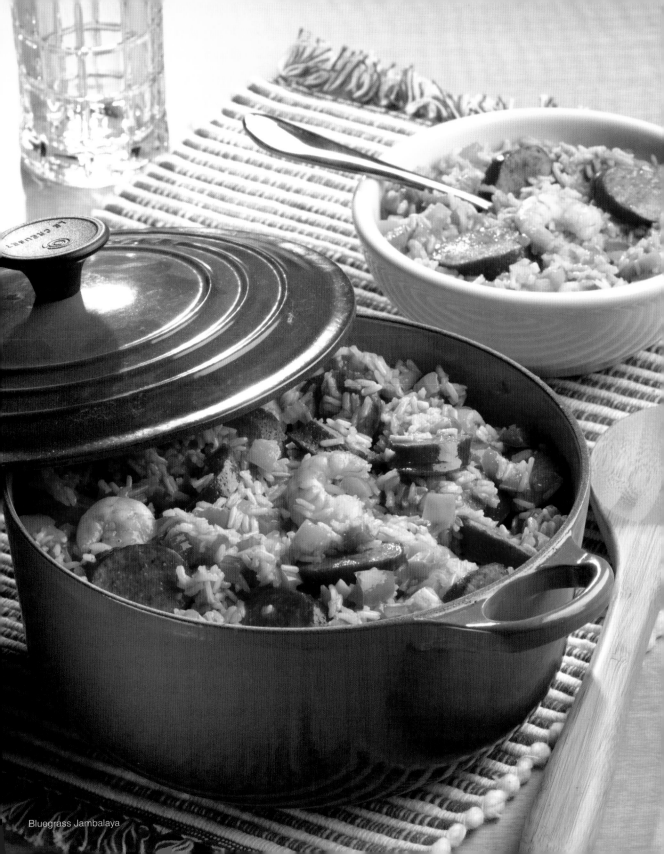

Bluegrass Jambalaya

Bluegrass Jambalaya

SLIM IT DOWN: Omit the rice and serve as a soup (180 calories).

No Cajun dish is more famous than the hearty stew called jambalaya. Chicken or shrimp, sometimes ham, always sausage, flavored with the "holy trinity" of Cajun cooking: celery, bell peppers, and onions. Rice cooks in the same pot to soak up every last bit of flavor.

Tasty as it is, traditional jambalaya is loaded with fat and can have a ½ teaspoon of salt in every cup! Most of the salt comes from the sausage. In this version, I've replaced it with lower-fat turkey sausage and swapped out the chicken thighs for lean shrimp. I added extra veggies, and kept the salt content as low as possible.

Sausage and cured meats should be seen as a condiment rather than the main source of protein in a dish. While a typical serving of meat is 3 ounces, that much sausage can have up to 800 milligrams of sodium, which is about 33 percent of your sodium limit for the day. I like to use small amounts of sausage and other fatty or salty meats to flavor a dish. Four ounces of sausage is enough to impart a smoky, rich flavor to this entire recipe.

Makes 4 Servings:
1 heaping cup per serving

1 Hour to Prepare and Cook

1 tbsp canola oil

1 cup finely diced onion

½ cup finely diced celery

2 cups finely diced bell peppers

2 cloves garlic, chopped

1 tsp ground cumin

¼ tsp cayenne pepper

2 tbsp no-salt-added tomato paste

4 ounces turkey sausage, cut into bite-sized pieces

3 cups homemade, low-sodium, or no-salt-added chicken stock

1 cup brown rice

8 ounces uncooked small (36/45 per pound) shrimp, peeled and deveined (about 1 cup)

4 green onions, sliced

1. Place a large saucepan over moderate heat and add the oil. Once hot, add the onions and celery, reduce the heat, and cook until the vegetables are softened, about 5 minutes. Add the peppers, garlic, cumin, and cayenne; and cook for 3 minutes more.

2. Add the tomato paste and sausage, and stir to combine. Slowly pour in the stock and bring the mixture to a boil. Stir in the rice, cover, and reduce the heat to low. Simmer, covered, for 40 minutes.

3. Remove the cover and add the shrimp. Cook until the shrimp is just cooked through and pink, about 5 minutes. Spoon into bowls, distributing the shrimp evenly, and garnish with the green onions. Serve warm.

Per Serving: 386 calories, 8.8 g total fat, 103.6 mg cholesterol, 371 mg sodium, 55.7 g total carbs, 7.1 g dietary fiber, 17.6 g protein

Chicken Creole

This dish is an easy introduction to the flavors of Creole cooking, which has its roots in the aristocratic society of New Orleans, and combines classic European cooking techniques with a range of flavor influences, especially African. Don't confuse Creole with Cajun cooking, which is based on the country-style cooking of Louisiana's Acadian settlers. Serve this with ½ cup brown rice.

Makes 4 Servings:
1 heaping cup per serving

45 Minutes to Prepare and Cook

1 tbsp canola oil

1 pound boneless, skinless chicken breasts, sliced into 1-ounce strips

½ green bell pepper, cored, seeded, and sliced into thin strips

1 red bell pepper, cored, seeded, and sliced into thin strips

1 small white or yellow onion, sliced into thin strips (½ cup)

2 small ribs celery, sliced on a diagonal (½ cup)

1 tbsp Creole Spice Blend (page 370)

1 can (14 ounces) low-sodium petite diced tomatoes, with juice

½ cup chili sauce

½ to ¾ cup homemade, low-sodium, or no-salt-added vegetable stock, or water, if needed

1. Place a deep sauté pan over moderate heat. Add the oil and, once hot, add the chicken. Sauté the chicken until no longer pink, about 5 minutes.

2. Add the peppers, onion, and celery. Stir to combine and continue to sauté for 3 to 4 minutes more. Sprinkle the spice blend over the mixture and sauté for 1 minute.

3. Reduce the heat to low and add the tomatoes and chili sauce; simmer for 15 additional minutes. If mixture seems too thick, thin out with vegetable stock or water.

Per Serving: 238.9 calories, 5.6 g total fat, 65.7 g cholesterol, 673.4 mg sodium, 19.5 g total carbs, 2.6 g dietary fiber, 27.8 g protein

Slow-Cooker Turkey Sausage and Bean Stew

SLIM IT DOWN: Use half the sausage (80 calories).

Beans and sausage is a match made in heaven. The velvety smooth beans really soak up all the flavor of the spicy sausage. This started as a member-submitted recipe with more than twice the calories and four times the sodium per serving. By switching to turkey sausage, we reduced the fat, and by cutting down on the amount of sausage, we were able to control the sodium. (See Bacon Is Back, page 322, for more ideas.) Serve this over brown rice for a complete meal.

This is a great slow-cooker recipe—it can be ready in as little as 4 hours or will hold for up to 8 hours if you're running late. If you're cooking for 4 hours, reduce the water to 1 cup. You have two options when it comes to seasoning this dish. If you're using a spicy sausage, use Taco Seasoning (page 371); if you use a sweet sausage, choose Italian Herb Seasoning (page 369).

Makes 4 Servings:
1½ cup per serving

20 Minutes to Prepare, 4 Hours to Cook

14 ounces Italian turkey sausage, cut into 1-inch slices

One 15.5-ounce can Great Northern beans, rinsed and drained (about 1½ cups)

1 medium onion, diced (1 cup)

1 cup baby carrots, cut into halves (about 20 carrots)

One 14.5-ounce can no-salt-added diced tomatoes

1 tbsp Taco Seasoning or Italian Herb Seasoning

1. Layer the sausage, beans, onions, carrots, tomatoes, and seasoning in a slow cooker. Add 1½ cups water. Cover, set on low, and cook for 4 to 8 hours.

2. Serve warm, with brown rice if desired.

Per Serving: 268.6 calories, 11.1 g total fat, 0 mg cholesterol, 236 mg sodium, 26.4 g total carbs, 6.7 g dietary fiber, 18.3 g protein

Slow-Cooker
White Bean Chicken Chili

Like clam chowder and wine, chili comes in red and white varieties. We use white beans and white meat, chicken in this case, instead of cheese and cream to achieve the white color. Mix it up and add corn, sweet potatoes, or black beans—and call it checkerboard chili. To save money and sodium, we used dried beans, but you could use canned beans that have been drained and rinsed.

· ·

Chef Meg's Tip: Did you forget to soak the beans before bed last night? No problem. You can still have this dish in the slow cooker before heading out the door. Give your dried beans a rinse, then place them in a saucepan. Add cold water to cover the beans by 3 inches, bring the water to a boil, turn off the heat, cover, and let stand for 1 hour. Drain the beans and proceed with your recipe as planned.

· ·

Makes 10 Servings:
1 heaping cup per serving

20 Minutes to Prepare, 8 Hours to Cook, plus overnight soaking

2 cups Great Northern beans, dried

1 pound boneless and skinless chicken breasts, cut into 1-inch cubes

1 tbsp ground cumin

1 tsp dark chili powder

2 cloves garlic, smashed

1 cup diced onions

1 cup diced carrots

1 cup low-sodium or no-salt-added canned diced tomatoes, drained

4 cups homemade, low-sodium, or no-salt-added chicken stock

2 tbsp chopped green chiles

1 tbsp chopped cilantro

1. Rinse the beans with cold water. Place in a large bowl, cover with water, and soak overnight in the refrigerator.

2. Preheat the oven to 375° F. Coat a roasting pan with nonstick cooking spray. In a mixing bowl, toss the chicken, cumin, chili powder, and garlic together, then place in the roasting pan. Roast for 10 minutes, stirring them halfway through.

3. Transfer the chicken to the slow cooker. Drain the beans, and add them to the slow cooker, along with the onions, carrots, tomatoes, and chicken stock. Cook on high for 4 hours or low for 8 hours.

4. Before serving, use an immersion blender or potato masher to puree about a quarter of the chili. This will thicken your chili and give it a creamy consistency. Add the chiles and cilantro before serving.

Per Serving: 143.3 calories, 1 g total fat, 26.3 mg cholesterol, 101.5 mg sodium, 16.8 g total carbs, 3.8 g dietary fiber, 15 g protein

Slow-Cooker Chicken Stew

The perfect meal for a cold winter's day, this recipe is from a SparkPeople member. Start it before work and dinner is ready when you walk in the door. It's simple and hearty, just what you'll crave. Change up the herbs and spices depending on your mood and your pantry. Feel free to swap chicken broth for the water.

Makes 8 Servings:
1 cup per serving

20 Minutes to Prepare, 8 Hours to Cook

2 pounds boneless, skinless chicken breasts, cubed

4 medium carrots, chopped (2 cups)

1 pound russet or Yukon gold potatoes, cubed (4 cups)

4 medium ribs celery, chopped (1 cup)

1 medium onion, chopped (1 cup)

8 ounces mushrooms, quartered

1 tsp garlic powder

1 tsp dried thyme

1 tsp dried oregano

1 tsp dried marjoram

1 tsp dried basil

1 tsp black pepper

1 bay leaf

1 tsp lemon juice

1. Place the chicken, carrots, potatoes, celery, and onion in the slow cooker. Scatter the mushrooms on top.

2. In a small bowl, mix together the garlic powder, thyme, oregano, marjoram, basil, and pepper. Sprinkle the seasonings over the chicken and vegetables, and add the bay leaf.

3. Add the lemon juice to 4 cups of water and pour it on top. Put the lid on the slow cooker. Cook on high for 4 hours, or on low for the day. Remove the bay leaf before serving.

Per Serving: 202.7 calories, 3.8 g total fat, 71.6 mg cholesterol, 124.3 mg sodium, 22.2 g total carbs, 4.2 g dietary fiber, 20.6 g protein

Chef Meg's Tip: Most slow-cooker dishes are based on dump-and-drop recipes. Open a can of this, drop in a pound of that, heat, and serve. You might also notice that your slow-cooker recipes have a duller flavor than you might expect—after all, it cooked all day. Many of our slow-cooker recipes require an extra step, which you might be tempted to skip if you're in a time crunch. Don't do it!

By roasting the chicken, spices, and garlic before putting them in the slow cooker, you're adding a layer of flavor. If you add dried spices to a liquid, you're not taking full advantage of their potential. They need a bit of dry heat to coax out their flavors. Ten extra minutes in the morning means a bit of browning on the chicken and garlic, and an extra kick from the spices. Trust me when I say this step is worth it.

MAIN DISHES WITH POULTRY, MEAT & FISH

When our boys were infants, I constantly worried about what "real foods" to feed them after they graduated from cereal. I read all the books, talked to their pediatrician, and took long walks at the zoo with them and my friend Theresa, who is a dietitian. All agreed: start with grains, add vegetables and fruits, and lastly meats. If it only stayed that easy! To this day I do try to arrange our meals around the same concept and encourage the boys to eat in that order. It works . . . sometimes.

We recently hosted 16 teenage boys and 10 adults for dinner on the fly. Each family brought a side dish; we provided salads and salmon, shrimp, and chicken. What a beautiful banquet table it was, filled with fresh fruit, salads of pesto and whole-wheat pasta, cherry tomatoes with avocados and a vinegar-based slaw. To stretch the meal and keep portions reasonable, salmon steaks were grilled then sliced into two-ounce servings, chicken breasts were grilled then sliced on an angle into one-inch strips, and the shrimp were divided into four per skewer. By doing this, the serving sizes were kept to two to three ounces and each person was able to have some variety.

Plates were filled high with vegetables and fruits and topped with few ounces of meat and everyone went home happy, with bellies that were satisfied—not stuffed. Meat was an equal partner in the meal—not the center of it.

PROTEIN PORTIONS

A little meat goes a long way, for a variety of reasons. According to the USDA, Americans' annual meat consumption per person has almost doubled in a generation—from 144 to 222 pounds. That's an increase from 6.3 ounces a day (between two and three servings) to 9.7 ounces a day (between four and five servings).

"Three ounces of meat is more than you think," says member DOWN2SEXY. On the rare occasions she and her husband dine out, she likes to order a 6-ounce filet. She eats half, takes half home, and says "since I'm eating more veggies, half a fillet is plenty for me."

Other families are taking the same approach.

BONDGIRL2010's beef-loving family—including her "Kansas-bred farm boy" husband—is gobbling up turkey these days. "Over time I have gone from cooking beef six days a week to maybe two or three times a month! Turkey products really helped me fool my family when I first started cutting us back. I didn't tell the family I was cutting back just in case they protested. They have so many different varieties (we had the turkey bratwurst yesterday) and they are all delicious!"

This Kentucky farm girl, like that Kansas farm boy, grew up eating plenty of beef. We butchered a cow every year. These days the boys have red meat once a week, and I have it once every two weeks. We eat plenty of chicken, but it's not my favorite. I prefer seafood, lean pork, and legumes.

Meat still appears on the dinner table at REVELATIONGIRL's (see her Success Story on page 63) house every night, but beef is appearing less often. Her husband and the rest of her family are on board, and they're all seeing results. The protein of choice is usually lean chicken cooked using a recipe from SparkRecipes.com. She's watching her portions, but her husband and son—who are always on the move and blessed with fast metabolisms—are still eating hearty portions but losing a bit of weight and feeling healthier.

GETFIT2LIVE eats "lots and lots of veggies and salads," then supplements with meat. "If it's a one-pot meal, it really takes very little meat to be satisfying," she says. Forty pounds down, she's "discovered new energy, enthusiasm, and strength within that I never knew were there" since joining SparkPeople.

Proteins are the star of the plate. If you go to a restaurant, you don't order mashed potatoes and asparagus with pork chops. When was the last time someone opened a broccoli house instead of a steakhouse? Meat, even when it's a lean cut, is full of flavor. It's the priciest item on that plate, too. So it's no wonder that that's what you order, that's the ingredient around which you base your meal. Plus, it's loaded with protein, which fills us up and sustains us.

According to Becky Hand, SparkPeople's dietitian extraordinaire, most of us meet and many actually exceed the amount of protein we need. Health organizations recommend limiting your protein intake to 10 to 35 percent of your total calorie needs, which for a 1,500-calorie meal plan is between 37.5 and 131 grams of protein. SparkPeople sets 20 percent as the baseline for protein consumption. Six ounces of meat has about 42 grams of protein, so you really don't need much, especially when you consider all the nonmeat sources of protein (see the next chapter for more on that topic).

You can eat meat every day, even a few times a day, as long as you're choosing the right ones. Our Nutritional Guidelines Chart (page 435) breaks meat down into three categories: choose often, limit, and avoid. The majority of the meats in this book are in the "choose often" category, meaning you can eat portion-controlled servings of them every day.

SparkPeople Cooking Challenge:
Swap a meat from the "limit" or "avoid" category with one from the "choose often" category. It can be as simple as choosing tuna packed in water instead of oil, turkey sausage instead of pork sausage, or lean sirloin instead of a prime cut of beef.

DECIPHERING A MEAT LABEL

When a meat label boasts that it's 95 percent fat-free, it sounds like a healthy choice since only 5 percent of it is fat. But fat contains a lot of calories (9 calories per gram), so check out the nutrition facts label for the actual number of calories and fat grams per serving.

Choose meat with the USDA labels Select (about 7 percent fat by weight) or Choice (15 to 35 percent fat by weight) rather than Prime (more than 35 percent fat by weight). What about the percentages you see on meat? A "lean" label means the meat contains fewer than 10 grams of total fat, 4.5 grams of saturated fat, and 95 milligrams of cholesterol in every 3.5 ounce (pre-cooked weight) serving. "Extra lean" means it has less than 5 grams of total fat, 2 grams of saturated fat, and 95 milligrams of cholesterol

in every serving. 93/7 beef is considered "lean"; extra-lean would be 95/5 beef or higher.

Switching even from extra-lean ground beef to lean turkey can have a significant impact on your meal.

3-Ounce Portion	Calories	Fat (g)
Ground beef	264	23
Lean ground beef	225	18
Extra-lean ground beef	199	15
Lean ground turkey	120	6
Extra-lean ground turkey	90	1

SparkPeople Cooking Challenge:
Swap your usual meat with one that's lower in fat at least once this week. Don't tell your family and see if they notice. If not, stick with it. If so, slowly make the switch, starting with ¾ of the higher-fat meat and ¼ of the leaner cut. Eventually, you'll become accustomed to the leaner meats.

Orange Chicken

When I first started thinking about this recipe, I envisioned a sauce made with honey and balsamic vinegar. Instead, I opted for rice-wine vinegar, which pairs well with oranges—and with this dish you get a serving of fruit in every portion. Dice the orange if you prefer smaller pieces and—if you're feeling creative—use a vegetable peeler to create curls of orange zest.

Makes 4 Servings:
   3–4 ounces of meat and
   ½ cup of fruit per serving

40 Minutes to Prepare and Cook

1 tbsp olive oil

1½ tsp dried thyme

½ tsp salt

¼ tsp white or black pepper

1 pound boneless, skinless chicken
   breasts

2 small to medium oranges

3 tbsp rice-wine vinegar

2 tbsp honey

1. In a glass dish, mix together the oil, thyme, salt, and pepper for a quick marinade.

2. Place the chicken flat on a cutting board, remove any fat, and slice each breast into quarters so that you have 1- to 1½-inch thick strips. Add the meat to the marinade and toss to coat. Cover and place in the fridge for at least 15 minutes. (You can also do this in the morning.)

3. Zest the orange by using a grater to remove just the orange part of the peel (not the white pith). Using a sharp knife, cut away the remaining peel and pith, then, holding the fruit over a bowl to catch the juice, cut sections from the orange, working in a V fashion to cut away any membrane. Reserve the fruit and juice for the sauce.

4. Preheat a nonstick skillet to moderate heat. Spray with nonstick cooking spray, then add the chicken once the pan is hot. Discard the marinade. Cook the chicken until firm and no longer pink, about 5 minutes.

5. While the meat is cooking, place the vinegar and honey in a small saucepan and bring to a boil. Lower the heat and simmer until the mixture is reduced by half. Add the orange, juice, and the zest to the sauce, stir, and remove from the heat. Divide the chicken onto 4 plates and pour the sauce over the meat.

Per Serving: 209.9 calories, 4.9 g total fat, 65.7 mg cholesterol, 364.9 mg sodium, 14.5 g total carbs, 1.3 g dietary fiber, 26.7 g protein

Make It a Meal:
Cook up whole-wheat couscous
and sautéed bell peppers
(330 calories) • Serve with brown
rice and broccoli (307 calories)

Slow-Cooker Marinara Chicken and Vegetables

We made over a versatile member recipe by adding extra vegetables and reducing the sodium. Serve with a side salad or over whole-wheat pasta or brown rice. Members say they love stuffing the leftovers into a baked potato or spooning them onto a piece of toasted whole-grain baguette as an appetizer. If you like your food a little spicy, add a dash of crushed red pepper or cayenne.

Makes 8 Servings:
1 heaping cup per serving

8 Minutes to Prepare, 6 Hours to Cook

2 pounds boneless, skinless chicken breasts

4 cloves garlic, peeled and crushed

4 tomatoes, chopped or one 14.5-ounce can low-sodium tomatoes, drained

4 medium ribs celery, diced (1 cup)

2 small zucchini, diced (2 cups)

1 bell pepper, cored, seeded, and diced

One 18-ounce jar low-sodium marinara sauce

1 tsp dried basil

1 tsp dried thyme

1. Place the chicken in the slow cooker; add the garlic, tomatoes, celery, zucchini, and pepper. Pour the marinara sauce over all, and sprinkle the basil and thyme on top.

2. Set the slow cooker on low and cook for 6 to 7 hours. Before serving, shred the chicken with a fork.

Per Serving: 164.2 calories, 2.1 g total fat, 65.7 mg cholesterol, 142.4 mg sodium, 7.9 g total carbs, 1.8 g dietary fiber, 27.3 g protein

> **Make It a Meal:**
> Pair with whole wheat spaghetti and steamed spinach (337 calories)
> • Serve over brown rice and roasted peppers (367 calories)

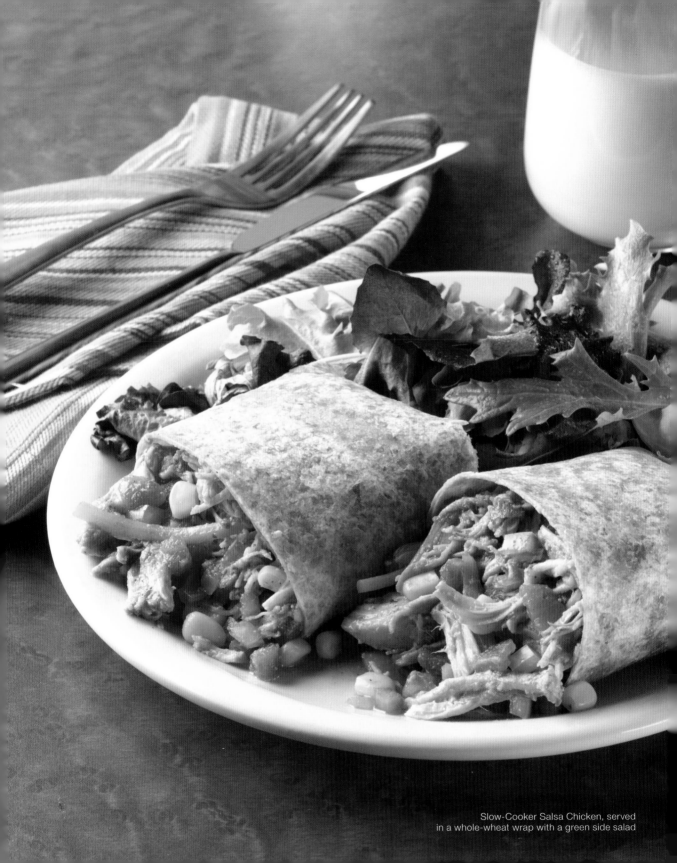

Slow-Cooker Salsa Chicken, served
in a whole-wheat wrap with a green side salad

Slow-Cooker Salsa Chicken

Birdie, one of our most successful members to-date, is a doctor and mother of five. (Chris introduced you to her at the beginning of the book.) Having lost 143 pounds on SparkPeople, she is always on the lookout for healthy recipe ideas, but they have to be quick and easy, like this one, which she found on SparkRecipes.com. "I'm not a good cook," she confesses, but this is one dish she serves regularly without worry. She's not the only member who's making this for dinner: the recipe has been rated more than 2,700 times! It's *the* most popular recipe on SparkRecipes. We've added more vegetables and reduced the sodium drastically to make it even better. Salsa Chicken is easy to make; just put all the ingredients in a slow cooker and let the machine do the work. To save even more time, chop your vegetables the night before, or use a 16-ounce bag of *mirepoix* (celery, carrot, and onion mix), found in your grocer's freezer. There are infinite variations, and your family is guaranteed to like each one.

Makes 8 Servings:
1 cup of chicken plus ½ cup brown rice

**15 Minutes to Prepare,
6 to 8 Hours to Cook**

2 pounds boneless, skinless chicken breasts

2 tbsp Taco Seasoning (page 371)

1 cup low-sodium petite diced canned tomatoes, with juice

1 medium onion, finely diced (1 cup)

½ cup finely diced celery

½ cup shredded carrots

1 cup salsa, homemade or purchased

3 tbsp reduced-fat sour cream

1. Place the chicken in a slow cooker (see Note). Sprinkle the Taco Seasoning over the meat then layer the vegetables and salsa on top. Pour ½ cup water over the mixture, set on low, and cook for 6 to 8 hours. The meat is cooked when it shreds or reaches an internal temperature of 165° F.

2. When ready to serve, shred the chicken with two forks, then stir in the sour cream.

Note: If you don't have a slow cooker, prepare a Dutch oven or heavy-bottomed saucepan with a generous coating of nonstick cooking spray, then place it over moderate heat to warm. Once warm, add the chicken and cook 4 to 5 minutes each side. Remove the chicken from the pan and set aside. Add the onion, celery, and carrots to the saucepan and cook, stirring constantly, for 2 minutes. Add the Taco Seasoning to the mixture, then stir to combine. Place the chicken over the vegetables, pour salsa and the entire can of tomatoes over the chicken, reduce heat to medium-low, cover, and cook for 45 minutes. Cool slightly, then shred the meat. Add the sour cream and stir to combine.

Per Serving: 164.9 calories, 2.5 g total fat, 67.9 mg cholesterol, 253.3 mg sodium, 7.3 g total carbs, 2.1 g dietary fiber, 27.6 g protein

Make It a Meal:
Dish it up with a whole-wheat tortilla and mixed greens (305 calories) • Serve with brown rice, low-fat Cheddar cheese, and bell peppers (335 calories)

Tasty Tips

Slow-Cooker Salsa Chicken really is an easy recipe and can be changed up in plenty of ways.

- If you like more spice or heat, add a few dashes of hot sauce or red pepper flakes.

- Garnish with chopped fresh cilantro.

- You can use fresh or jarred salsa in this recipe, but try to choose a low-sodium variety.

- If you're really trying to reduce the salt in this recipe, make your own salsa using fresh onions, tomatoes, and peppers.

- Stretch the recipe by adding a can of drained and rinsed black beans or pinto beans to the slow cooker an hour before serving.

Here are just a few of the ways SparkPeople members have made this dish their own.

- "I shredded the chicken after I removed it from the slow cooker and served it as a burrito with a low-carb, whole-wheat tortilla filled with the chicken, sauce, brown rice, and fresh veggies!" — 1EVILANGEL

- "I used jarred salsa and it was fantastic! I used chicken breast tenders and served over brown rice. Even my picky boyfriend loved it!" — BLUESTARMOM

- "I cooked this on the stovetop with homemade taco seasoning and then added fat-free plain yogurt. It was amazing!" — KIKILEBEAU

- "I did add a can of corn and some peppers for added nutrition." — ELPHABA12

- "Eat this while watching the game. We used baked nachos for scooping instead of rice." — BILLALEX70

- "Didn't add the sour cream to the cooker. Placed a spoonful on top of chicken breast just before eating." — LSMOTHERS

Slow-Cooker Rosemary Chicken Breasts

Looking for an easy dinner for entertaining? This dish, from a SparkPeople member, features sophisticated flavors, and tender and delicious chicken courtesy of the slow cooker. Chicken and rosemary is a classic combination; serve this with brown rice and a salad, and you're ready for guests anytime.

This dish is easily adapted. Swap tarragon or Italian seasoning mix for the rosemary, swap broth for the wine, and add any vegetables you have in the fridge. For more flavor, use low-sodium broth instead of water.

Makes 4 Servings:
1 piece of chicken per serving

10 Minutes to Prepare,
3 to 6 Hours to Cook

4 boneless, skinless chicken breast halves

1½ tsp balsamic vinegar

1 tsp granulated garlic, or garlic powder

1 tbsp lemon juice

¼ tsp salt

⅛ tsp black pepper

½ cup dry white wine

½ tsp dried rosemary

1 tomato, diced (½ cup)

1. Place the chicken in the slow cooker in a single layer.

2. In a small bowl or glass measuring cup, mix together the vinegar, garlic, lemon juice, salt, pepper, and wine. Pour the mixture over the chicken.

3. Cover. Cook on low for 6 hours or high for 3 hours. A half hour before the chicken is done, sprinkle the rosemary over the chicken and stir in the tomato. Shred the chicken before serving.

Per Serving: 164.4 calories, 1.6 g total fat, 68.4 mg cholesterol, 226.9 mg sodium, 3.5 g total carbs, 0.6 g dietary fiber, 27.8 g protein

Make It a Meal:
Cook up bulgur and sautéed carrots (295 calories) • Serve with roasted potatoes and steamed broccoli (265 calories)

Lemon Herb-Roasted Chicken

Placing roasted chickens near the checkout is a smooth move by supermarkets. That smell is irresistible, and the meat has infinite uses. Picking up a precooked chicken is much better than driving through a fast-food restaurant after work, but you're still throwing money away—and supermarket rotisserie chicken is loaded with sodium. Buying a whole chicken and cooking it yourself is affordable and manageable, even for a novice cook.

Makes 4 Servings:
3 ounces of mixed white and dark meat per serving (see Note)

**5 Minutes to Prepare,
90 Minutes to Cook**

1 lemon, zested and cut in half

2 tsp olive oil

1 tsp thyme

1 tsp black pepper

1 bay leaf

4½- to 5-pound whole chicken

1. Preheat the oven to 425° F. Combine the lemon zest, oil, thyme, and pepper in a small bowl.

2. Pat the chicken dry and rub the herbed oil over the breasts and under the skin (gently break the membrane under the skin with your hands to coat the breast meat), so the bird will self-baste. Place both lemon halves and the bay leaf into the chicken cavity.

3. Place the chicken in a roasting pan on a roasting rack or on bed of vegetables (1 roughly chopped carrot and 1 chopped onion). Tie the legs together with kitchen string.

4. Roast the chicken for 20 minutes at 425° F, then reduce the oven temperature to 375° F. Continue to roast the chicken until a meat thermometer inserted into the thickest part of the inner thigh registers 180° F; about 1 hour, 10 minutes more.

5. Remove the pan from the oven; lift the chicken and tilt slightly so the juices from the cavity run into the pan. The juices should be clear. If the juice is still pink, return the chicken to the oven and cook until done.

6. Transfer the chicken to a cutting board. Cover the chicken with aluminum foil to keep warm. Allow it to rest for 15 minutes before removing the skin and carving. If you roasted the chicken on a bed of vegetables, discard them.

Note: Serving sizes will vary. A 4.8-pound chicken will yield approximately 16 ounces of white meat and 6 ounces of dark. Feel free to calculate using the amount and type of chicken you eat. You will save about 125 calories and 11 grams of fat per serving by removing the skin before serving.

Per Serving: 156.9 calories, 4.5 g total fat, 76.9 mg cholesterol, 84.5 mg sodium, .5 g total carbs, .2 g dietary fiber, 26.9 g protein

> **Make It a Meal:**
> Put it in a whole-wheat pita with cucumbers, tomatoes, and Honey-Mustard Dressing (page 382) (389 calories) • Add a baked potato with butter, and green beans with lemon (367 calories)

- Always truss, or tie up, the legs of the chicken to promote even cooking. Trussing is like a push-up bra for birds—it plumps up the breasts.

- Chicken is one meat you never want to undercook. When fully cooked, the juices should run clear, the joints should be loose, and the flesh firm. Look for an internal temperature of 180° F in the inner thigh of the chicken.

- Use a roasting rack or a bed of vegetables to allow the fat and juices to drain from the chicken while cooking.

Chew on This: A Chicken in Every Roasting Pan

Roasted chicken is not just a special-occasion meal, it's one of the most versatile foods you can make. Save time and energy by roasting two chickens at once. Carve the second chicken, let cool, and then freeze the meat and bones separately.

Instead of buying expensive deli meats, which can be full of sodium and fillers, use homemade roasted chicken. Use the meat in soups, throw it on pasta, or pair it with a simple salad. Use the bones to make homemade, low-sodium chicken stock (page 148).

Parmesan Chicken with Tomato-Basil Salad

While Chicken Parmesan is traditionally fried and served with a heavy topping of mozzarella cheese, this lighter version is delightful atop a hearty green salad. I've substituted a lighter coating of Parmesan cheese, and a variation on *fines herbes,* a traditional French herb blend, adding flavor to the dish with no fat. Look for this mixture in the spice aisle or mix your own—or try combining ⅓ teaspoon each of any 3 of these dried herbs: parsley, chives, basil, and tarragon.

Makes 4 Servings:
 3–4 ounces chicken with 1 cup mixed greens and ¼ cup tomato mixture per serving

25 Minutes to Prepare and Cook

1 pound boneless, skinless chicken breasts (2 breasts)

¼ cup all-purpose flour

2 egg whites, beaten

6 tbsp grated Parmesan cheese

1 tsp *fines herbes,* dried (mixture of dried chives, parsley, basil, and tarragon)

3 plum (Roma) tomatoes, seeded and chopped

2 tsp shredded fresh basil leaves

1 lemon, juiced

Dash of black pepper

2 tbsp extra-virgin olive oil

4 cups mixed baby salad greens (mesclun mix)

1. Trim any visible fat from the chicken breasts and slice them into four 4-ounce servings. Place the chicken between two sheets of wax paper or plastic wrap. Pound with the bottom of a pan or rolling pin until the meat is ¼- to ½-inch thick.

2. Prepare three pie plates or flat-bottomed bowls and place the flour, egg whites, and Parmesan in each respectively. Toss the dried herbs in with the cheese. Working with one piece of chicken at a time, dip the meat into the flour, then the egg white, and finally the cheese. Shake off any excess egg white before coating with the cheese. It is best to use one hand for the dry coatings and one for the wet to avoid clumping the batter.

3. Spray a nonstick skillet with nonstick cooking spray and place over moderate heat. Sauté the chicken until cooked through, 5 to 6 minutes per side.

4. While the chicken is cooking, combine the tomato and basil in a small bowl. In a separate bowl, combine the lemon juice and pepper. Slowly whisk in the oil, then pour the mixture over the tomatoes.

5. To serve, toss the greens with the tomato and dressing and divide among four plates. Top with the chicken.

Per Serving: 340.5 calories, 14.0 g total fat, 82.5 mg cholesterol, 507.3 mg sodium, 13 g total carbs, 2.7 g dietary fiber, 39.4 g protein

Make It a Meal:
Add on whole-wheat breadstick and roasted garlic (420 calories) • Enjoy with whole-grain bread and margarine (450 calories).

Green Chicken Curry

Like a stoplight, curry has three colors: red, yellow, and green. Yellow curries are usually associated with Indian cooking, while green and red often hail from Southeast Asia. This is a mild green curry that's full of Thai influences. It's a curry that's great for beginners. You can add any vegetables you'd like: eggplant, broccoli, cauliflower, carrots, onions, and spinach are all good in curries. This goes great with Baked Lemon-Spiced Rice (page 288).

If you chop your vegetables the night before, this dinner can be on the table in about 20 minutes.

Makes 4 Servings:
   1¼ cup per serving

45 Minutes to Prepare and Cook

½ cup cilantro leaves

1 lime, juiced

2 tbsp sweetened flaked coconut

1 pound boneless, skinless chicken
   breasts, cut into ½-inch cubes

1 large or 2 small shallots, minced (¼ cup)

1 cup chopped red bell pepper

1 cup chopped yellow bell pepper

1 tbsp green curry paste

¼ tsp salt

½ cup light coconut milk

2 cups frozen peas

1. Place the cilantro, lime juice, and coconut in a blender or small food processor and puree. Add one or two tablespoons of water as needed: The mixture should be saucelike in consistency, not thick like pesto. Set aside.

2. Heat a large sauté pan over moderate to high heat and coat with nonstick cooking spray. Add the chicken to pan and sauté for 3 to 4 minutes. Add the shallots and peppers and cook for 2 minutes more. Add the curry paste, salt, coconut milk, and peas; stir to combine and simmer for 2 minutes. Add the cilantro mixture and simmer until heated through, about 3 minutes.

3. Serve 1¼ cup of the chicken mixture over ½ cup of rice.

Per Serving: 248.6 calories, 5.1 g total fat, 65.7 mg cholesterol, 400.8 mg sodium, 19.9 g total carbs, 4.5 g dietary fiber, 31.4 g protein

Make It a Meal:
Serve atop whole-wheat couscous
with pineapple (399 calories) •
Eat with whole-wheat pasta and
a side of mango (389 calories).

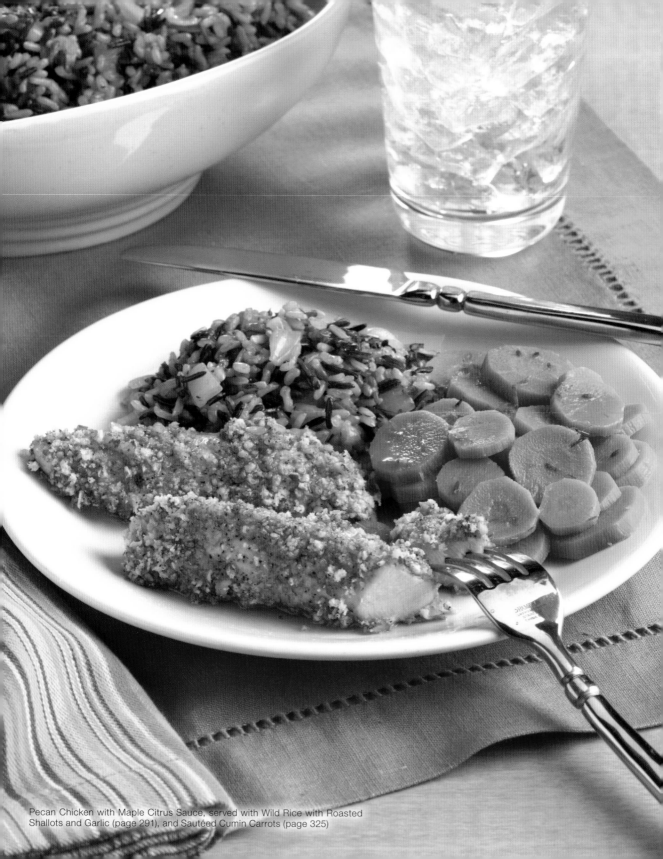

Pecan Chicken with Maple Citrus Sauce, served with Wild Rice with Roasted
Shallots and Garlic (page 291), and Sautéed Cumin Carrots (page 325)

Pecan Chicken with Maple Citrus Sauce

SLIM IT DOWN: Pass on the pecans (50 calories).

Consider this a riff on that Southern favorite, chicken and waffles—only our chicken is baked and we ditched the waffles. We use decidedly Southern pecans and real maple syrup to evoke that "breakfast for dinner" feeling.

This is a makeover of a member's recipe. The original used sugar-free artificial pancake syrup, which we swapped for real maple syrup. We also use panko (Japanese breadcrumbs) to give the chicken a crispier crunch. It's better than fried chicken!

Since this dish doesn't contain any fruits or vegetables, be sure to serve it as part of a balanced meal. Add a cup of skim milk, a serving of steamed or roasted broccoli, and a side of fruit. Or, if you really miss the waffles, serve it along with a whole-grain version.

Makes 4 Servings:
3–4 ounces of meat with 1½ tbsp of sauce per serving

45 Minutes to Prepare and Cook

¼ cup pecans, halved or pieces

¼ cup panko (Japanese breadcrumbs)

½ tsp black pepper

¼ cup pure maple syrup

1 pound boneless, skinless chicken breasts

½ lemon, juiced

½ cup orange juice

1 tsp finely chopped parsley

1. Preheat the oven to 350° F. Spray a baking dish with nonstick cooking spray.

2. Chop the pecans by hand or in a food processor until they are the same size as the breadcrumbs; set aside 2 tablespoons for use in the sauce. Combine the chopped pecans with the breadcrumbs and the pepper; place in a flat-bottomed bowl.

3. Pour 2 tablespoons of the maple syrup into a plastic bag or onto a dish. Trim any fat from the chicken, and cut each breast into three slices.

4. Dip the chicken in the syrup, then coat in the nut mixture. Place the chicken in the prepared baking dish and bake until the meat is no longer pink, about 30 minutes.

5. About 10 minutes before the chicken is done, start preparing the sauce. Pour the remaining 2 tablespoons syrup, and the lemon and orange juice into a small saucepan. Bring the mixture to a simmer and cook until reduced by half. Just before serving add in the reserved 2 table-spoons chopped pecans and the parsley. Pour the sauce over the meat or serve it on the side.

Per Serving: 283 calories, 9.6 g total fat, 65.8 mg cholesterol, 84.2 mg sodium, 22 g total carbs, 1.4 g dietary fiber, 27.9 g protein.

Make It a Meal:
Pair with roasted sweet potatoes with steamed broccoli and bell peppers (445 calories) • Eat with a whole-grain toaster waffle and add a side of sautéed collard greens (393 calories).

Cornish Hens with Apple-Pecan Stuffing

Cornish hens are very young chickens that usually weigh between one and two pounds each; their meat is very tender and delicate in flavor. This is an easy recipe to make for company—and Cornish hens are a great option for a small holiday meal as well. They make for an impressive display—and allow each diner to have a bit of light and dark meat.

While most people think of bread when they think of stuffing, this recipe instead uses fruits and vegetables for a light, fiber-rich filling. You can use prunes or raisins instead of dried cherries in the fruit butter.

> **Chef Meg's Tip:** This type of poultry is the only variety that I will stuff. Stuffing large birds is dangerous. With a large bird that might take 3 or 4 hours to roast, the stuffing inhibits the flow of air within the bird, which can yield a bacteria breeding ground and gummy stuffing. You'll notice that I didn't use a bread-based stuffing, which would take longer to cook, and the stuffing is loosely packed, which will allow more air flow and a safely cooked bird.

Makes 4 servings:
 ½ Cornish hen and ½ cup stuffing

1 Hour, 15 Minutes to Prepare and Cook

For the Stuffing:

1 tsp canola oil

½ cup chopped celery

1 leek, white and pale green parts
 only, chopped

1 Granny Smith apple, cored,
 and chopped

½ tsp fennel seeds

¼ tsp black pepper

¼ tsp salt

1 tbsp apple-cider vinegar

1 tbsp chopped pecans or walnuts

For the Fruit Butter:

2 tbsp chopped dried cherries

1 tbsp unsalted butter, softened

2 Cornish hens, about 1½ pounds each,
 thawed and patted dry

1. Preheat oven to 400° F.

2. Make the stuffing. Heat the oil in a sauté pan over moderate heat, then add the celery and leeks and cook until tender, about 5 minutes. Add the apple, fennel seeds, pepper, and salt. Cook for another 2 minutes, then pour in the vinegar. Add the nuts, stir well, and remove from heat to cool.

3. Make the fruit butter. Place the cherries and butter in a small bowl and use a wooden spoon to blend them into a paste.

4. If the Cornish hens have a package of giblets in the cavity, remove them and discard. Place the hens in a roasting pan and divide the stuffing into the cavity of each bird. Rub the fruit butter above the breast area and underneath the skin of each bird. Tie the legs together using two 12-inch long pieces of kitchen string. (See Perfect Poultry for more information on cooking whole birds, page 185.)

5. Roast, breast side up, for 50 minutes, then check the internal temperature at the point where the leg meets the thigh. The temperature should be at least 180° F. Remove the hens from the oven and allow to rest for 5 minutes.

6. Cut each bird in half down the center of the breast bone with kitchen shears or a sharp knife.

Per Serving: 252.8 calories, 10 g total fat, 116.5 mg cholesterol, 241.4 mg sodium, 15.9 g total carbs, 2.7 g dietary fiber, 25 g protein

Make It a Meal:
Serve with brown rice with sautéed mushrooms and green beans (392 calories) • Enjoy with whole-wheat bread with mixed vegetables and roasted garlic (390 calories)

Chew on This: Dark Meat vs. Light Meat

One 3-ounce serving of light or white meat typically contains 140 calories and 3 grams of fat. Dark meat is more caloric (160 calories and 7 grams of fat) but it also contains twice as much iron—about 15 percent of your daily recommended intake.

Buffalo Chicken

Buffalo wings and game day are an inseparable pair. I hate to rain on your parade, but have you ever checked out the nutrition info on those wings? For just three wings, they have 10 grams of fat and 650 milligrams of sodium. Wing sauce, which is pretty much equal parts fat and hot sauce, has an addictive taste and texture, but all that salt and fat will leave you feeling awful.

I set out to keep the spicy, tangy flavor while cutting the fat and salt. I added mustard and vinegar to the sauce and used leftover white-meat chicken (you could use the Lemon Herb-Roasted Chicken from page 184 or plain grilled chicken).

Of course, no one eats wings without blue-cheese dressing. I made a quick sauce from nonfat Greek yogurt and blue cheese. Tangy and cool, it's a perfect companion to the spicy chicken. Don't forget the celery sticks!

Makes 4 Servings:
3 ounces chicken with about 2 tsp of sauce per serving

15 Minutes to Prepare and Cook

For the Buffalo Sauce:

3 tbsp hot sauce

2 tbsp apple-cider vinegar

1 tbsp mustard

1 tbsp honey

12 ounces skinless cooked chicken, diced into 1-inch cubes

For the Dipping Sauce:

2 tbsp nonfat Greek yogurt

1 tbsp crumbled blue cheese

1. Make the Buffalo Sauce. In a small saucepan, stir together the hot sauce, vinegar, mustard, and honey. Heat over moderate-low heat until warmed.

2. Add the cooked chicken to the sauce and toss to coat. Heat until the chicken is warmed through.

3. Prepare the Dipping Sauce. While the chicken is warming, stir the yogurt and blue cheese together in a small bowl.

Per Serving: 169.6 calories, 4 g total fat, 65.3 mg cholesterol, 96.9 mg sodium, 5.8 g total carbs, 0 g dietary fiber, 24.1 g protein

> **Make It a Meal:**
> Place in a whole-wheat wrap with chopped tomatoes and lettuce (321 calories) • Serve atop baked tortilla chips with chopped celery and tomatoes (299 calories)

Paprika Chicken

Like Better-for-You Beef Stroganoff (page 214), Paprika Chicken is a classic comfort food. Whether you call it Chicken Paprikash, Goulash, or Paprika Chicken, it's a hearty and flavorful dish that evokes the feeling of home—perfect for a winter's night. Marinate the chicken in the morning or the night before, and dinner will be ready in less than a half hour.

Traditionally, the dish is served with spaetzle or egg noodles. I prefer it with Baked Lemon-Spiced Rice (page 288) or plain brown rice, and sliced cucumbers with our Tomato-Basil Vinaigrette (page 387). Caramelized Onions (page 310) work well on the side, too.

Makes 4 Servings:
3–4 ounces cooked chicken per serving

45 Minutes to Prepare and Cook

For the Spice Marinade:

1 tbsp sweet or hot paprika

¼ tsp salt

¼ tsp black pepper

1 tsp chili powder

1 tsp onion powder

1 lemon, zested and juiced

½ cup low-fat plain yogurt

1 pound boneless and skinless chicken breasts

1. In a small mixing bowl, stir together the paprika, salt, pepper, chili powder, onion powder, lemon zest, juice, and yogurt.

2. Trim any remaining fat from the chicken, add it to the bowl, and completely cover with the marinade. Cover the bowl, refrigerate, and marinate for 30 minutes or up to 8 hours.

3. Preheat the oven to 350° F. Prepare a baking dish with nonstick cooking spray.

4. Remove the chicken from the marinade and place in the prepared baking dish. Bake for 20 minutes, or until the internal temperature reaches 165° F.

Per Serving: 154 calories, 2.2 g total fat, 67.7 mg cholesterol, 248.3 mg sodium, 4.2 g total carbs, 0.9 g dietary fiber, 28.2 g protein

Make It a Meal:
Pour over whole-wheat pasta and serve with peas and carrots (395 calories) • Enjoy with whole-wheat couscous and roasted tomatoes (294 calories).

Baked Chicken Tenders

 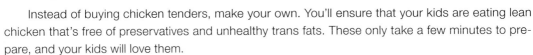

Instead of buying chicken tenders, make your own. You'll ensure that your kids are eating lean chicken that's free of preservatives and unhealthy trans fats. These only take a few minutes to prepare, and your kids will love them.

By combining the milk and vinegar, you're creating a buttermilk-like mixture that will tenderize and flavor the chicken. (If you have low-fat buttermilk on hand, you can use that instead.) There are two tricks to getting a crusty coating. First, use panko (Japanese breadcrumbs), which will crisp up great and brown well in the oven. (You can use regular breadcrumbs if that's all you have.) Second, bake the tenders on a rack—I used a pizza screen. Make sure the rack you choose is ovenproof and does not have any type of plastic coating.

Makes 4 Servings:
3 chicken tenders per serving

30 Minutes to Prepare and Cook

½ cup skim milk

1½ tsp white vinegar

1 pound chicken tenders, or boneless skinless chicken breasts, each cut into 4 strips

1½ cups panko (Japanese breadcrumbs)

¼ cup shredded Parmesan cheese

1 tbsp dried basil, thyme, or oregano

1. Preheat oven to 400° F. Combine the milk and vinegar in a small mixing bowl. Stir to combine and let rest on the counter for 5 minutes. Add the chicken tenders to the milk mixture and soak for 5 minutes.

2. While the chicken is soaking, combine the panko, cheese, and herbs in a shallow baking dish. Place a pizza screen or an ovenproof cooling rack on top of a sheet pan.

3. Using one hand, remove the meat from the milk mixture, shake off any excess liquid, and place into the breadcrumb mixture. With a dry hand, pat into the breadcrumbs to coat and then place on the wire rack. Bake for 20 minutes, until outside is crispy and inside is no longer pink.

Per Serving: 159.2 calories, 2.9 g total fat, 69.9 mg cholesterol, 174.8 mg sodium, 2.5 g total carbs, 0.5 g dietary fiber, 29.3 g protein

> **Make It a Meal:**
> Add on roasted potatoes, carrot sticks, and Spicy Yogurt Sauce (page 380) (351 calories) • Serve on a whole-wheat bun with mustard, lettuce, tomato, and pickles, alongside cucumbers with hummus (363 calories)

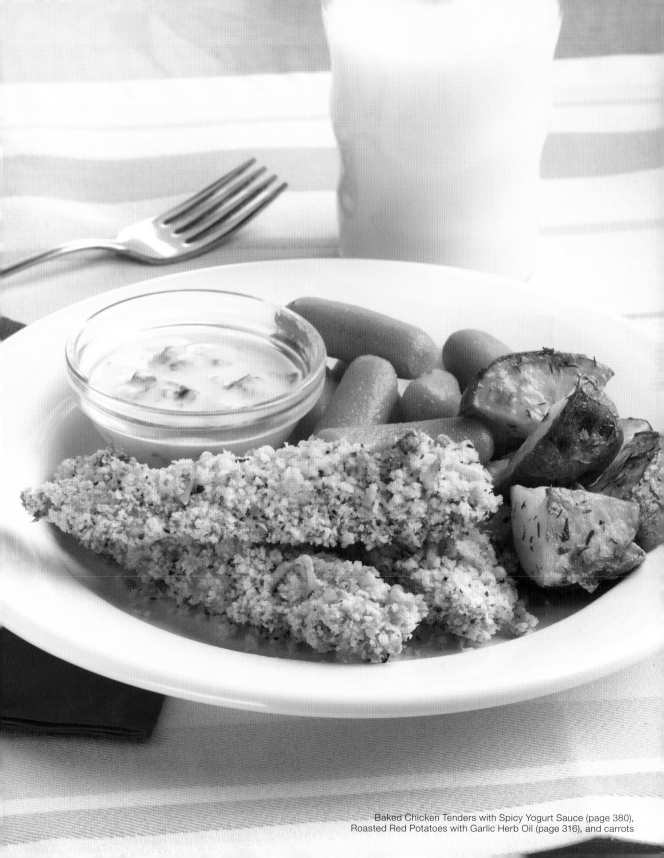

Baked Chicken Tenders with Spicy Yogurt Sauce (page 380),
Roasted Red Potatoes with Garlic Herb Oil (page 316), and carrots

Spinach-Stuffed Chicken with Cheese Sauce

We made over this great, member-submitted recipe by replacing a mayonnaise-based sauce with an easy cheese sauce; it reduced the fat and cut the amount of salt in half.

We use fresh instead of frozen spinach, although the recipe works just fine with one cup of frozen; just be sure to thaw it and squeeze it dry before sautéing. Serve the chicken with brown rice and a side salad.

Makes 4 Servings:
1 stuffed chicken breast with ¼ cup sauce per serving

1 Hour to Prepare and Cook

For the Cheese Sauce:

2 tbsp butter

2 tbsp all-purpose flour

1½ cups skim milk

¼ tsp grated nutmeg

½ cup shredded low-fat Swiss cheese

Four 4-ounce boneless, skinless chicken breasts

4 cups fresh spinach

¼ cup lemon juice

½ tsp white or black pepper

2 tbsp shredded Parmesan cheese

1. Preheat oven to 350° F.

2. Make the Sauce. Place the butter in a small saucepan over moderate heat and heat until melted. Add the flour and stir to combine. Cook the mixture for 2 minutes, stirring constantly with a wooden spoon. Do not let it brown. Gradually pour in the cold milk and whisk to combine. Simmer for 20 minutes, stirring occasionally.

3. While the sauce is cooking, pat the chicken breasts dry with a paper towel. Cut a horizontal slit into the side of each chicken breast to create a pocket.

4. Coat a large ovenproof sauté pan with non-stick cooking spray and place over moderate heat. Add the spinach to the pan and sauté until wilted. Season spinach with the lemon juice and pepper. Remove the spinach from the sauté pan, place in a bowl. Add the Parmesan to the spinach and mix to combine.

5. Generously coat the sauté pan with nonstick cooking spray again. Place a quarter of the spinach filling into the pocket of each chicken breast, folding over the chicken so the filling is completely inside. Place the chicken in the sauté pan and sear the meat on both sides until nicely browned, 3 to 4 minutes.

6. Place the sauté pan in the preheated oven, and bake until the internal temperature reaches 165° F, about 25 minutes.

7. Finish the sauce by adding the nutmeg and Swiss cheese; heat until cheese has melted. Remove chicken from the oven and serve each piece with ¼ cup of cheese sauce.

Per Serving: 288.8 calories, 11.3 g total fat, 95.2 mg cholesterol, 212.3 mg sodium, 10.6 g total carbs, 1.7 g dietary fiber, 34.9 g protein

Make It a Meal:
Serve over whole-wheat pasta with grilled zucchini and eggplant (424 calories) • Enjoy with whole-wheat couscous with roasted tomatoes and peppers (449 calories)

Chicken Breasts with Red-Wine Sauce

This is a lighter take on the classic Italian preparation of Chicken Cacciatore (or Chicken Hunter Style). Our made-over version uses white meat rather than dark and less oil to cut almost 60 calories per serving and reduce the fat and sodium of the traditional recipe. Mushrooms cut in quarters bulk up the recipe and increase the serving size.

Makes 4 servings:
    3–4 ounces of chicken and
    1 cup vegetables per serving

1 Hour to Prepare and Cook

1 pound boneless, skinless chicken breasts

½ tsp black pepper

2 tbsp canola oil

1 yellow or white onion, sliced

1 cup mushrooms cut into quarters

1 clove garlic, minced

½ cup (4 ounces) red wine (see Note)

One 14.5-ounce can stewed tomatoes, with liquid

1 tbsp Worcestershire sauce

2 tsp chili powder

1 tsp thyme

2 tsp Dijon mustard

1 tbsp chopped fresh parsley

12 pearl onions, peeled and halved (optional, see Note)

1. Slice the chicken breasts in half and pat dry with a clean cotton cloth or paper towel. Season with pepper.

2. Place the oil in a medium saucepan with a heavy bottom and a lid; once the oil is hot, add the chicken. Lightly brown the chicken on all sides, remove from the pan, and set aside.

3. Add the onions, mushrooms, and garlic to the hot pan. Cook, stirring occasionally, until the onions turn light brown, 4 to 5 minutes.

4. Add the wine; stir to combine with the vegetables and scrape the bottom of the pan to loosen the browned bits. Simmer until the wine reduces by half in volume, 3 to 4 minutes. Stir in the tomatoes, Worcestershire, chili powder, thyme, and mustard;, then return the chicken to the pan. Bring to a simmer and then reduce heat to low. Cover with a lid and simmer for 35 to 40 minutes. Garnish with the chopped parsley and pearl onions (if desired) before serving.

Note: In choosing a wine for cooking, always use one that's good enough to drink. Never buy "cooking wine," which is full of additives and sodium. Keep a four-pack of small wine bottles on hand for cooking.

Halved pearl onions is a classic garnish for this dish. To serve them, peel and lightly brown them in a small sauté pan just before the chicken is done cooking. Add to the dish just before serving.

Per Serving: 179.7 calories, 6.4 g total fat, 49.3 mg cholesterol, 214 mg sodium, 5.8 g total carbs, 1.1 g dietary fiber, 20.8 g protein

Make It a Meal:
Serve over whole-wheat penne, and add on spinach with vinaigrette (345 calories) • Enjoy with a Multigrain Roll (page 302), and cucumbers with dill and Greek yogurt (337 calories).

Herb-Roasted Turkey

For perfect results try using a V-rack in your roasting pan. This rack lifts your bird and allows it to roast rather than braise in its own juices. If you do not have a V-rack, you can create a similar platform for the bird by placing roughly chopped carrots, celery, and onions (about ½ cup each), under the turkey.

The flavorful herb rub makes basting the bird with additional fat unnecessary. If you want to reduce the sodium amount, look for a fresh turkey rather than a frozen one.

Makes 15 Servings: 3–4 ounces of mixed light and dark meat without skin per serving

10 Minutes to Prepare, 4 Hours to Cook

One 12-pound turkey

1 orange

2 tbsp olive oil

1 tbsp dried rosemary

1 tsp dried thyme

1 tsp dried sage

½ tsp black pepper

1. Preheat the oven to 400° F. Remove the giblets and neck if they are encased within the turkey, then rinse out the cavity and pat the turkey dry. Slice the orange in half and stuff it inside the bird.

2. In a small bowl, combine the oil with the rosemary, thyme, sage, and pepper. Rub the seasoning mixture under the skin and on top of the breast of the turkey. Rub any remaining seasonings over the entire turkey. If the legs are not secured with a wire, tie them together with kitchen string. Place the turkey on a V-rack in a roasting pan, tucking the wings under the bird.

3. Roast the turkey at 400° F for 30 minutes; reduce the oven temperature to 325° F and continue cooking the turkey until an internal temperature of 165° F is reached for the breast or 180° F for the leg. Also look for other indications of doneness: loose joints and juices running clear. If turkey begins to turn dark brown before the internal temperature is met, cover the breast with foil and continue to roast until done.

Per Serving: 154.6 calories, 3.1 g total fat, 63.8 mg cholesterol, 57.4 mg sodium, 8.4 g total carbs, 0.4 g dietary fiber, 28.8 g protein

> **Make It a Meal:**
> Serve on a baguette with tomatoes, cucumbers, and Dijon mustard (307 calories) • Enjoy with roasted potatoes and Brussels sprouts (325 calories).

Slow-Cooker Pulled Tom

What's pulled tom, you ask? Well, it's a lighter version of pulled pork. We use turkey and a slow cooker to achieve that same finger-licking, fork-tender meat, but with a whole lot less fat. Three ounces of pulled pork has 13.5 grams of fat, and when was the last time you were served only three ounces of meat at a barbecue restaurant?

Our version has less than a gram of fat per serving. Made with a Low-Sodium Barbecue Rub (page 374) it's perfect topped with Sweet and Spicy Barbecue Sauce (page 383). This would be a great dish to make for a nontraditional Thanksgiving meal or a potluck.

This recipe makes enough for two meals. For the second go-around, use the turkey to top off a salad, or eat it with some low-fat Cheddar as a midday snack. Serve with whole-wheat pita, Bibb lettuce, and extra cranberry sauce for a great sandwich.

Makes 14 Servings:
½ cup per serving

15 Minutes to Prepare; 7 Hours to Cook

3-pound boneless turkey breast, rinsed (see Note)

1½ cups sliced onions

2 tsp Low-Sodium Barbecue Rub

2 tbsp chili sauce

¼ cup cranberry sauce with whole cranberries

1. Layer the turkey breast, onions, rub, chili sauce, and cranberry sauce in the slow cooker. Set the cooker on low and cook for 7 hours.

2. Remove the lid from the cooker and, using two forks, shred the meat. Remove the meat from the cooker and serve.

Note: Closely examine your turkey before you buy it. Is it packaged in a salt solution? If so, ask your butcher for a brine-free turkey. If there is no other option, give the bird a good rinse, which will reduce some of the salt.

Per Serving: 121.2 calories, 0.7 g total fat, 0 mg cholesterol, 61.8 mg sodium, 64.3 g total carbs, 0.4 g dietary fiber, 24.8 g protein

Make It a Meal:
Serve with polenta with rosemary, and steamed cauliflower with lemon and butter (262 calories) • Eat with a baked potato with Greek yogurt and chives, and sautéed carrots (335 calories)

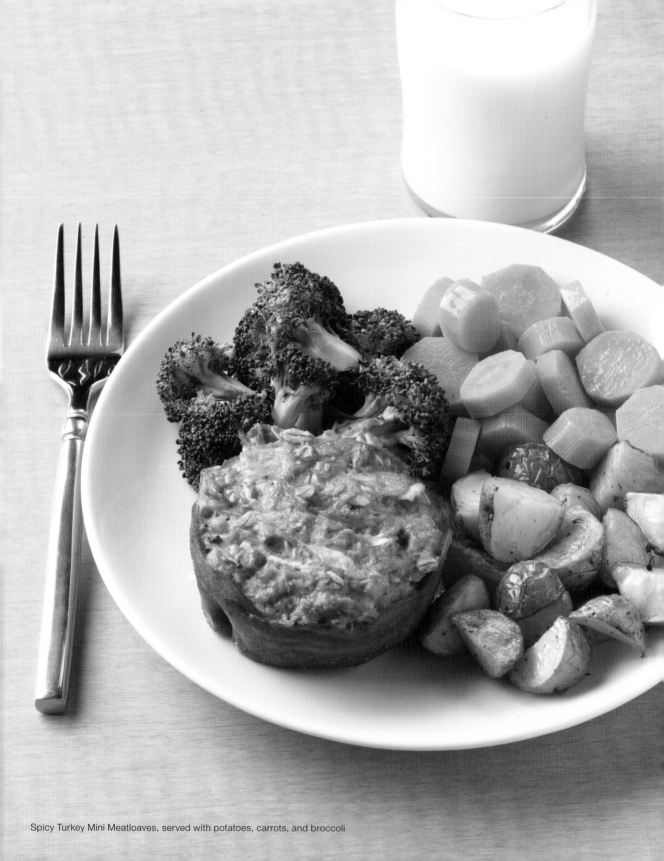

Spicy Turkey Mini Meatloaves, served with potatoes, carrots, and broccoli

Spicy Turkey Mini Meatloaves

SLIM IT DOWN:
Skip the bacon (35 calories, plus 180 mg sodium).

Your family will never suspect that there is a quarter cup of vegetables (a half serving) hiding in each mini meatloaf. I use an oversized muffin tin for this recipe, but if you don't have one, you can use mini loaf pans or regular muffin tins, which will yield twice as many loaves.

My boys like these with a side of homemade Three-Cheese Macaroni, a heaping serving of steamed broccoli, and a cup of milk. I prefer to serve them with roasted potatoes, a green salad, and, of course, a cup of milk. Make meatloaf sandwiches if you have leftovers: top a toasted whole-wheat bun with one mini meatloaf, chili sauce, lettuce, and pickles.

Makes 6 Servings:
    1 meatloaf per serving

50 Minutes to Prepare and Cook

1 pound ground turkey, 93% lean

1 medium onion, finely diced (1 cup)

1 cup old-fashioned oats

¾ cup shredded carrots

2 large eggs, beaten

½ tsp salt

½ tsp black pepper

½ to 1 tsp chipotle pepper powder (or the chili powder of your choice)

2 tbsp chili sauce

2 tsp Dijon mustard

6 slices turkey bacon

1. Preheat oven to 350° F. In a large mixing bowl, combine the turkey, onions, oats, carrots, eggs, salt, pepper, chili powder, chili sauce, and mustard.

2. Prepare large muffin tins with nonstick cooking spray. Line the inside of each tin with one slice of bacon. Drop ¾ cup of the meat mixture into each turkey bacon–lined cup.

3. Bake until an internal temperature of 165° F is reached, about 40 minutes.

Per Serving: 234.2 calories, 8.9 g total fat, 53.4 mg cholesterol, 566.7 mg sodium, 17 g total carbs, 2.9 g dietary fiber, 20.1 g protein

Make It a Meal:
Cook up some Three-Cheese Macaroni (page 265) with broccoli (459 calories) • Add a baked potato with Sweet and Spicy Barbeque Sauce (page 383) and green salad with Homemade Ranch Dressing (page 367) (432 calories).

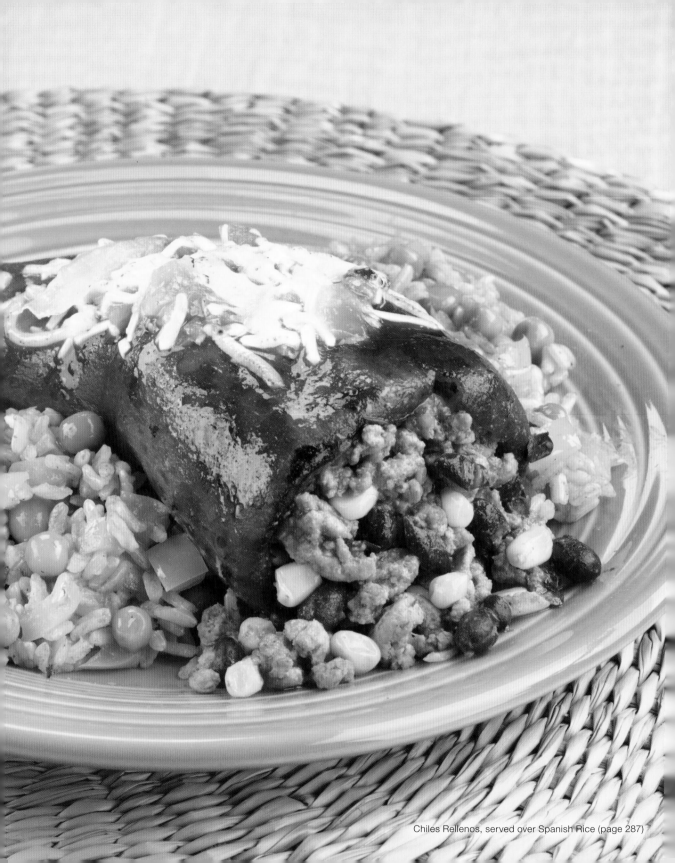

Chiles Rellenos, served over Spanish Rice (page 287)

Chiles Rellenos

SLIM IT DOWN: Leave off the cheese (52 calories).

Chiles Rellenos are stuffed peppers. Common in cuisines from Bulgaria to Peru, this is our healthy take on the Mexican dish that is usually filled with a high-fat cheese and then fried.

You might be accustomed to stuffed bell peppers, but I really encourage you to use a poblano in this recipe. They're slightly darker than a bell pepper, with a slimmer shape and a wonderful smoky and mild flavor. They're perfect for stuffing. Instead of relying on a fried coating for flavor, I roasted the peppers. Roasting and removing the charred skin leaves behind a pepper that will melt in your mouth. It also reduces the time in the oven for baking from 1 hour to just 15 minutes.

Depending on the size of the peppers you use, you may have some stuffing left over. You can freeze it, or use it in an omelet the next day.

Look for queso asadero or quesadilla cheese in the refrigerated case of the Mexican food aisle. Any mild white Mexican cheese will work in this recipe, or you could substitute reduced-fat Monterey or pepper Jack cheeses.

Online bonus: Learn how to roast a pepper. Visit SparkRecipes.com for Chef Meg's videos.

. . . .

Chef Meg's Tip: If you have a plantain (like a savory banana) on hand, dice it up and add it to the stuffing. You will be so surprised to find that it balances with the heat of the spice and the flavor of the salsa.

. . . .

Makes 4 Servings:
1 stuffed pepper per serving

45 Minutes to Prepare and Cook

4 poblano peppers, stems removed

6 ounces ground turkey, 93% lean

½ cup finely diced onion

½ tsp ground cumin

1 tsp chili powder

1 cup black beans, drained and rinsed

½ cup corn, fresh or frozen

6 tbsp salsa verde, canned or fresh (see Note)

¼ cup shredded queso asadero or queso quesadilla (Mexican melting cheese)

1. Preheat the oven to 350° F. Prepare a baking dish with nonstick cooking spray.

2. Roast the Peppers. Preheat a grill or turn on the oven broiler. Place the whole peppers onto the grill or onto a sheet pan if using broiler. Roast them on all sides until the skin is charred and brown, about 5 minutes. Place the peppers in a mixing bowl and cover the bowl with a lid

or foil. Let the peppers stand to steam for 10 minutes.

3. While the peppers are steaming, coat a sauté pan with nonstick cooking spray and place over moderate heat. Once hot, add the ground turkey and onion, and cook until turkey is no longer pink. Add the cumin and chili powder and stir, then add the beans, corn, and 2 tablespoons of salsa; stir to combine. Cook until the filling is warm, about 5 minutes.

4. Remove the peppers from the bowl and pull off the charred skin (it may help to run the peppers under cool water).

5. Pat the peppers dry, slice off the tops, and pull out any inner membrane or seeds, then stuff with the turkey mixture.

6. Arrange the peppers in the prepared baking dish. Pour the remaining 4 tablespoons of salsa over the peppers and then top with cheese. Bake for 15 minutes. Serve warm.

Note: Salsa verde is made from tomatillos, peppers, onions, cilantro, and lime. Contrary to popular belief, tomatillos aren't green tomatoes; these little husk-covered fruits are in the same family though. If you buy a salsa verde, look for one with low sodium.

Per Serving: 191.1 calories, 7.6 g total fat, 44.8 mg cholesterol, 264.8 mg sodium, 13.6 g total carbs, 3.2 g dietary fiber, 14.7 g protein

> **Make It a Meal:**
> Serve atop brown rice with chopped tomatoes and peppers (341 calories) • Enjoy on a corn tortilla with shredded red cabbage, lime juice, olive oil, and cilantro (421 calories)

Turkey Meatballs

Everyone's mom has a meatball recipe. Pork, veal, and beef, secret seasonings, and hours of work later, those huge orbs of meat would top mounds of spaghetti. But four regular meatballs can top 400 calories, with 23 grams of fat. So we've given meatballs a makeover. Not only are they ready in less than 30 minutes, this version has half the calories and a third of the fat—and they're also just as delicious when made with lean turkey.

The mixture couldn't be simpler—just ground turkey and Italian seasoning—but the results are delicious. And by baking the meatballs instead of simmering them in sauce, you are keeping all of that extra fat out of your sauce.

Serve these for the family with Weeknight Spaghetti (page 256) or, for your next potluck, serve these meatballs in a slow cooker with Sweet and Spicy Barbecue Sauce (page 383) or your favorite tomato sauce. Make the meatballs smaller (use a teaspoon instead of a tablespoon to measure) and add them to the sauce after baking.

Makes 4 Servings:
4 meatballs per serving

30 Minutes to Prepare and Cook

1 pound ground turkey, 93% lean

2 tbsp Italian Herb Seasoning Blend (page 369)

1. Preheat the oven to 375° F. Prepare a sheet pan with nonstick cooking spray.

2. In a mixing bowl, combine the ground turkey and Italian seasoning. Scoop out the meat mixture in tablespoon-size servings, roll into a compact ball, and place 1 inch apart on the sheet pan. Bake 20 minutes.

Per Serving: 160.7 calories, 8 g total fat, 80.1 mg cholesterol, 85.1 mg sodium, 0.1 g total carbs, 0.1 g dietary fiber, 22 g protein

Make It a Meal:
Serve atop whole-wheat pasta with pesto, zucchini, and peppers (352 calories) • Enjoy on a whole-wheat bun with tomato sauce, part-skim mozzarella, and grilled onions (435 calories).

Mama's Red Beans and Rice

Mama knows best, especially when it comes to making over member recipes! This New Orleans–style one pot meal is hearty, tasty, and healthy—and it feeds a crowd. We load up on the beans and chop the sausage fine to spread the flavor throughout the dish.

Vegetarian smoked sausage (found in the refrigerated health-food section of most supermarkets) makes a great substitute for the turkey sausage.

Makes 12 Servings:
    1 heaping cup per serving

1 Hour to Prepare and Cook

1 pound smoked turkey sausage

2 tbsp canola oil

1 large onion, diced

1 yellow or red bell pepper, seeded and diced

2 cloves garlic, minced

1 bunch green onions, sliced, green part reserved for garnish

½ tsp red pepper flakes

1 tbsp dried oregano

1 tsp fresh thyme, or pinch dried

Pinch of salt

1 tsp black pepper

Three 15-ounce cans of kidney beans, drained and rinsed

One 14.5-ounce can diced tomatoes with basil and garlic

1 bay leaf, whole

1 cup brown rice, uncooked

Hot sauce to taste

1. Slice the sausage links in half lengthwise and then in half again. Cut crosswise to dice.

2. Heat the oil in a large Dutch oven or heavy saucepan with lid. Once hot, add the onions, bell pepper, garlic, and the white parts of the green onion. Cook until the vegetables are soft, about 5 minutes.

3. Add the sausage to the pan and cook just until browned. Add the red pepper, oregano, thyme, salt, and black pepper and stir to combine. Then stir in the beans and tomatoes, and add the bay leaf.

4. Add the rice, stir, and let cook for 1 minute to coat the rice. Add 1½ cups of water. Bring to a boil and immediately reduce to a simmer. Cover and continue to cook until the rice is tender, about 40 minutes. Before serving, remove the bay leaf and garnish with a dash or two of hot sauce, if desired, and the sliced green onions.

Per Serving: 212.1 calories, 6.3 g total fat, 23.3 mg cholesterol, 967 mg sodium, 27 g total carbs, 8.3 g dietary fiber, 12 g protein

Make It a Meal:
Pair with whole-wheat toast with low-fat Cheddar cheese and cole slaw (445 calories) • Serve on a Multigrain Roll (page 302), with stewed okra and tomatoes with Creole seasoning (page 370) (355 calories)

Roasted Pork Tenderloin with Mustard Dill Sauce

Of all the recipes in the book, this is one of my favorites. The sauce is an example of how easily you can trim fat and still achieve the taste and texture you crave.

Usually a mustard sauce like this one would be made from a béchamel, the classic creamy white sauce. Not only does such a sauce contain gobs of fat, but it also takes about 30 minutes to prepare. This recipe is low in fat and made in a flash. Mustard can be quite high in sodium. If you're concerned about your sodium intake, you can cut back on the amount of mustard you use or experiment with dried mustard. If you don't have the Lemon-Pepper Rub on hand, just zest a lemon, then add ½ teaspoon of black pepper.

Pork tenderloins are quite affordable cuts of meat, and they're usually leaner than a beef roast. Serve this roast with Braised Spinach with Pine Nuts (page 329) and Baked Lemon-Spiced Rice (page 288). Use the leftover pork and any leftover sauce on a sandwich. Add sliced tomatoes and spinach for one tasty lunch.

Makes 4 Servings:
3–4 ounces meat with
1 tbsp sauce per serving

25 Minutes to Prepare and Cook

For the Sauce:

¼ cup plain low-fat yogurt

¼ cup Dijon mustard

1 tbsp dried dill

1½ tbsp lemon juice

1-pound pork tenderloin, fat trimmed

½ tsp Lemon-Pepper Rub (page 375)

1. Preheat the oven to 375° F.

2. Make the Sauce. In a small mixing bowl, combine the yogurt, mustard, dill, and lemon juice. Chill.

3. Place a flat-bottomed, ovenproof skillet over high heat. Lightly spray the pork roast with nonstick cooking spray and rub Lemon-Pepper Rub all over the meat. Sear the meat on all sides in the hot skillet, then transfer the pan to the oven.

4. Roast the pork until the internal temperature reaches 150° F, 15 to 20 minutes. Remove the meat from the oven, and let rest for 5 minutes before carving into thin slices. Serve with mustard sauce.

Per Serving: 198.7 calories, 7.3 g total fat, 68.1 mg cholesterol, 419.2 mg sodium, 1.8 g total carbs, 2.1 g dietary fiber, 26 g protein

Make It a Meal:
Serve with brown and wild rice with roasted broccoli (345 calories) • Enjoy with roasted sweet potatoes and green beans with Lemon-Pepper Rub (page 375) (361 calories).

Spinach and Mushroom-Stuffed Pork Tenderloin

Pork tenderloin is an affordable and lean protein that's easy to cook. Many home cooks shy away from larger cuts of meat, but they are both economical and practical—and tenderloins offer all the elegance of a roast with much less cooking time. Tenderloins often come two to a package, so cook both if you have a crowd or freeze one for later.

I prefer to use fresh spinach, but you can use frozen. Just be sure to thaw, drain, and squeeze it dry before cooking. This restaurant-quality dish is perfect for a special occasion. Serve the pork with brown rice and a nice salad.

Makes 4 Servings:
¼ of the tenderloin with stuffing per serving

1 Hour to Prepare and Cook

2 tbsp olive oil or butter, divided

½ cup finely diced onion

8 ounces baby bella mushrooms, chopped

½ tsp black pepper

2 tbsp lemon juice or white wine

10 ounces fresh spinach, washed and stems trimmed

½ cup crumbled reduced-fat feta cheese

½ tsp dried thyme

1 pound pork tenderloin

1. Preheat oven to 375° F. Place a large, oven-proof sauté pan over moderate heat. Add one tablespoon of the oil and heat until warm.

2. Add the onions to the pan and sauté until tender, about 3 to 4 minutes. Add the mushrooms to the pan, season with pepper, and continue to sauté for 2 to 3 minutes more. Add the lemon juice and spinach to the pan and cook until wilted, about 2 minutes.

3. Remove the pan from the heat, stir in the feta cheese and thyme, then allow mixture to cool slightly.

4. Pat the tenderloin dry with paper towels. Slice the meat lengthwise almost to the other side, then open as you would a book. Place the meat between two sheets of plastic wrap or waxed paper and, using the flat side of a meat mallet, a rolling pin, or a heavy-bottomed pan, pound the meat to flatten it until it is ½- to ¾-inch thick. Remove the top piece of plastic wrap.

5. Place the mushroom mixture along the center of the meat and roll it up like a jelly roll, using the plastic wrap to press it into a tight log. Secure the roll at intervals with 16 inches of kitchen string.

6. Place the second tablespoon of oil into the sauté pan and, when hot, add the meat and sear it on all sides. Move the pan into the oven and roast the meat until the thickest part reaches 150° F, about 30 minutes. Let the meat rest for 10 minutes before slicing.

Per Serving: 300.2 calories, 14.6 g total fat, 97.9 mg cholesterol, 225.6 mg sodium, 6 g total carbs, 2.2 g dietary fiber, 36.1 g protein

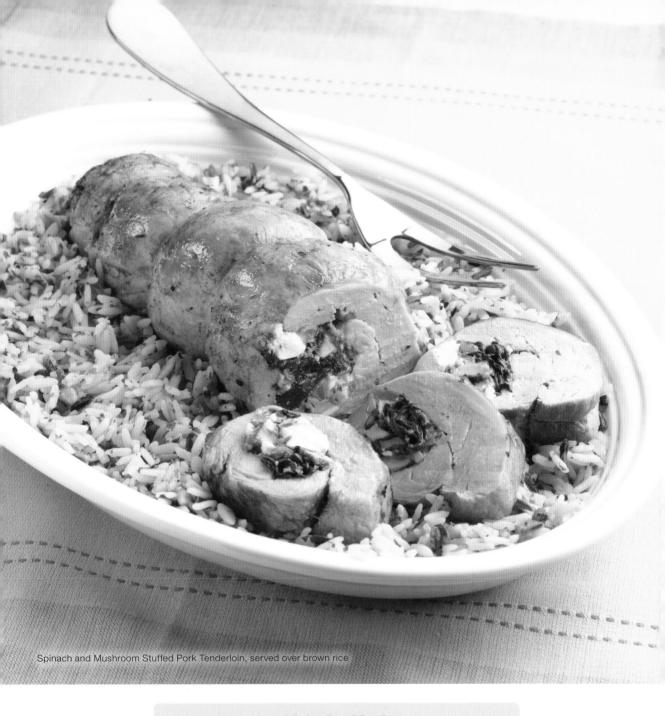

Spinach and Mushroom Stuffed Pork Tenderloin, served over brown rice

Make It a Meal:
Add whole-wheat couscous with grilled summer
squash (415 calories) • Pair with roasted beets, and
Romaine and tomato salad with vinaigrette (440 calories)

Grilled Pork Chops with Apple Chutney

Pork chops and applesauce, as any *Brady Bunch* fan knows, are a great combination. My mother was British, so rather than applesauce, I grew up eating chutneys and I love them. They're a great way to add flavor to cooked meats and add fruit to the meal.

All chutneys are not alike. Some are sweet; others are spicy. Some are chunky, others smooth, and they can be made with everything from mint or cilantro to peanuts or yogurt. Indian in origin, colonialism brought the chutney to Britain, where they continue to be popular. Traditionally, most contain curry powder. In this recipe, I swapped out the curry for allspice because of the tartness of the apples. European-style chutneys are mostly fruit, vinegar, and sugar cooked down to a paste. I cut the sugar and added more fruit. This chutney could also be used on grilled chicken or as an addition to a cheese and fruit tray.

Makes 4 Servings:
3–4 ounces pork with
¼ cup chutney per serving

1 Hour to Prepare and Cook

For the Chutney:

½ cup finely chopped onion

3 Granny Smith apples, peeled, cored, and diced

1 tbsp brown sugar

2 tbsp golden raisins

1 large orange, zested and juiced

½ cup red-wine vinegar

½ tsp allspice

1 pound boneless pork chops

¼ tsp black pepper

1. Make the Chutney. Prepare a saucepan with nonstick cooking spray and place the pan over moderate heat. Add the onion and cook until tender, 3 to 4 minutes. Do not let them brown. Add the apples, brown sugar, raisins, orange zest and juice, vinegar, allspice and ½ cup of water. Cook over low heat for 30 minutes.

2. Preheat a grill to medium heat. Scrape the hot grill with a grill brush to remove any cooked food. Pat chops dry, sprinkle with pepper. Place the chops on the grill to cook until the internal temperature reaches 150° F, 3 to 4 minutes per side.

3. Remove the meat from the grill and let it rest on a plate for 2 minutes before serving. Garnish each chop with ¼ cup of chutney.

Per Serving: 290.4 calories, 8.7 g total fat, 68.9 mg cholesterol, 57.9 mg sodium, 27.9 g total carbs, 3.4 g dietary fiber, 26.9 g protein

Make It a Meal:
Cook up brown rice with sautéed zucchini (425 calories) • Pair with Broccoli and Spaghetti Squash with Lemon Pepper (page 243) (340 calories)

Beef Roast

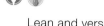

Lean and versatile, this recipe is the little black dress of your healthy recipe arsenal. Cook this roast on a Sunday and enjoy it throughout the week. We used no salt, just pepper for a truly flavorful roast.

Searing the roast before roasting it will seal in the juices and add another layer of flavor. At the same time, allowing the meat to rest for 10 minutes after cooking will give the juices time to redistribute. If you cut into the meat as soon as it comes out of the oven, all the juices will run out, and your meat will be dry.

Use the leftover roast to make a Beef and Blue Sandwich (page 136).

Makes 12 Servings:
    3–4 ounces per serving

20 Minutes to Prepare, 1 Hour to Cook

1 top-round beef roast (2½ pounds)

1 tsp cracked black pepper

1. Preheat the oven to 400° F. Remove meat from the refrigerator; allow to stand at room temperature for 20 minutes.

2. Pat meat dry with paper towels to remove any moisture. Sprinkle and then rub the pepper over the meat.

3. Place a cast-iron skillet or heavy ovenproof sauté pan over moderate heat. Do not add cooking spray or any oil to the pan. Sear the meat on all sides, then move the pan to the oven.

4. Immediately reduce the oven temperature to 350° F and roast until the internal temperature reaches 125° F, about 50 minutes. Remove the meat from the oven, cover loosely with foil, and let stand for 10 minutes before carving into thin slices.

Per Serving: 191.2 calories, 7.6 g total fat, 84.1 mg cholesterol, 62.4 mg sodium, 0.1 g total carbs, 0 g dietary fiber, 28.7 g protein

Make It a Meal:
Serve with a baked sweet potato with goat cheese, and sautéed spinach (452 calories) • Enjoy with roasted potatoes and broccoli with pesto (406 calories)

Peppercorn Steak with Herbed Blue Cheese

Think we're crazy to include this recipe in a collection of healthy dishes? Truthfully, this recipe is right at home here, and it illustrates our philosophy of satisfaction and eating what you love.

This recipe calls for one 12-ounce fillet, but it serves four. That's not a typo. You might be served that 12-ounce fillet as a single portion at a restaurant, and you'd be eating almost 80 grams of fat—more than what most of us eat in a day! What happens when you eat that huge steak? You end up feeling sick to your stomach and lethargic. You clutch your belly, loosen your pants, and let guilt wash over you.

You can eat steak while losing or maintaining your weight. It's all about moderation and balance. At many steakhouses, chefs finish steaks with a flavored butter to add richness and shine to the steak. Here we use an herbed blue cheese to achieve the same effect.

· ·

Chef Meg's Tip: The key to eating rich foods without going overboard is balance. If you're ordering the steak, choose simple sides like steamed asparagus or a baked sweet potato. If you want the lobster mac and cheese, skip dessert. If it's crème brûlée you crave, choose the grilled fish and vegetables as your main course. This is the same principle I use to balance all that heavy food I taste at school.

· ·

Makes 4 Servings:
  3–4 ounces of meat per serving

30 Minutes to Prepare and Cook

3 tbsp crumbled blue cheese

¼ cup chopped parsley (⅓ of a bunch)

2 tsp of black, red, and pink peppercorns,
  cracked (see Note)

1 beef fillet (12 ounces), cut into 3-ounce
  steaks

1. Preheat the oven to 375° F. In a small bowl, combine the blue cheese and parsley and use a wooden spoon to loosely work into a paste. Cover and refrigerate.

2. Spread the cracked peppercorns onto a plate. Pat the meat dry and roll in the peppercorns to coat on all sides.

3. Place a cast-iron skillet or heavy-bottomed ovenproof sauté pan over moderately high heat. (Do not use nonstick cooking spray or any type of oil to prepare the pan.) Once hot, place steaks into the dry pan and sear the top and bottom of each steak (see Note), 1 to 2 minutes per side.

4. Place 1 tablespoon of the blue cheese mixture on top of each steak and transfer the pan to the oven. Roast 6 to 7 minutes for rare, 7 to 8 minutes for medium.

Note: To crack whole peppercorns, pour the desired amount into a sturdy plastic bag and then spread them flat on a dish towel or cutting board (to protect your countertop). Then, with the smooth side of a meat mallet, a rolling pan, or the bottom of a heavy pan, pound the peppercorns into a very coarse grind.

When searing a steak (or any meat), you want to achieve a nice, crispy, well-caramelized crust. To do so, don't be tempted to pull the meat from the pan's surface too early. The meat will release easily once completely seared; any resistance and it's not done yet.

Per Serving: 245.8 calories, 18.2 g total fat, 65.3 mg cholesterol, 159.1 mg sodium, 1.2 g total carbs, 159.1 mg sodium, 1.2 g total carbs, 0.4 g dietary fiber, 18.5 g protein

Make It a Meal:
Pair with roasted potatoes and green beans with tarragon (415 calories) • Serve with a Multigrain Roll (page 302), and arugula with lemon juice and olive oil (399 calories).

Better-for-You Beef Stroganoff

SLIM IT DOWN: Leave out the noodles (72 calories).

Beef Stroganoff has its roots in Russia, but it's a recipe that's synonymous with American childhood. There are plenty of variations: with or without red wine, tomato paste, onions, and even its trademark mushrooms; but whether Mom's recipe served the sour cream in the sauce or on the side, Beef Stroganoff has cemented its reputation as a comfort food. Unfortunately, the traditional version is as caloric as it is comforting, with up to 40 grams of fat per serving. Discomforting, isn't it?

With lean sirloin cut against the grain to maximize taste and texture, and reduced-fat sour cream, our version has less than half the calories and a third of the fat of the original.

Makes 4 Servings:
1 cup beef-mushroom mixture with 1 cup cooked noodles per serving

1 Hour to Prepare and Cook

1 pound beef top-sirloin roast, fat trimmed

1 tbsp canola oil

1 pound mushrooms, quartered

1 medium onion, finely diced (1 cup)

2 tsp tomato paste

2 tsp mustard, Dijon or stone-ground

½ tsp black pepper

1 tsp dried thyme, or 1 tbsp fresh

1½ cups homemade or low-sodium beef broth

2 cups whole-wheat egg noodles

½ cup reduced-fat sour cream

1 tbsp chopped parsley

2 tsp chopped dill

1. Slice the meat into 2-inch thick slices against the grain. Pat dry.

2. Place a sauté pan over moderately high heat and, once hot, add the oil. When the oil is hot, add the meat to the pan and sear on all sides. Do not crowd the pan; brown the meat in batches if necessary. Remove the meat from the pan and set aside. Once it has cooled slightly, carve into ½-inch slices.

3. Add the mushrooms and onions to the pan. Sauté until the onions are tender, the mushrooms start to caramelize, and the pan is somewhat dry, about 10 minutes.

4. Add the tomato paste, mustard, pepper, and thyme to the vegetables. Stir to combine and cook for 1 minute. Deglaze the pan by pouring ½ cup of the stock into the hot pan and quickly scraping the bottom to remove the cooked bits.

5. Add the remaining stock and the beef, reduce the heat to a simmer, and cook for 10 minutes.

6. Meanwhile, cook the noodles according to package directions, but don't salt the water.

7. Remove the beef and sauce from the heat and place in a serving dish.

8. Place the sour cream in a small bowl, then whisk in ½ cup of the sauce to prevent the cream from seizing up and separating, then gradually add the sour-cream mixture back into the beef mixture. Garnish with parsley and dill and serve over the noodles.

Per Serving: 336.3 calories, 12.2 g total fat, 75.7 mg cholesterol, 215 mg sodium, 26.7 g total carbs, 4.8 g dietary fiber, 32 g protein

Make It a Meal:
Just add fruit and milk—
it's already a meal!

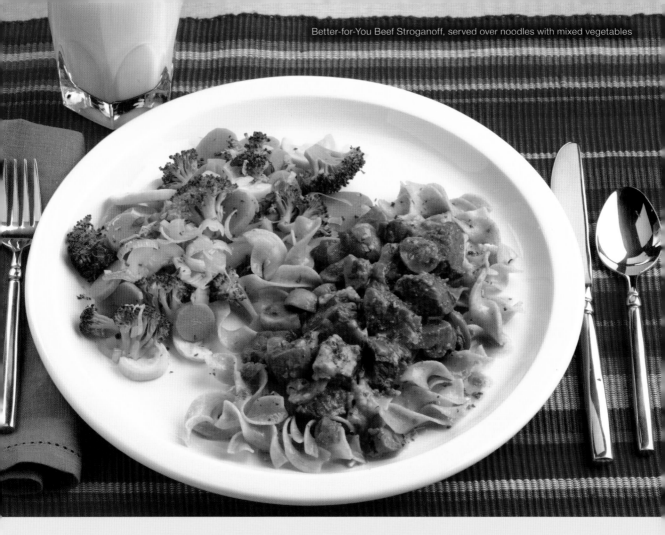

Chew on This: Cutting Against the Grain

Saving money by buying cheaper cuts of meat is a great tip for any home cook, but the trick is turning those tougher cuts of meat into delectable dinners. It can be done, and all you need is a knife and a few minutes.

Like an onion or a piece of wood, meat has a very distinct grain. Pick up a piece of beef and take a close look at it. You should see lines running in one direction. As we know, meat is muscle, and those lines are the muscle fibers. If we cut along the lines, or "with the grain," our meat is tougher and more fibrous. Each bite of meat will contain long strings of muscle fiber that require more work to tenderize and chew. By cutting "against the grain," or perpendicular to the lines, we shorten those long fibers, making the meat easier to chew and more tender. The fastest way to ruin a piece of meat—cheap or expensive—is to cut with the grain, even if you cooked it perfectly.

Liken it to a piece of celery. If you chomp on a stalk of celery, those tough fibers get stuck in your teeth. With a chopped piece of celery, those fibers are shorter and already cut.

The next time you carve a cut of beef, whether it's a tenderloin or a flank steak, take the time to slice against the grain. Use long knife strokes to achieve thin slices, and you'll enjoy your meat that much more.

Spring Garden Stir-Fry

When most people think stir-fry, they think soy sauce, sesame oil, and ginger. As tasty as that combination is, there are plenty of other ways to flavor a stir-fry with a lot less salt than soy sauce.

Use this recipe as a guide: any combination of veggies or meat will work; just keep the ratio of meat to veggies at 3 ounces of cooked meat to 2 cups of vegetables per serving. Add the vegetables that will take longer to cook first.

Often you will see stock or soy sauce used in a stir-fry. Though it's rare in my kitchen that I use premade flavorings, I do like to use recaito (cilantro cooking base) in stir-fries. You'll find it in the Hispanic food aisle of most supermarkets. It has less salt than most stocks you buy and considerably less than even low-sodium soy sauce. It lasts for months and can be used in any dish that could benefit from a burst of fresh cilantro flavor. If you can't find it, substitute additional cilantro or a quarter cup of fresh parsley.

This is also a great recipe for leftover cooked or raw meat. If it's cooked, add at the end of cooking just to heat through.

Escarole is a hearty green that's a member of the endive family. Substitute fresh spinach if you can't find it.

. . . .

Chef Meg's Tip: Check your local butcher's for stir-fry meat. Mine offers meat already sliced into thin strips ready to go into the wok! It saves time and clean up. If you purchase a larger cut of meat, freeze it for 10 minutes before you slice it. You'll be able to slice thinner strips.

. . . .

Makes 4 Servings:
1 cup per serving

30 Minutes to Prepare and Cook

1 tbsp canola oil

1 pound beef sirloin, sliced into thin strips, patted dry

3 cloves garlic, minced

1 bunch green onions, white part cut to 4-inch lengths, remaining green parts sliced for garnish

1 lemon, zested into large strips and juiced

2 tbsp rice-wine vinegar

2 tbsp recaito (cilantro cooking base)

1 bunch thin asparagus, sliced at an angle into 3- to 4-inch pieces (about 3 cups)

1 tsp cornstarch or arrowroot (optional)

2 cups roughly chopped escarole

2 tbsp roughly chopped cilantro leaves

1. Heat a wok or flat-bottomed skillet over high heat. Add the oil and, once hot, add half of the meat to the skillet. Stir-fry until no longer pink on the outside. Remove with a slotted spoon or tongs, set aside. Repeat with remaining meat. Set all meat aside and keep warm.

2. Add the garlic and green onions to the skillet. Stir-fry for 1 to 2 minutes. Add the lemon zest and juice, vinegar, and recaito to the pan and stir. Add the asparagus and continue to stir-fry for 1 to 2 minutes.

3. If the sauce is too thin, combine the cornstarch with 1 tablespoon of water and stir into skillet. Allow the liquid to come to a boil, then return the meat to the pan.

4. Top the mixture with the escarole and cook just until the greens have wilted, 1 or 2 minutes more. Garnish with chopped cilantro and the sliced green onion tops. Serve with brown rice, if desired.

Per Serving: 332.7 calories, 13.1 g total fat, 100.9 mg cholesterol, 284.1 mg sodium, 16.3 total carbs, 6.4 g dietary fiber, 38.9 g protein

Make It a Meal:
Add brown rice and a side of Fruit Salad with Poppy Seed Dressing (page 346) (492 calories) • Serve with whole-wheat pasta and a side of strawberries (443 calories)

Chew on This: Arrowroot

Arrowroot is a starch derived from the tuber of a South American plant. In cooking, it is used as a thickener in place of cornstarch or flour. It is excellent for making clear sauces or fruit jellies, and its taste is completely neutral: it won't carry the bitter aftertaste that sometimes comes with cornstarch and, because it's gluten-free, it is easier to digest than wheat flours. Make a slurry of arrowroot and a cooler liquid before mixing it into hot food. Arrowroot will thicken at a cooler temperature than cornstarch or flour, but overheating can cause the resulting sauce to break, so remove your sauce from the heat as soon as it thickens. Substitute 2 teaspoons of arrowroot for 1 tablespoon of cornstarch, or 1 teaspoon of arrowroot for 1 tablespoon of wheat flour.

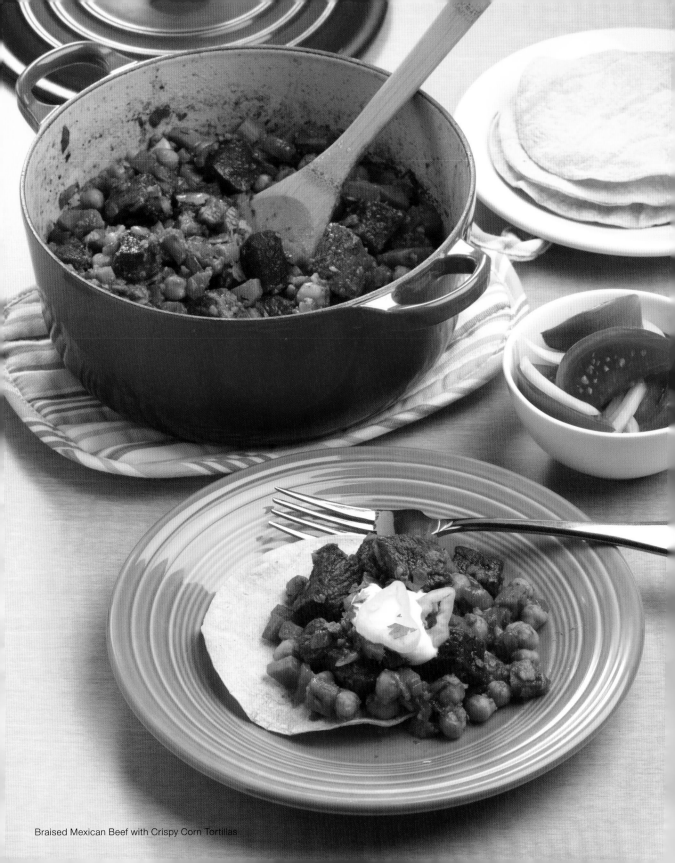

Braised Mexican Beef with Crispy Corn Tortillas

Braised Mexican Beef with Crispy Corn Tortillas

Stews and other braised dishes are usually heavy on meat and skimpy on the vegetables. For this recipe, I reduced the meat to 12 ounces, included 2 servings of vegetables per portion, and added chickpeas as a healthy and fiber-rich protein source.

Braised dishes often use a thickener, like flour, in the sauce. With the Mexican influences in this recipe, masa (corn) flour would be my first choice, but it's only available in large bags. I improvised by baking, then crushing two corn tortillas. Why buy a lot of one ingredient if you only need a small amount?

Makes 4 Servings:
1 heaping cup per serving

10 Minutes to Prepare; 1 Hour, 15 Minutes to Cook

12 ounces beef chuck roast (stew meat), excess fat trimmed, cut into 1-inch cubes

1 red onion, diced (about 1½ cups)

3 large carrots, peeled and cut into ¾-inch dice (2 cups)

4 garlic cloves, peeled and halved

2 tbsp no-salt-added tomato paste

¼ cup red-wine vinegar or leftover red wine

1½ cups low-sodium beef stock

1 tsp chili powder

1 tsp dried thyme or 3 fresh sprigs

6 corn tortillas, baked until crispy

1 cup canned chickpeas, rinsed and drained

1 tbsp chopped cilantro

1 banana pepper, diced

2 tbsp low-fat Greek yogurt

1. Preheat oven to 325° F.

2. Place an ovenproof, heavy-bottomed, lidded saucepan over moderate heat. Pat the meat dry with a paper towel, then add to the saucepan to sear on all sides. Remove the meat from the saucepan and set aside.

3. While the pan is still hot, add the onions and sauté for 2 to 3 minutes. Add the carrots and garlic and continue to sauté for 3 minutes more. Add the tomato paste and vinegar, then slowly add the stock, stirring with a wooden spoon to remove the browned bits at the bottom of the saucepan.

4. Add the chili powder and thyme, then return the meat to the pan. Bring to a simmer, cover, and place in the preheated oven. Braise for 1 hour.

5. Place 2 of the baked tortillas in a sandwich bag and crush—using a rolling pin or a heavy-bottomed pan—until they are crumbs.

6. Remove saucepan from oven (remember the handles get hot!). Stir in the chickpeas and crushed tortillas. Replace the cover and return to the oven for 15 minutes more.

7. Place 1 heaping cup of stew onto a tortilla, top with the chopped cilantro, peppers, and one tablespoon of Greek yogurt. Serve warm.

Per Serving: 338.4 calories, 7.2 g total fat, 55.3 mg cholesterol, 221.9 mg sodium, 45.9 g total carbs, 10.7 g dietary fiber, 25.2 g protein

Make It a Meal:
Just add a piece of fruit and a cup of milk!

Grilled Southwest Flat-Iron Steak

This is a meal that will have your guests begging for your secrets. I'll spill: it's the cut of the meat and the flavorful marinade. The only way to mess this up is to forget to cut it against the grain (see Cutting Against the Grain, page 215).

I call this steak a "flat iron," but it answers to other names. Your butcher will probably call it a top blade as it comes from the top of the shoulder blade of the cow; it's quite a tender cut, with less connective tissue and a tight grain that makes it perfect for marinating, as I did here. This cut is great for kebobs, stir-fries, or on the grill.

Serve this over an arugula salad with a garnish of Avocado Cherry-Tomato Salsa (page 313).

Makes 4 Servings:
3–4 ounces of beef per serving

2 Hours to Marinate, 30 Minutes to Prepare and Cook

For the Marinade:

1 clove garlic, smashed and chopped

2 tbsp chopped cilantro

1 tsp cumin

1 tsp Dijon mustard

1 lime, zested and juiced

1 tbsp canola oil

1 chipotle pepper in adobo sauce, chopped (see Note)

1 flat-iron steak (16 ounces)

1. In a baking dish large enough to hold the steak, combine the garlic, cilantro, cumin, mustard, lime zest and juice, oil, and chipotle pepper. Add the meat and turn to coat evenly. Cover and refrigerate for 2 to 8 hours.

2. Preheat the grill to 350° F. Remove the meat from the marinade and grill for 10 minutes on one side, then flip and continue to cook until the meat reaches 130° F for rare or 140° F for medium, about 15 minutes.

3. Remove the meat from the grill and let it rest for 5 minutes before carving in thin strips against the grain.

Note: You'll have leftover chipotle peppers in the can. To freeze them: place in a plastic bag and roll them up tight (as you would a roll of cookie dough). Label and date the bag; the peppers will keep in the freezer for up to 6 months. Just slice off peppers as needed.

Per Serving: 227.8 calories, 14.6 g total fat, 71 mg cholesterol, 129.1 mg sodium, 1.4 g total carbs, 0.2 g dietary fiber, 21. 2 g protein

Make It a Meal:
Serve with a corn tortilla, and grilled peppers and onions (388 calories) • Pair with brown rice with cilantro and lime, and tomatoes and cucumbers with vinaigrette (455 calories)

Slimmer Sloppy Joes

SLIM IT DOWN: Skip the bun (100 calories) or halve the portion (145 calories).

If ever there was a kid-friendly recipe, this is it! My three boys love these—and my husband does, too. Instead of opening a can, you can create your own sloppy joe sauce in no time. Dinner will be on the table in less than 20 minutes—and our version has a quarter of the fat and 100 fewer calories than a standard loose-meat sandwich.

I like to use whole-wheat sandwich thins instead of buns, but you can also serve this over a baked potato. We like to serve this with sweet potato fries, a serving of green beans, and a cup of milk.

Makes 4 Servings:
1 cup meat mixture with 1 sandwich thin per serving

20 Minutes to Prepare and Cook

1½ cups no-salt-added tomato puree

One 14.5-ounce can red beans, rinsed and drained

8 ounces ground beef, extra lean, at least 91% lean

1 medium onion, finely diced (1 cup)

3 cloves garlic, minced

1 cup finely diced red or orange bell pepper

1 tsp chipotle or dark chili powder

½ tsp salt

¼ tsp black pepper

2 tbsp canned chopped green chiles

4 whole-wheat sandwich thins, toasted (see Note)

1. Place the tomato puree and beans in a blender with ½ cup of water. Puree until most of the mixture is blended. Set aside.

2. Place a large sauté pan over moderate heat. When the pan is hot, add the beef, stir, and cook until light brown.

3. Add the onions and continue to cook for 2 minutes, then add the garlic and peppers and cook for 2 minutes more. Add the chili powder, salt, and pepper; stir to distribute and cook for 1 minute more.

4. Add the tomato and bean mixture and the green chiles to the beef, stir, and cook for an additional 10 minutes. Divide the mixture evenly among 4 sandwich thins.

Note: Use homemade Multigrain Rolls (page 302) to cut the sodium in this recipe. Store-bought bread contains a great deal of salt.

Per Serving: 389.7 calories, 6.3 g total fat, 35 mg cholesterol, 608.3 mg sodium, 56.3 total carbs, 9.9 g dietary fiber, 28 g protein

Make It a Meal:
Pair with carrots and cucumbers with Homemade Ranch Dressing (page 367) (467 calories) • Serve with green beans with margarine and Lemon Pepper Rub (page 375) (444 calories)

CHEF MEG'S TIPS:

- If you prefer a thicker, less sloppy sauce, add a couple of tablespoons of tomato paste with the spices.

- Adding a can of pinto, black, or kidney beans thickens the sauce and adds fiber and protein to the dish. When you're trying to stretch your meat, beans are a great help.

- Swap lean ground turkey for the beef.

SOMETHING'S FISHY

- If the skin is still attached to your fillets, it should have a bright shiny appearance. The scales should be firmly attached and not flaking.

- If the skin is off the fish when you buy it, the flesh should be firm and moist, not slimy or squishy.

- Ask to smell and touch the fish at the fish counter. If they won't let you, make chicken for dinner instead. Don't risk wasting your money on spoiled fish.

- Let your nose be the guide when purchasing any seafood; you should smell the essence of the sea, not ammonia.

- How do you tell when fish is cooked? The flesh will begin to flake and feel firm, and it will go from transparent to opaque.

- If you live in the middle of the country, IQF (Individually Quick Frozen) seafood is a convenient option. The fillets are frozen in individual packages, which means easy portion control and dinners in a flash. At my supermarket, they're often near the fish counter in a freezer. Thaw frozen fish overnight in the fridge or under cold running water—not in the microwave.

- If you're buying a whole fish, look him in the eye first. A sunken, cloudy eye means that the fish is not fresh.

Grilled Fish with Mango Salsa

If there is one protein that people are afraid to cook, it's fish. Fish is lean, quick-cooking, and versatile; there's no need to fear it. Just keep in mind this rule of thumb: fish requires 10 minutes per inch of thickness no matter the cooking method. I sometimes use fluke in this recipe, but grouper is another good choice. Other good options are sole or summer flounder.

Fish doesn't need much seasoning—just a squeeze of lemon will do. The fruit salsa can be made ahead of time. It's a great low-calorie topping that's very versatile: use it on chicken or with baked tortilla chips as an appetizer.

Online bonus: Learn how to cut a mango and how to buy fish. Visit SparkRecipes.com for Chef Meg's videos.

Makes 4 Servings:
3–4 ounces of fish with ¼ cup of salsa per serving

20 Minutes to Prepare and Cook

For the Salsa:

1 lime

1 mango, peeled and diced

½ jalapeño pepper, seeded and minced (see Note)

1 tbsp chopped cilantro

For the Fish:

1 lemon, zested and juiced

1 pound firm, white-fleshed fish fillets

1. Make the Salsa. Zest the lime, then, with a sharp knife and holding it over a bowl to catch the juice, cut away the remaining pith. Segment the lime by cutting away the sections in a V, leaving behind the membrane. Put the lime zest and the segmented fruit in a bowl and add the mango, jalapeño, and cilantro. Mix well and set aside.

2. Preheat the grill to high. Sprinkle half of the lemon zest over the fish. Place the fish on the grill, skin side up if skin is still on the fillet. Grill for 4 minutes, then turn. Squeeze the lemon juice over each fillet along with a pinch of lemon zest. Grill for an additional 5 minutes, until the fish is no longer transparent and cooked through. Serve with the salsa on top of the fish.

Note: Most of the heat in a jalapeño pepper is in the seeds and white ribs. Remove them and you'll eliminate most of the pepper's punch. Leave them in for a spicier salsa.

Per Serving: 122.4 calories, 1.7 g total fat, 55 mg cholesterol, 91.2 mg sodium, 8.9 g total carbs, 1.3 g dietary fiber, 21.4 g protein

Make It a Meal:
Add on baked tortilla chips with tomato salsa (250 calories) • Serve with brown rice with tomato and onion salad with vinaigrette (286 calories)

Easy Steamed Fish Packets

Cooking fish or chicken in parchment-paper packets is a technique known as *en papillote*. The protein stays moist without any added fat, and the herbs and fish lend flavor to the vegetables. Be sure to slice your vegetables thinly to ensure even cooking. We used peppers, mushrooms, and leeks here; but you can choose your favorite vegetables. Thinly sliced peppers, asparagus, carrots, celery, onions, zucchini, and green beans are all good choices. Switch up the herbs and spices, too: garlic, basil, or oregano will all work well.

The best thing about this recipe: because everything is cooked in the parchment, cleanup is a breeze!

Makes 4 Servings:
3–4 ounces fish with 1 cup of vegetables

30 Minutes to Prepare and Cook

2 leeks, thinly sliced

2 red or yellow bell peppers, cored, seeded, and thinly sliced

1 cup thinly sliced button mushrooms

1 tbsp chopped fresh parsley, or 1 tsp dried

1 tsp chopped fresh thyme

1 pound sole fillets (or another white-fleshed fish), cut into 4-ounce portions

2 lemons, zested and cut in half

1. Preheat the oven to 450° F. In a small bowl, mix together the leeks, bell pepper, and mushrooms. In another small bowl, mix together the parsley and thyme.

2. Fold four sheets of 15" x 15" parchment paper in half. Coat one half with nonstick cooking spray and place on a baking sheet, uncoated side down (if you have a griddle that fits across two burners, you can use that in place of the baking sheet). In the center of the sprayed side of each piece of parchment, place 1 fish fillet, one-quarter of the vegetables, lemon zest, and herbs. Juice 1 lemon half over each mixture. Fold over the left side of the parchment. Crimp the edges to form a packet.

3. Place the baking sheet across two burners on the stovetop and set to moderate heat. Once the liquid inside each packet starts to bubble, transfer the pan to the oven. Bake for 8 to 10 minutes, depending on the thickness of the fish. A general rule of thumb is 10 minutes per inch of thickness.

Per Serving: 158.4 calories, 1.5 g total fat, 50 mg cholesterol, 103 mg sodium, 16.6 g total carbs, 4.8 g dietary fiber, 23.4 g protein

Make It a Meal:
Serve with brown rice (268 calories) • Pair with a baked potato (278 calories)

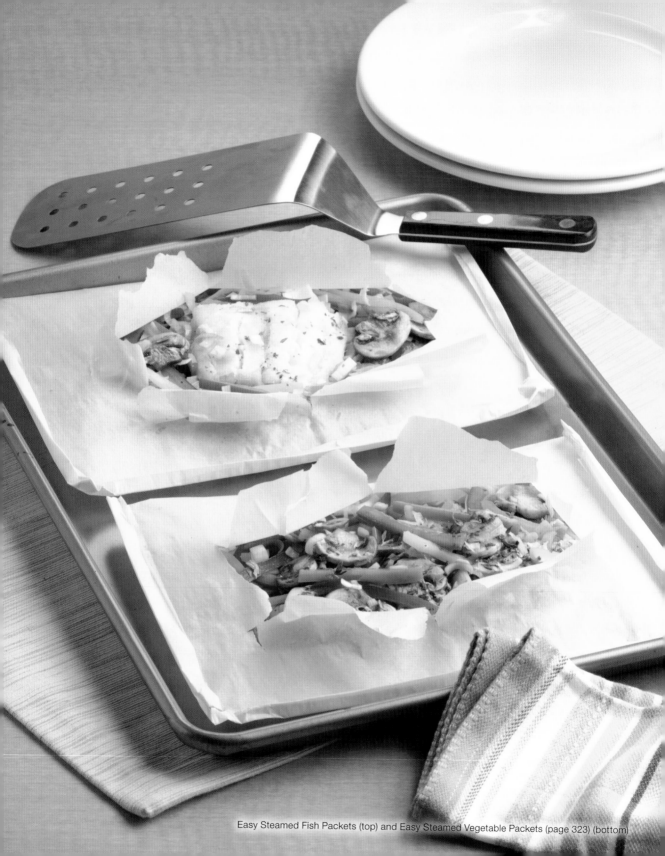

Easy Steamed Fish Packets (top) and Easy Steamed Vegetable Packets (page 323) (bottom)

Maple-Glazed Roasted Salmon

SLIM IT DOWN:
Use half the marinade (25 calories).

Like tuna, salmon is a fatty fish—but it's a good-for-you fish that's filled with omega-3 fatty acids (the heart-healthy fats). A 4-ounce serving of sockeye salmon will provide more than 100 percent of the required daily amounts of vitamin D. Whenever possible, choose wild salmon over farm-raised to minimize exposure to contaminants. Wild salmon is also more flavorful than farmed.

Salmon is an easy fish to cook, and it's delicious poached, baked, roasted, or grilled. Want to add a little more zest to this dish? Try adding 1 teaspoon of Dijon mustard to the marinade.

Makes 4 Servings:
3–4 ounces per serving

1 Hour to Prepare and Cook

¼ cup pure maple syrup

1 tbsp light soy sauce

½ lemon, juiced

1 garlic clove, minced

Dash of black or white pepper

1 pound fresh salmon fillets

1. In a small bowl, stir together the syrup, soy sauce, lemon juice, garlic, and pepper.

2. Place the salmon in a glass baking dish; pour the marinade over the fish and turn to coat both sides. Cover and refrigerate for 20 minutes.

3. Preheat the oven to 400° F. Pour off the excess marinade, and bake the salmon, uncovered, until the fish becomes firm and flakes easily with a fork, 18 to 20 minutes.

Per Serving: 295.7 calories, 11.1g total fat, 96.6 mg cholesterol, 308 mg sodium, 12.3 g total carbs, 0.5 g dietary fiber, 35.2 g protein

Make It a Meal:
Pair with broccoli and brown rice (430 calories) • Enjoy with whole-wheat couscous and peas (438 calories)

The Downies' Honey-Ginger Salmon

This recipe comes from SparkPeople founder Chris Downie and his wife, Karina. She says, "This is one of our family's absolute favorite dishes. It got our boys eating salmon at a very young age. They cheer every time I make it and they even ask for seconds! This tastes great with cooked millet and Brussels sprouts." Tamari is a very flavorful, wheat-free soy sauce. If you are watching your sodium, choose a light variety.

Makes 4 Servings:
3 ounces per serving

15 Minutes to Prepare and Cook

¼ cup grapeseed or canola oil

½ tsp toasted sesame oil

¼ cup honey

1 lemon, juiced

2 tbsp tamari soy sauce

1-inch piece of fresh ginger, finely grated
   (about 1 tbsp)

1 pound salmon, cut into four portions
   (approximately 4 ounces each)

1. In a small bowl, whisk together the oils, honey, lemon juice, tamari, and ginger. With a spoon or brush, spread about a third of the sauce on the salmon.

2. Spritz a heavy-bottomed skillet with oil or nonstick cooking spray and place over high heat. Once the pan is hot, add the salmon and cook for 1 minute, then lower the heat to medium and cook for 2 minutes more. Turn the fish and cook for 3 minutes for medium rare or slightly longer if you like it cooked through. (I leave it for 4 minutes since my family likes it more well done.) When the salmon is cooked, remove it from the pan, place on a plate, and cover to keep warm.

3. Pour the remaining sauce into the same pan and cook over moderate heat until it becomes a syrup, 3 to 4 minutes. Stir frequently, being careful that it doesn't burn.

4. Spoon the sauce over the salmon and serve.

Per Serving: 408.4 calories, 23.4 g total fat, 80.5 mg cholesterol, 567.9 mg sodium, 19.9 g total carbs, 0.3 g dietary fiber, 30 g protein

Make It a Meal:
Serve with whole-wheat couscous and tri-colored peppers (572 calories)
• Pair with Brussels sprouts and cooked millet (541 calories)

CHEF MEG'S TIPS:

- Measure the oil, then measure the honey in the same measuring cup. The residual oil will allow the honey to slide out easily.

- No grapeseed oil? Use canola instead.

Salmon Patties with Spicy-Sweet Yogurt Dressing

Apple in a fish cake—who knew it could taste so good? But they taste great in this sophisticated take on the lunch-room classic. The apple keeps the cake moist and replaces the need for heavy mayo. The tangy yogurt dressing adds a kick of spice that's balanced by the sweetness of the fruit.

Makes 4 Servings:
1 cake and 2 tbsp dressing per serving

20 Minutes to Prepare and Cook

For the Dressing:

1 tbsp capers, rinsed and drained

6 dill pickle slices, drained

1 shallot, cut into half

1 tsp Dijon mustard

⅛ tsp hot sauce

½ lemon, juiced

¼ cup low-fat plain yogurt

For the Salmon Cakes:

10 ounces canned pink salmon

1 Granny Smith apple, peeled and cut into
¼-inch pieces

½ cup panko (Japanese breadcrumbs)

1. Make the Dressing. Place the capers, pickles, shallot, and mustard into the bowl of a food processor and pulse to chop. Remove 1 tablespoon of the mixture, place it in a small bowl, and set aside.

2. Place the remaining mixture into a larger bowl, and add the salmon, apple, and panko. Toss to combine. To the small bowl with the reserved relish, add the hot sauce, lemon juice, and yogurt. Stir to combine. (If you like, you could cover and place in the refrigerator to chill overnight to make the next day.)

3. Divide the fish mixture into four ½-cup rounds, then flatten to form cakes. Preheat a nonstick skillet over moderate heat. When the pan is heated, coat with nonstick cooking spray. Add the fish cakes and cook until nicely browned and heated through, about 4 minutes on each side. Serve each cake with 2 tablespoons of the yogurt dressing on the side.

Per Serving: 166.7 calories, 4.7 g total fat, 39.9 mg cholesterol, 321.2 mg sodium, 13.6 g total carbs, 1.1 g dietary fiber, 15.9 g protein

> **Make It a Meal:**
> Serve on a Multigrain Roll (page 302) with a side of carrots and hummus (360 calories) • Enjoy atop a whole-wheat baguette with cucumbers and Homemade Ranch Dressing (page 367) (387 calories)

Warm Tuna with Two-Bean Salad

SLIM IT DOWN: Use half the oil (40 calories).

This is a quick and tasty warm salad that also works great as a cold leftover the next day. I simply add 2 more cups of cold torn lettuce, toss, and—lunch! Use the thin French green beans known as haricots verts if you can find them. If not, regular green beans work just fine.

Makes 4 Servings:
1½ cups per serving

20 Minutes to Prepare and Cook

2 tbsp olive oil

½ cup finely diced red onion

1 clove garlic, minced fine

1 can (15 ounces) cannellini beans, drained and rinsed

2 cups green beans, ends trimmed and cut into half

4 cups torn leaf lettuce

½ tsp black pepper

1 lemon, zested and juiced

10 ounces low-sodium canned tuna, packed in water and drained

1. Heat a sauté pan over medium heat, then add the oil. Once hot, add the onion and garlic, and cook, stirring constantly, for 1 to 2 minutes. Do not let them brown.

2. Add the cannellini and green beans and continue cooking for 1 minute. Add the lettuce just to wilt, then season with pepper and lemon zest and juice. Add the tuna and toss to combine. Serve warm or cold.

Per Serving: 266.4 calories, 8.6 g total fat, 31.3 mg cholesterol, 176.9 mg sodium, 24 g total carbs, 7.6 g dietary fiber, 23.9 g protein

Make It a Meal:
Pair with a whole-wheat baguette (406 calories) • Serve with whole-grain crackers (386 calories)

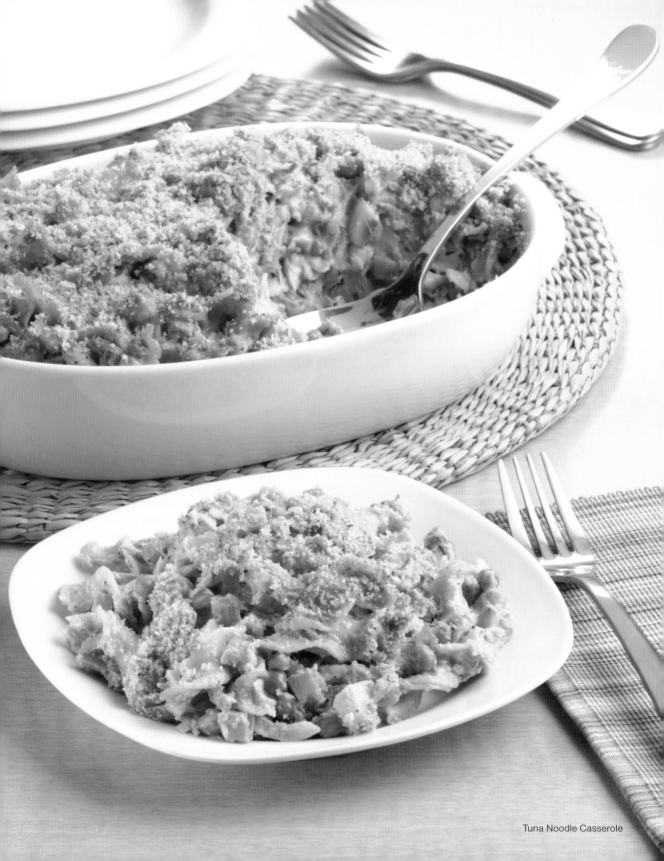

Tuna Noodle Casserole

Tuna Noodle Casserole

Tuna noodle casserole is one of those pour-and-dump recipes left over from the 1950s. Traditional versions, made with condensed soup and white pasta, are laden with fat and sodium. Vegetables were scarce. The base for this casserole is a lower-fat white sauce made with skim milk, and although we still take shortcuts from the pantry and freezer, it has whole-wheat noodles and two servings of vegetables in every portion. Use frozen vegetables (no need to thaw them) in this recipe to save time. Instead of peas and carrots, try chopped broccoli, green beans, corn, or a mix of your favorites.

Because the casserole is hot going into the oven, this is a quick weekday meal—25 minutes from cutting board to table! If you're in a real hurry, you could serve it from the stovetop, but I like how thick and creamy the sauce gets in the oven, and the layer of breadcrumbs adds a satisfying crunch.

Makes 4 Servings:
1½ cups per serving

25 Minutes to Prepare and Cook

4 ounces whole-wheat noodles

½ slice whole-wheat bread (3 tbsp breadcrumbs)

2 tbsp unsalted light butter

½ cup finely diced onions

1½ cups finely diced mushrooms

2 tbsp flour

1 tsp fresh thyme or ⅓ tsp dried

½ tsp white or black pepper

1½ cups nonfat milk

12 ounces reduced-sodium canned tuna, packed in water, drained

¼ cup shredded Swiss cheese

2 cups frozen peas and carrots

1. Preheat the oven to 350° F. Prepare an 8" x 10" baking dish with nonstick cooking spray. Cook the noodles according to package directions (you'll want 2 cups of cooked noodles); place ½ slice of whole-wheat bread into a small food processor to grind into crumbs.

2. Place the butter into a medium saucepan over moderate heat. Once the butter is melted and hot, add the onions and mushrooms. Cook, stirring, until soft, about 2 minutes. Do not let the onions brown. Sprinkle the flour over the vegetables and stir to combine; cook for 1 minute. Add the thyme and pepper, and then add the milk. Stir until the mixture comes to a boil, then reduce to a simmer and cook for 2 to 3 minutes more.

3. Add the tuna, cheese, peas and carrots, and noodles to the pan and stir to combine. Transfer to the prepared baking dish and top with the breadcrumbs. Bake for 15 to 20 minutes until bubbly. Serve warm.

Per Serving: 307 calories, 6.5 g total fat, 43 mg cholesterol, 234.5 mg sodium, 36.4 g total carbs, 6 g dietary fiber, 30.1 g protein

> **Make It a Meal:**
> Just add a serving of fruit
> and a cup of milk!

Tilapia with Roasted Tomatoes and Lemon

The No. 1 reason why people don't cook fish is because they're afraid of messing it up. They think it's too expensive to experiment with in the kitchen. Tilapia is as easy to cook and as versatile as chicken, and this recipe really proves that simplicity and satisfaction are within reach. You can substitute your favorite white-fleshed fish—such as cod, pollock, or haddock—for the tilapia. This is such a beautiful meal! Your family will wonder what they've done to deserve it.

Online Bonus: Learn how to thinly slice (chiffonade) basil. Visit SparkRecipes.com for Chef Meg's video.

. . . .

Chef Meg's Tip: I am a big believer in saving dishes, but don't try to roast the tomatoes in the same baking dish as the fish. It will make the fish watery.

. . . .

Makes 4 Servings:
3 ounces fish with ½ cup tomatoes

30 Minutes to Prepare and Cook

1 lemon, zested into ½-inch strips (see Note) and juiced

12 ounces tilapia fillets

1 tbsp chopped shallot

2 cups grape tomatoes

½ tsp black or white pepper

2 tbsp shredded fresh basil leaves

1. Preheat the oven to 425° F.

2. Place the lemon zest into a small saucepan, cover with water, and bring to a boil. Drain the water and repeat the process one more time to soften the lemon zest, then slice it into thin, matchstick-style strips.

3. Prepare a baking dish with nonstick cooking spray. Place the fillets in the dish, sprinkle with the chopped shallot, and pour the lemon juice over each piece.

4. Place the tomatoes into a separate baking dish and sprinkle with the pepper.

5. Roast both dishes together in the oven until the fish starts to flake, 9 to 10 minutes. Remove from the oven, sprinkle each fillet with lemon zest and basil, and serve warm alongside the tomatoes.

Note: Use a vegetable peeler to zest the lemon peel into large strips.

Per Serving: 105.4 calories, 2.4 g total fat, 34.3 mg cholesterol, 71.5 mg sodium, 4.5 g total carbs, 1 g dietary fiber, 17.9 g protein

Make It a Meal:
Serve with Quick Herbed Couscous with Vegetables (page 293) (248 calories) • Add on whole-wheat pasta and sautéed spinach (340 calories) • Pair with a roasted sweet potato with margarine and steamed green beans (260 calories)

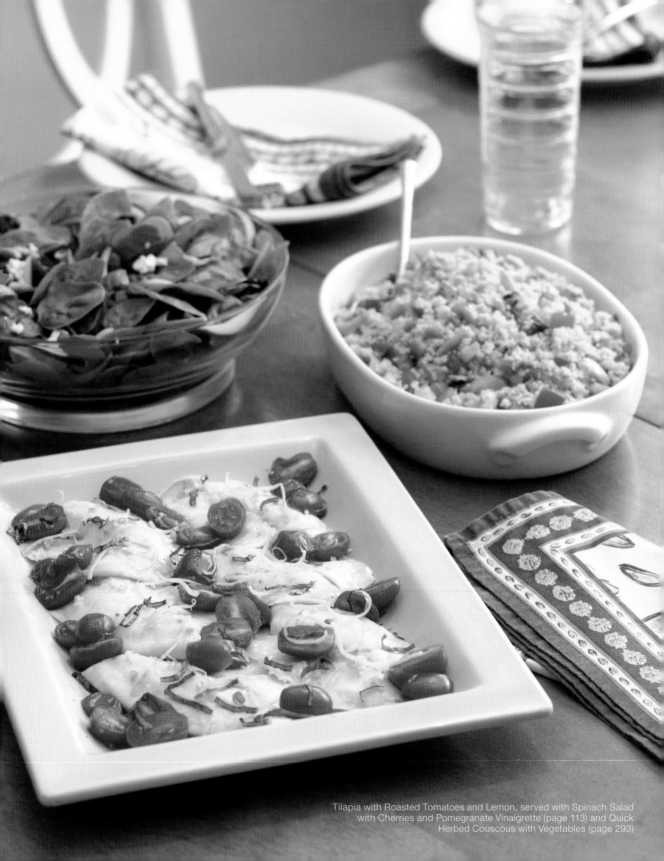

Tilapia with Roasted Tomatoes and Lemon, served with Spinach Salad with Cherries and Pomegranate Vinaigrette (page 113) and Quick Herbed Couscous with Vegetables (page 293)

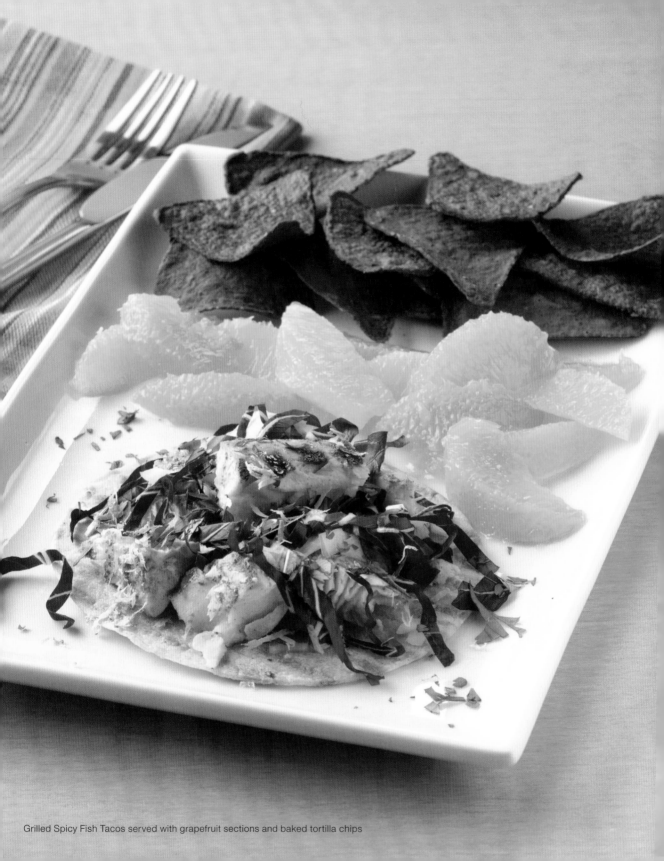

Grilled Spicy Fish Tacos served with grapefruit sections and baked tortilla chips

Grilled Spicy Fish Tacos

Fish tacos are a fresh and tasty alternative to the beef or turkey filling that we're all accustomed to. Because the fish is grilled, I prefer to use a firmer-fleshed fish like mahi-mahi, but you could use any white-fleshed fish.

When making tacos, we tend to pile on the ingredients—especially cheese and sour cream. Traditionally, tacos have just a few ingredients. I simplified this recipe to cut the fat and let the fish be the star of the dish. You can swap Romaine for the radicchio and lemons for the limes, depending on what's in your fridge. You could also substitute chicken for the fish, but give these a try. They're a great way to introduce fish to your kids' diet.

Makes 4 Servings:
   1 tortilla with about 3 ounces fish per serving

15 Minutes to Prepare and Cook

12 ounces mahi-mahi fillets, cut into 4 pieces

1 tbsp Creole Spice Blend (page 370)

Four 6-inch corn tortillas

2 limes, zest removed and reserved

½ red onion, finely diced (¾ cup)

1 cup shredded radicchio

½ bunch roughly chopped cilantro leaves

1. Heat gas grill to medium. Scrape the grill with a wire brush to remove any residue. Wash and pat fish dry, then spray the fillets with non-stick cooking spray and dust with Creole Spice Blend. Place fish on grill and cook 1 minute per inch of thickness (approximately 2 minutes).

2. Spray the tortillas with nonstick cooking spray and place them on grill just to mark with grill marks. Toss zested limes on grill and heat to warm. Turn the fish and continue to cook for 2 to 3 minutes. Toward the end of cooking, remove one lime from grill, cut it in half, and squeeze lime juice over fish. Remove fish and tortillas from grill. Place one-fourth of the fish on top of each tortilla and garnish with the diced onion, radicchio, reserved lime zest, and cilantro. For extra flavor and moisture, squeeze juice from the second lime over dish just before serving.

Per Serving: 171.1 calories, 1.9 g total fat, 80 mg cholesterol, 111 mg sodium, 18.3 g total carbs, 3.2 g dietary fiber, 22.2 g protein

> **Make It a Meal:**
> Serve with cucumber salad with cilantro and vinaigrette (231 calories)
> • Enjoy with baked tortilla chips and tomato salsa (313 calories)

Chew on This: Radicchio

Radicchio (pronounced rah-DEE-kee-oh) looks like a small red cabbage and has a bitter edge when eaten raw, but once wilted or cooked the flavor mellows. Also called Italian chicory, it is often grilled with olive oil or shredded for salads. When buying radicchio, look for firm leaves with no signs of browning.

Coconut-Lime Shrimp

SLIM IT DOWN:
Skip the coconut (62 calories).

Coconut Shrimp are on the menu at every seafood restaurant. Coated in coconut, then deep-fried, those crispy and addictive shrimp are often served by the platterful—sometimes more than a pound of shrimp at a time. Most of the flavor comes from the sweetened coconut and the grease in which it's fried. Here, we add lime zest for a burst of freshness and use unsweetened coconut to keep the sugars low.

Though shrimp is a lean protein, the coconut does contain saturated fat, so this is a meal you probably won't serve every week. Our shrimp are baked, which cuts the fat in half, and we've also reduced the salt. These are great alone or dipped in Coconut-Cilantro Pesto (page 376).

I like to keep the tails on the shrimp; that way if you use them for appetizers they are finger food. Just be sure to keep a bowl nearby for the tails. As a cocktail party food, this dish serves 16 to 20, depending on the size of your shrimp. As a plated first course, I like to serve two on a plate, with the aforementioned pesto and a lightly dressed spinach salad. Or go ahead and serve the shrimp atop a spinach salad. Use the Mango Salsa that we pair with grilled fish (page 223) instead of a dressing.

Makes 4 Servings:
    4 to 5 shrimp per serving

30 Minutes to Prepare and Cook

⅓ cup cornstarch

½ tsp cayenne

3 egg whites, at room temperature

¼ tsp salt

½ cup unsweetened coconut

½ cup panko (Japanese breadcrumbs) or whole-wheat breadcrumbs

2 limes, zested

1 pound extra jumbo (16/20 per pound) shrimp, deveined, tails left on, rinsed and patted dry

1. Preheat oven to 375° F. Prepare a sheet pan with nonstick cooking spray. Set out three pie plates or other flat-bottomed bowls. Combine the cornstarch and half of the cayenne in the first; whip together the egg whites and salt until frothy in the second; and combine the coconut, breadcrumbs, the remainder of the cayenne, and the lime zest in the third.

2. Working with one shrimp at a time, coat the shrimp in the cornstarch, shake off the excess, then dip it in egg mixture, shake off any excess liquid, and finish with the coconut blend.

3. Place on the prepared sheet pan and bake for 8 minutes. Flip the shrimp over and cook until golden brown, 6 to 8 minutes more. Serve warm.

Per Serving: 258.1 calories, 7.7 g total fat, 172.3 g cholesterol, 234.9 mg sodium, 17.6 g total carbs, 1.1 g dietary fiber, 28 g protein

Make It a Meal:
Add brown rice and mixed vegetables (398 calories) • Enjoy with couscous with extra pesto and chopped broccoli (402 calories)

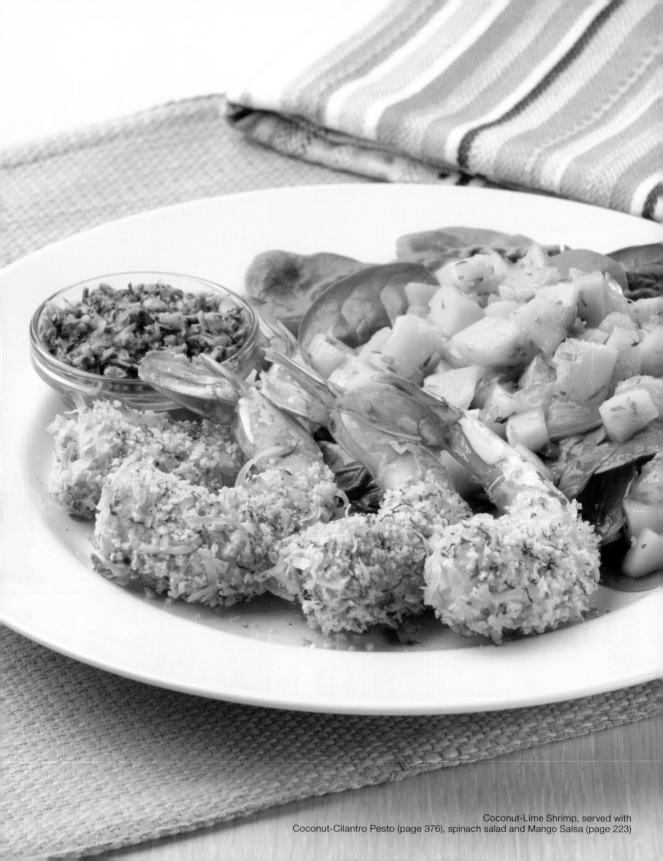

Coconut-Lime Shrimp, served with
Coconut-Cilantro Pesto (page 376), spinach salad and Mango Salsa (page 223)

Skimpy Shrimp Scampi

"Scampi" is the culinary name for a type of lobster, but most of us think of a buttery, garlic shrimp dish when we think of the word. This dish is on most seafood menus and for good reason. It's delicious! Butter, garlic, parsley, and lemon or wine pair well with shrimp, but we've swapped the butter for heart-healthy olive oil (or you could use canola oil).

I really like garlic, but feel free to tone it down by using only two cloves. This is an easily adaptable dish: Try adding 1 minced shallot, 1 cup of halved grape tomatoes, or ¼ cup sliced roasted peppers instead of garlic. You could also serve alongside sautéed spinach.

Make it easier on yourself and buy deveined shrimp. If you can't find them, just follow the directions for cleaning shrimp in the Note.

Online bonus: Learn how to peel and devein shrimp. Visit SparkRecipes.com for Chef Meg's video.

Makes 4 Servings:
about 6 shrimp per serving

30 Minutes to Prepare and Cook

2 tbsp olive oil

2 to 3 cloves garlic, peeled and chopped

1 pound headless raw shrimp, peeled and deveined (21–25 count per pound) (see Note)

1 lemon, juiced

1 large bunch flat-leaf parsley, washed, dried, and chopped (¾ cup)

¼ tsp red pepper flakes

1. Place a large sauté pan over moderate heat and add the oil. Once warm, add the garlic and sauté until soft, about 1 minute. Do not let it brown.

2. Add the shrimp and sauté until cooked (the shrimp will be firm and pink), 3 to 4 minutes. Stir in the lemon juice and parsley. Cook just 3 to 4 minutes longer (do not overcook or the shrimp will be tough). Remove from heat and season with the red pepper flakes.

Note: If shrimp is not deveined prepare over a sink under running cold water. Using a paring knife, run the tip of the blade just under the surface down the back of the shrimp and remove the vein. Discard the vein. It is very important to wash hands and all utensils when you've finished cleaning the shrimp.

Per Serving: 191.7 calories, 9.1 g total fat, 172.3 mg cholesterol, 174.5 mg sodium, 3.2 g total carbs, 0.5 g dietary fiber, 23.5 g protein

Make It a Meal:
Add to whole-wheat pasta with roasted tomatoes and steamed spinach (442 calories) • Serve with whole-wheat couscous with artichokes and roasted peppers (340 calories)

MEATLESS MAINS, PASTA & PIZZA

MEATLESS MAINS

Here's the thing about labels: they're meant to fit us all into tidy little boxes, but that's like trying to squeeze a square peg into a round hole. "Flexitarian," "vegetarian," "vegan," or "omnivore." They're all just names. If you choose to align yourself with a specific way of eating and that label suits you, use it. But don't feel obligated or pressured to define yourself based on your food preferences. Eat what you like, and eat what satisfies you—and keeps you healthy.

Although there are 5 million vegetarians in America, my family is not among them. We do, however, eat meat-free meals at least a few times a week.

We're not swapping beef burgers for soy patties or turkey for Tofurky. Our meatless meals, like all of our meals, are based on natural, satisfying, delicious foods that don't come from a box or the freezer. In addition to beans in soups, stews, burritos, and salads, we enjoy omelets and frittatas, veggie pizzas, grilled vegetable sandwiches, pasta, hearty salads, and

lasagna. You probably already have a few meat-free dishes in your recipe box—you just don't think about them as being "vegetarian."

SparkPeople Cooking Challenge:
Make a meat-free meal for dinner this week, but don't draw attention to the fact that it's "vegetarian." Did anyone notice?

Though it sounds trendy, a less meat-dependent lifestyle is one that's been around for generations, and remains the norm in many parts of the world. Back in the day, meat was most often eaten in side-dish portions, while other food groups took up the rest of the plate. Beans, vegetables, and grains were the bulk of a meal, while the meat added flavor. Many nutrition experts agree that our health would benefit if we took this "old-fashioned" approach to eating.

According to experts, vegetarians have lower rates of cancer, heart disease, hypertension, diabetes, and asthma. You don't have to forgo meat for the rest of your days on earth to enjoy many of the health benefits of a meatless diet.

The trick to healthy vegetarian meals is to replace the meat with other forms of lean protein. French fries with a side of onion rings would technically constitute a meat-free meal, but no one would argue that it's more nutritious than a portion of pork tenderloin over herbed couscous with broccoli and green beans. Giving up meat simply to lose weight is a plan that often backfires, as people tend to substitute high-fat cheesy entrées and unhealthy vegetable side dishes.

Eating less meat and more grains, beans, fruits, and veggies means you'll be consuming fewer calories, less saturated fat and cholesterol, and higher amounts of vitamins, minerals, and fiber. And that adds up to a lot of health benefits.

OUBACHE is three pounds from her weight-loss goal and embracing a "flexitarian" attitude of eating meat on rare occasions. "We eat several meatless meals per week," says the avid gardener from Indiana. "I find the less meat I eat, the less I want. I will probably never be a vegetarian but I feel good about eating less meat."

The 2010 USDA Dietary Guidelines for Americans includes diet plans for vegetarians and vegans for the first time, and they encourage swapping out proteins high in solid fat for those that are lower in solid fat, including legumes and soy products. Research has shown that eating a few meatless meals per week can lower the risk of heart disease and may even prolong life. Why? Well, vegetarian meals are usually rich in unrefined carbohydrates, vitamins, minerals, and fiber, while low in cholesterol and saturated fat.

During the warmer weather months meat-free meals are really my favorite way to cook, or should I say *not* cook. How wonderful is it, after a long, hot day spent in the garden, to wash tomatoes, peppers, and cucumbers and give them a whirl in a food processor, add some vinegar and whole-wheat bread and—can you say gazpacho?

SparkPeople Cooking Challenge:
A national health campaign known as Meatless Monday, in association with the Johns Hopkins Bloomberg School of Public Health, promotes cutting out meat one day each week. Join the campaign. If Mondays don't work for you, pick another day of the week. Start with build-your-own-burrito, an omelet bar, or pasta-as-you-like-it, before branching out to more adventurous meat-free meals.

You'll notice that vegetarian cooking opens your eyes to an entire world of new ingredients and cooking techniques. Without the flavor of meat dominating the meal, you'll really taste the other components. You might find that it's the cumin you use in your taco seasoning that satisfies you, rather than the ground beef. Or that the peanut sauce in your chicken stir-fry is just as good on tofu. Or that the tomatoes from your garden really shine in a meat-free pasta dish.

With 70 pounds gone, JULIEIRENE has completely transformed her eating habits and discovered her meat-free side. She went from eating meat regularly to just eating fish and seafood a couple of times a week. "It became a long-term lifestyle for me, for a variety of reasons," she says. "One is that I feel like reducing my meat consumption has actually enhanced my creativity in the kitchen and challenged me to think outside of the traditional plate, which can be a lot of fun!" Far from feeling deprived, she says her new way of eating truly satisfies her, and she has more energy than ever.

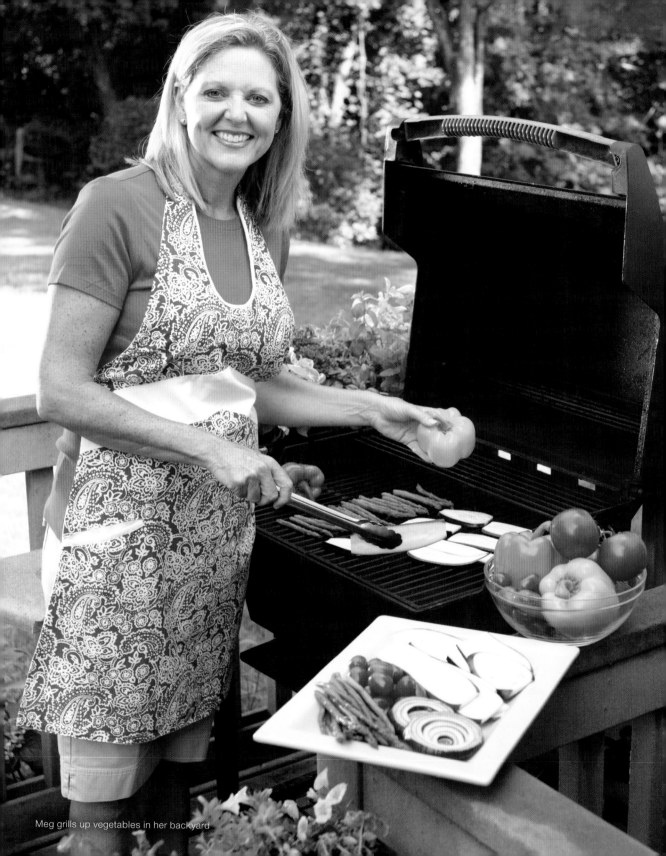

Meg grills up vegetables in her backyard

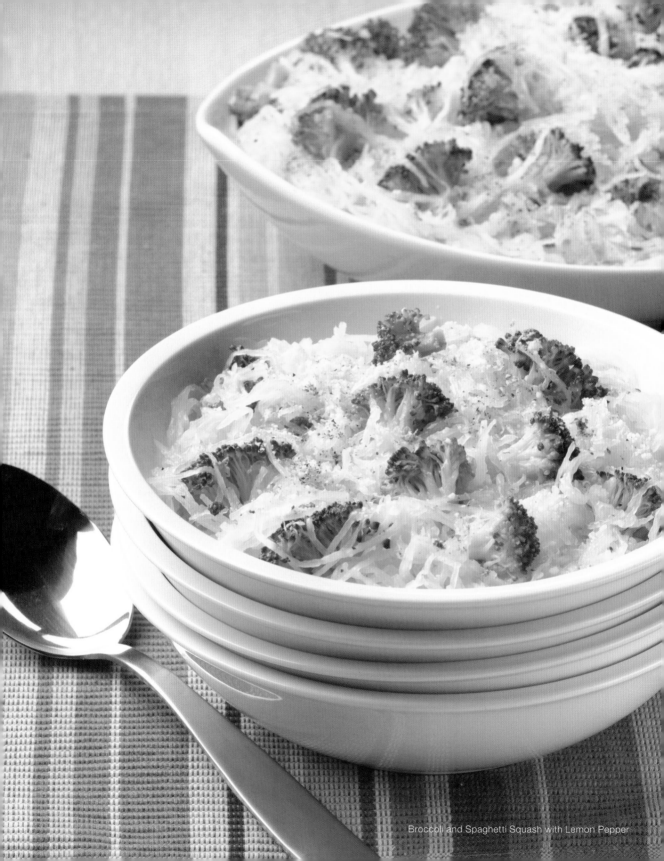

Broccoli and Spaghetti Squash with Lemon Pepper

Broccoli and Spaghetti Squash with Lemon Pepper

If you are constantly on the search for the perfect pasta replacement, look no further than the garden. The spaghetti squash is a great stand-in for the real thing, for about a quarter of the calories. Simple, quick, and tasty, this "pasta" is ready in less time than it takes to boil water. You can serve it with your favorite tomato sauce—I like to use the Weeknight Spaghetti sauce (page 256) and top it with some Turkey Meatballs (page 205).

It's even better as we serve it here: with broccoli, a bit of lemon pepper, and Parmesan for a side dish or light supper. Use the florets from one head of broccoli or a 10-ounce bag of frozen broccoli. You could also make the squash without the broccoli. It's just as tasty. If you don't have any of our Lemon-Pepper Rub (page 375) on hand just add ½ teaspoon pepper and zest of one lemon.

Makes 4 Servings:
2 cups per serving

30 Minutes to Prepare and Cook

1 spaghetti squash, stem end trimmed, halved lengthwise (about 2½ to 3 pounds)

1 head broccoli, large stalks removed, florets cut into bite-size pieces

¼ cup grated Parmesan cheese

1 tsp Lemon-Pepper Rub

1. Scoop out the seeds of the squash with a spoon.

2. Pierce the skin of the squash with a fork, place it cut-side down in a dish, and microwave on high for 6 to 8 minutes. Remove, and set aside until cool enough to handle.

3. Using a fork, scrape out the flesh of the squash into a serving bowl. Toss in the broccoli, Parmesan, and Lemon-Pepper Rub. Serve warm.

Per Serving: 113.8 calories, 2.8 g total fat, 4.9 mg cholesterol, 185.4 mg sodium, 18.4 g total carbs, 6.8 g dietary fiber, 8.2 g protein

> **Make It a Meal:**
> Pair it with roasted chicken and a Multigrain Roll (page 302) (312 calories)
> • Enjoy with cannellini beans and whole-wheat pasta (318 calories)

Slow-Cooker Vegetable Curry

Slow cookers aren't just for meat! This is a tasty, affordable one-pot vegetarian meal that's filling and perfect for your slow cooker. You can also add shrimp during the last 20 minutes of cooking, if you like. If the dish is a little too spicy for the kids, add 1 tablespoon of plain yogurt to their serving. Serve with a glass of milk and a cucumber salad.

Makes 8 Servings:
1½ cups per serving

25 Minutes to Prepare; 6 Hours to Cook

1 tbsp canola oil

4 medium carrots (about 2 cups), sliced ¼-inch thick

1 onion, thinly sliced

3 garlic cloves, peeled and thinly sliced

2 tbsp curry powder

½ tsp cayenne

½ tsp turmeric

4 to 5 Yukon Gold or red potatoes, quartered

8 ounces fresh or frozen green beans

3 cups canned chickpeas, drained and rinsed

2 large tomatoes, diced (1 cup)

2 cups vegetable stock

½ cup frozen peas

½ cup light coconut milk

1. In a sauté pan, heat the oil until moderately hot. Add the carrots and onion and sauté for 3 to 4 minutes. Add the garlic, curry powder, cayenne, and turmeric to the pan. Continue to cook for 2 minutes more or until the spices become fragrant.

2. Remove the vegetables from the pan and transfer to a slow cooker. Add the potatoes, green beans, chickpeas, tomatoes, and vegetable stock to the slow cooker.

3. Set the slow cooker on low and cook for 5 ½ hours. Add the peas and coconut milk and cook for 15 minutes more.

Per Serving: 179.1 calories, 5.3 g total fat, 0 mg cholesterol, 349.8 mg sodium, 27.2 total carbs, 7.3 g dietary fiber, 6.4 g protein

> **Make It a Meal:**
> Serve atop brown rice (358 calories)
> • Pair with whole-wheat pasta
> (352 calories).

TAKE ON TOFU

I don't cook tofu very much, but Stepfanie is a vegetarian and prepares it often. She lived in South Korea for a year and even learned how to make it from scratch. She offers suggestions for learning to like tofu, a versatile and affordable protein.

Few foods are as polarizing as tofu: say the word and watch as noses crinkle or mouths water. I fall on the tofu-lover side of the spectrum, but I think we might be of the minority.

Tofu, also known as soybean curd, is made by soaking, boiling, blending, and straining soybeans, then adding a coagulating agent and pressing it. Think of it like this: cheese is to milk as tofu is to soy milk.

Really whets the appetite, doesn't it?

Scratch that. Think of tofu as the other white meat. Like chicken, it's a versatile protein, a blank canvas upon which to test your culinary prowess. I have substituted tofu in just about every chicken recipe I have.

There are basically two kinds of tofu: soft and firm. Let's just focus on firm tofu, which is easier for beginners to cook. You'll find "firm" and "extra-firm" styles, but actual textures vary greatly by brand. Firm-style tofu is best for stir-fries or for replacing meat in a recipe. These varieties take on the flavor of the dish into which they are incorporated. So you can spice, sauce, or marinate to your heart's content—you decide the flavor. Firm varieties of tofu are available in both refrigerated and shelf-stable packages. Just open, drain the water, slice, and cook as desired. If you don't use the whole block at once, cover the rest with water and store (tightly covered) in the refrigerator for up to five days, changing the water daily.

Three Terrific Tofu Tips

1. *Press it.* Tofu is packed in water, which needs to be drained before using. I also recommend pressing it for a crispier finished product and to prevent watering down your flavorings. Slice the tofu as desired, then place on a lint-free dish towel and top with another towel. Place a heavy object atop the tofu (I use my cutting board), and let it sit for up to 30 minutes. For a quicker version, you can use your hands to gently press down on the tofu to squeeze out the water

2. *Freeze it.* Freezing then thawing tofu changes the texture. It becomes denser and chewier. I crumble and sauté thawed blocks of tofu with onions and garlic, then throw them into tomato sauce, chili, or soup. It adds a texture similar to ground meat. (Place in a lint-free towel and squeeze out excess water before using.)

3. *Crisp it.* When sautéed with a bit of nonstick cooking spray or broiled in the oven, tofu gets slightly crispy and crunchy on the outside just like meat does. The texture makes a big difference in the taste. Use just a bit of oil because tofu is like a sponge; it will soak up as much oil as you give it!

Pad Thai

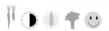

SLIM IT DOWN: Leave off the peanuts (40 calories).

The freezer section of the grocery store is your friend! In as much time as it would take to call and order Thai takeout, you can make a healthier version of Pad Thai at home. It only requires one specialty item, tamarind paste, which is available in the Asian food section of most larger supermarkets. Tamarind is a fruit with a sweet-and-sour taste that is native to Asia. The paste will keep in your pantry for months, but if you can't find it, substitute an equal amount of grated fresh ginger.

This version is vegetarian, but you could easily swap chicken for the tofu. I used whole-wheat pasta noodles instead of the traditional rice noodles. Not only are they easier to find, they contain more fiber. Likewise, you can substitute whatever vegetables you like for the Asian-style frozen medley; broccoli, shredded carrots, broccoli slaw, and peas are good choices.

Makes 4 Servings:
1½ cups per serving

30 Minutes to Prepare and Cook

For the Sauce:

1 lime, zested and juiced

1 tbsp light soy sauce

1 tbsp rice-wine vinegar

¼ tsp cayenne

¼ cup chopped cilantro

4 garlic cloves, smashed and chopped

2 tbsp tamarind paste (1 ounce)

1 tbsp smooth natural peanut butter

1 block firm tofu, drained and cubed (see page 245 on working with tofu)

1 tbsp canola oil

One 12-ounce bag Asian medley frozen vegetables (green beans, broccoli, onions, and mushrooms)

6 ounces whole-wheat spaghetti, cooked

2 tbsp peanuts, unsalted (see Note)

1. In a small bowl, combine the lime zest and juice, soy sauce, vinegar, cayenne, cilantro, garlic, and tamarind paste. Pour half of this mixture into another bowl. Add the peanut butter to one bowl and the tofu to the other. Mix the peanut butter into the sauce until smooth.

2. Heat the oil in a wok or flat-bottomed skillet. Once hot, add the tofu and cook over high heat until crispy on all sides. Remove from skillet and set aside.

3. Add the vegetables to the heated wok and stir-fry for 1 to 2 minutes. Return the tofu to the pan and continue to stir-fry for 2 minutes more. Add the peanut-butter sauce and the cooked noodles, then stir well and cook just to heat through. Garnish with the peanuts and serve hot.

Note: Concerned about peanut allergies? Stepfanie makes Pad Thai with almonds and almond butter. Soynut or sunflower seed butter is also a good substitute for peanut butter.

Per Serving: 312.8 calories, 14.8 g total fat, 0 mg cholesterol, 169.4 mg sodium, 42.7 g total carbs, 8 g dietary fiber, 21.8 g protein

> **Make It a Meal:**
> Just add fruit and a cup of milk.

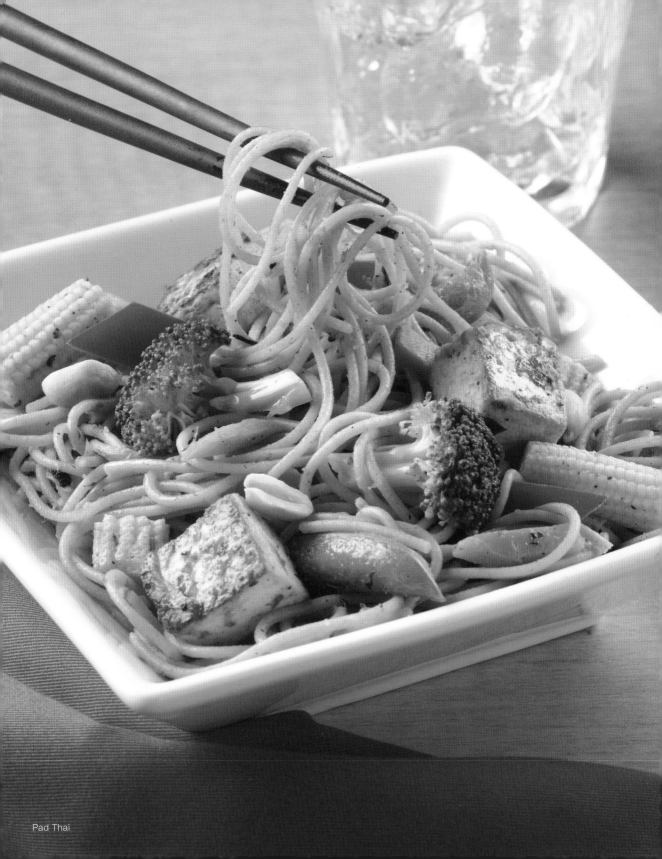

Pad Thai

Stepfanie's Quinoa–Black Bean Casserole

This recipe came about because Stepfanie had just made vegetable enchiladas and had leftovers, plus quinoa from earlier in the week. Her experiment yielded a hearty, delicious meal. She cooked up a batch of dried black beans seasoned with onions, garlic, chiles, and spices. If you use canned beans, you might need more spices. Serve this with steamed broccoli or wilted spinach and a dollop of light sour cream or plain Greek yogurt. (For more on quinoa, see Chew on This on page 296.)

Makes 8 Servings
1 heaping cup per serving

40 Minutes to Prepare and Cook

1 cup cooked quinoa

3 cups cooked black beans (or two 15-ounce cans, drained and rinsed)

2 large sweet potatoes, shredded

1 cup shredded low-fat cheddar cheese

1 tbsp ground cumin

Liberal pinches salt and pepper

2 eggs

1 cup salsa

2 tbsp fresh cilantro, chopped, for garnish

1. Preheat oven to 350° F. Prepare a 9" x 9" casserole dish with nonstick cooking spray.

2. In a large bowl, mix together the quinoa, black beans, sweet potato, ½ cup of the cheese, and the cumin, salt, and pepper. In a small bowl, mix together the eggs and the salsa. Pour the salsa mixture over the vegetables, then pour everything into the prepared casserole dish.

3. Sprinkle the remaining cheese over the top and bake, uncovered, for 30 minutes. Garnish with the cilantro.

Per Serving: 257.4 calories, 4.3 g total fat, 72 mg cholesterol, 301.8 mg sodium, 40.9 g total carbs, 9.6 g dietary fiber, 15.4 g protein

Make It a Meal:
Serve over wilted spinach (264 calories) • Enjoy with a tomato salad (283 calories)

Baked Egg Cups

SLIM IT DOWN:
Skip the cheese (35 calories).

Eggs aren't just for breakfast. They make a great, quick, affordable supper, too. This dish is a variation on the classic shirred eggs, which are eggs baked in a casserole. Traditionally, shirred eggs are cooked with butter, milk, or cream; but I saved calories by using tomatoes instead, and ramekins in a water bath, to keep the eggs from drying out while cooking. Just turn on your tea kettle when you start the tomatoes, then pour the hot water into a baking dish around the outside of the ramekins. Try changing up the recipe by including spinach, turkey bacon, eggplant, asparagus, cheese, fresh basil—your possibilities are endless.

Makes 4 Servings:
1 egg per serving

30 Minutes to Prepare and Cook

1 can (14.5 ounces) diced tomatoes, drained, or 4 plum (Roma) tomatoes, chopped

1 tsp dried basil or 1 tbsp fresh basil, chopped

Pinch of salt

¼ tsp pepper

2 slices reduced-fat mozzarella cheese

4 eggs

1. Preheat oven to 350° F; fill a tea kettle with water and set to boil. Place the tomatoes in a sauté pan and season with the basil, salt, and pepper. Sauté for about 5 minutes, allowing the moisture to evaporate and the flavors to concentrate.

2. Prepare four ½-cup ramekins with nonstick cooking spray. (If you don't have ramekins, which are straight-sided ceramic baking dishes, any ovenproof ½-cup baking containers will do.) Place one-fourth of the tomato mixture into each ramekin, top with half a slice cheese, then crack 1 egg over the mixture.

3. Place the ramekins in an ovenproof baking dish and place the dish in the oven, setting it toward the front of the rack. Pour hot water into the pan until the water reaches halfway up the ramekins and then carefully push the pan to the center of the oven. Bake for 15 minutes, until whites are set but the yolks are still soft. Serve the eggs in the ramekins.

Per Serving: 123.3 calories, 7.5 g total fat, 220 mg cholesterol, 113.1 mg sodium, 3.7 g total carbs, 0.8 g dietary fiber, 9.8 g protein

Make It a Meal:
Serve with sautéed spinach and whole-wheat toast (253 calories) • Eat with steamed cauliflower with pesto and whole-wheat pasta (285 calories)

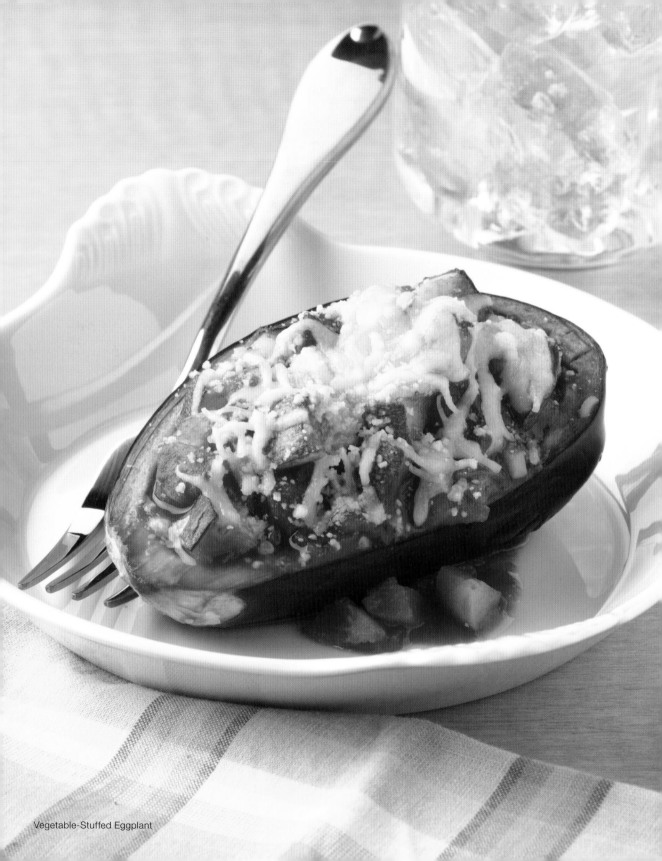

Vegetable-Stuffed Eggplant

Vegetable-Stuffed Eggplant

This was an excellent member-submitted recipe that required very few tweaks to improve its healthy profile. I reduced the oil to 1 tablespoon, added more herbs, and left out the salt. I also added another vegetable: zucchini. This dish is surprisingly filling. I recommend serving it with a side salad for a vegetarian meal. (You'll never miss the meat!) You can also add ½ cup pitted and chopped green olives to the vegetable mixture before baking. However, you shouldn't do this if you're watching your sodium intake.

Makes 4 Servings:
½ eggplant per serving

45 Minutes to Prepare and Cook

2 small eggplants (see Note)

1 tbsp olive oil

1 onion, finely chopped

1 garlic clove, peeled and minced

1 small zucchini, chopped

Pinch of black pepper

½ cup tomato sauce

1 cup low-sodium petite diced canned tomatoes (or 4 plum [Roma] tomatoes, peeled, deseeded, and diced)

½ teaspoon dried thyme

1 tsp dried basil

1 cup shredded Monterey Jack cheese

4 tbsp grated Parmesan cheese

1. Preheat oven to 375° F. Prepare a baking pan with nonstick cooking spray.

2. Trim the stems from the eggplant, and cut them in half lengthwise. Cut the pulp from the center of each half, leaving about ½-inch shell of flesh.

3. Cube the eggplant pulp into ½-inch pieces. Place a large sauté pan over moderate heat, then add the oil. Once the oil is hot, add the onion, garlic, zucchini, black pepper, and the cubed eggplant. Cook, stirring until very tender, about 5 to 7 minutes. Add the tomato sauce, tomatoes, thyme, and basil; and heat through.

4. Lightly spray the cut edges of the eggplant with nonstick cooking spray, then spoon one-quarter of the vegetable mixture into each shell. Top each eggplant with one-fourth of the Monterey Jack and Parmesan.

5. Place the stuffed eggplants in the prepared baking pan and bake until the eggplant is hot and the cheese is bubbly, 20 to 25 minutes.

Note: Use small eggplants of about ½ pound each if you can. The larger the eggplant, the more bitter it will be. The small, thin Japanese eggplants would also work well here.

Per Serving: 208.8 calories, 9.8 g total fat, 16.6 mg cholesterol, 194.2 mg sodium, 24.4 g total carbs, 8.3 g dietary fiber, 9.6 g protein

Make It a Meal:
Cook up some roasted chicken with whole-wheat couscous (426 calories) • Enjoy with sautéed tofu with pesto and whole-wheat pasta (455 calories)

GOOD-FOR-YOU PASTA

Talk about satisfaction: a bowl of pasta on a cold night is the definition of comfort food. In our house, we reach for pasta on our busy nights, or the rare nights when the pantry and fridge seem almost bare. If we're low on fresh produce, I know I can always make a healthy and delicious pasta dish from the pantry. Though most us associate pasta with jarred sauce, a pound of ground beef, and a box of noodles, it can be so much more. With or without meat, depending on your budget, food preferences, and inventory, pasta is a blank canvas for a novice or advanced cook.

Look beyond the Italian borders, like KALORIE-KILLAH did. Two monthlong meat-free challenges helped her feel more comfortable in the kitchen. Having lost 37 pounds using SparkPeople, she's still a meat lover but says vegetarian pasta is a go-to meal. Some of her favorite creations: pasta with spicy peanut tofu and veggies and a makeover of spicy Southwestern cream pasta from one of her favorite restaurants.

Our family has made the switch to whole-wheat pasta, and yours can, too. Whole-wheat pasta is packed full of fiber, which makes you feel fuller, and it's a whole grain, which takes longer to digest. Making the switch to whole-wheat pasta is a simple one, but it adds a boost of nutrition and fiber to your meal.

For some people, the nutty taste takes some getting used to, but not for SLIMKIM2B's family. "The switch to whole-wheat pasta was easy for my family. I bought it once and they were hooked," she said. "We like it much more than regular white pasta." Down to 150 from an all-time high of 275 pounds, the Connecticut resident now bulks up the family's pasta dishes with plenty of veggies to compensate for smaller, controlled portions. No one complains!

	Whole-wheat Spaghetti	Regular Spaghetti
Calories	174	197
Fat (g)	1	1
Fiber (g)	6	2
Carbs (g)	37	40

SparkPeople Cooking Challenge:
Swap half whole-wheat pasta for white the next time you make spaghetti. Add more whole-wheat each time you cook pasta, eventually weaning yourself off the white variety.

PASTA 101

A few small swaps will lighten up even Mom's spaghetti and meatballs and bring pasta back onto the healthy cook's menu; but before you take on that recipe, here are a few tips for successful healthy pasta.

Oil and water don't mix. If you add oil to water—even pasta cooking water—it will float on the surface, no matter what Momma and Grandma told you. The oil does not coat the pasta until you drain the water, then it clings to the pasta and prevents the sauce from sticking. Save the calories and skip the oil—and the salt. If you really want to keep your pasta from sticking, use ample amounts of water—at least 3 parts water to 1 part pasta.

Listen to the Italians—pasta should be cooked *al dente,* which means "to the tooth." Cooking should stop when the pasta feels firm to the bite. Throwing pasta against your refrigerator is not a good test for doneness; it only makes a mess of your refrigerator.

If you like to roll and twirl your spaghetti around on a spoon, ignore this suggestion, but I prefer to break my long pasta in half before cooking. I really don't want to sweep up dry pasta off my kitchen floor, so I roll the pasta into a kitchen towel, snap it in half, and then drop it in the boiling water to cook.

The most difficult decision when cooking pasta is penne or linguini, rigatoni or orzo. For dishes with thin or smooth sauces, I prefer long pasta such as spaghetti, fettuccine, or angel hair. For chunky sauces, I like shorter pastas like penne, farfalle (bowties), or fusilli (twists). For creamy sauces, I choose pasta with nooks, crannies, and ridges, like elbow macaroni, penne rigate, or shells, to catch more sauce. In soups and pasta salads where the pasta is not the main ingredient, I reach for orzo, ditalini, or another mini pasta. Of course, I always buy the whole-wheat varieties. Look at the ingredient list. It shouldn't have more than whole-wheat flour and eggs or water on the list. If your "whole-grain" pasta has ingredients you can't pronounce, swap it for another kind.

Busy Night? Pasta to the Rescue!

Pasta is quite the versatile whole grain, and your topping choices aren't limited to white or red sauce. For those truly busy nights when there's no time to open a cookbook, pasta is a lifesaver.

When dinner emergencies arise, have a plan ready. For REKAREKS, that plan has just five ingredients: "I always cook pasta, throw in a protein, spinach, goat cheese, and top with olive oil." A healthy dinner is on the table in 20 minutes or less.

Here are some great tips for no-recipe pasta meals. For four servings, you'll need:

- 2 to 4 cups of cooked vegetables (try tomatoes, zucchini, spinach, mushrooms, peppers, or broccoli)

- 1 pound of protein (grilled chicken, extra-lean ground turkey or beef, pork loin, or shrimp)

- 2 cups uncooked pasta

- ¼ cup grated cheese or pesto

Add a drizzle of good olive oil, a squeeze of lemon juice, or a sprinkle of fresh herbs to the pasta, top with your ingredients, and dinner is served—no "recipe" needed.

Ten Healthy Ways to Top Pasta

You don't have to rely on sauce to top your pasta. Think about flavor combinations you've tried in restaurants or in other dishes. If blue cheese, spinach, dried cranberries, and walnuts work on a salad, why not in pasta? Here are our favorite healthy toppings.

1. Grilled vegetables, including eggplant, shallots, tomatoes, peppers, and summer squash.

2. Grilled chicken, roasted peppers, and artichokes.

3. Steamed zucchini and summer squash with parsley pesto.

4. Sautéed portobello or shiitake mushrooms with baby spinach and Parmesan shavings.

5. Grilled or broiled shrimp with grape tomatoes, fresh basil, and feta cheese.

6. Roasted chicken with sautéed radicchio and asparagus.

7. Arugula with yellow tomatoes and fresh mozzarella.

8. Turkey sausage with cannellini or fava beans and arugula.

9. Steamed broccoli rabe with sautéed lean ham, shallots, and garlic.

10. Roasted butternut squash, spinach, and toasted pumpkin seeds or slivered almonds.

Spinach and Tomato Pasta Salad

SLIM IT DOWN:
Ditch the pasta (140 calories) or the feta (100 calories).

Most pasta salads are heavy on the pasta and light on everything else. This version, which can be served warm or cold, includes a hefty portion of vegetables, and a full serving of cheese to boost the protein content. If you're watching your sodium intake, we suggest replacing the feta with a naturally lower-sodium cheese like mozzarella.

Makes 6 Servings:
2 cups per serving

15 Minutes to Prepare and Cook

8 ounces small whole-wheat pasta, such as ditalini or orzo

4 cups baby spinach

8 ounces feta cheese, crumbled

2 tbsp capers, drained

1 pound grape tomatoes

¼ tsp black pepper

2 tbsp shredded Parmesan or Manchego cheese

1. Cook pasta according to package directions until it is al dente (firm to the bite). Do not add salt to the pasta water.

2. While the pasta is cooking, place the spinach, feta, and capers in a large bowl. Before draining pasta, add ¼ cup of the pasta cooking liquid to the bowl; toss to combine.

3. Place the tomatoes in the bottom of a colander. Once the pasta is cooked, drain it over the tomatoes for a quick blanch.

4. Toss the tomatoes and pasta with the spinach mixture. Season with black pepper and garnish with shredded cheese. Serve warm or cold.

Per serving: 267.1 calories, 8.9 g total fat, 35 mg cholesterol, 559.8 mg sodium, 33 g total carbs, 2.6 g dietary fiber, 12 g protein

Make It a Meal:
Add a serving of rotisserie chicken (417 calories) • Dish it up with cannellini beans (387 calories).

Weeknight Spaghetti

SLIM IT DOWN:
Swap spaghetti squash for the pasta (138 calories).

Be honest: do you make your own tomato sauce? It's okay, most of us don't. In a pinch, low-sodium jarred sauces can be a lifesaver. But even on busy nights, it doesn't take much time to make a from-scratch sauce, and the taste is incomparable.

When you cook from scratch, you are in control. No sugar, no salt, no corn syrup. Extra garlic, no hot pepper flakes, a sprinkle of oregano. Your sauce will be exactly how you like it, and you won't have to scrutinize the label and wonder what additives and preservatives you're eating.

This is a great basic sauce, and it is ready in the same time as your pasta. My boys love it with Turkey Meatballs (page 205). My husband prefers a bit of Italian sausage in his, and I like adding sautéed vegetables.

I like to use a vegetable peeler to create strips of Parmesan. Grated cheese can melt into the sauce, but the strips (or shreds) keep their bite so you really taste the cheese's pungent, salty flavor.

Makes 4 servings:
¾ cup pasta and sauce per serving

30 Minutes to Prepare and Cook

1 tbsp olive oil

½ onion, finely diced (½ cup)

4 cloves garlic, smashed and chopped

One 28-ounce can low-sodium petite diced tomatoes

¼ tsp red pepper flakes

1 tsp dried basil or 1 tbsp fresh, shredded

8 ounces whole-wheat spaghetti

¼ cup grated Parmesan cheese

1. Place 2 quarts of water in a large pot and bring to a boil. Heat a large sauté pan over moderate heat, then add the oil. Once warm, add the onion and garlic to the pan and sauté until the onion becomes soft, 3 to 4 minutes.

2. Add the tomatoes, pepper flakes, and basil. Simmer, stirring occasionally, for 15 minutes. Cook the spaghetti according to package directions, but do not salt the water.

3. Remove the sauce from the heat. Puree if preferred or leave chunky. Serve over the pasta with the Parmesan.

Per serving: 303.4 calories, 57.3 g total fat, 4.9 mg cholesterol, 117.5 mg sodium, 47 g total carbs, 3 g dietary fiber, 10.6 g protein

Make It a Meal:
Serve with chickpeas and sautéed spinach (450 calories) • Pair with Turkey Meatballs (page 205) and roasted peppers (460 calories).

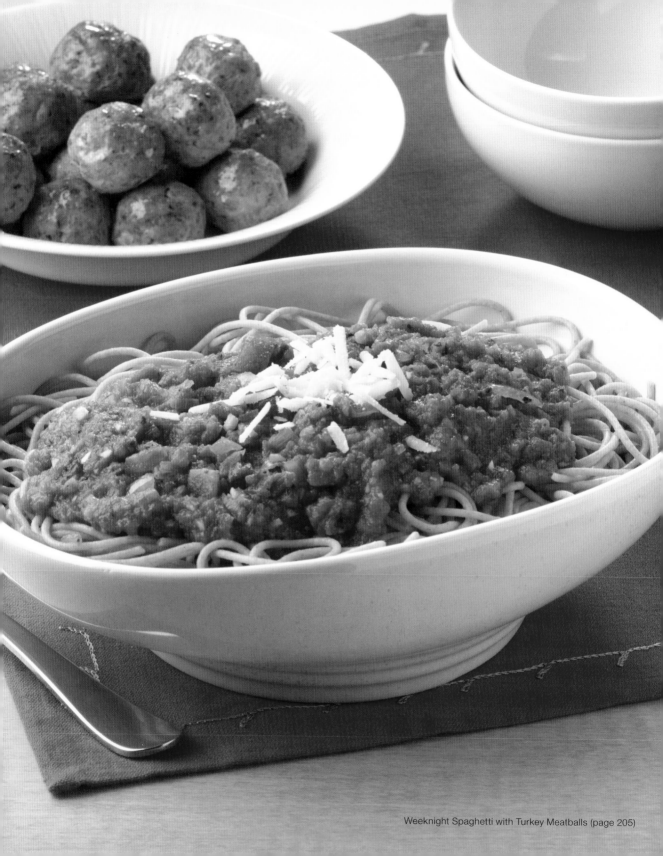

Weeknight Spaghetti with Turkey Meatballs (page 205)

Ratatouille with Whole-Wheat Pasta

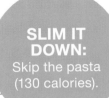

SLIM IT DOWN: Skip the pasta (130 calories).

This traditional French dish has a great history and was a favorite long before the animated movie came along. We've adjusted the seasonings and made a few other tweaks to make it healthier while keeping the authentic flavor. Served over whole-wheat penne, this is a fiber-rich, filling meal.

One bite and it won't be hard to imagine you are in the Provence region of France! It's a wonderful dish to make ahead—the flavors marry well into the second day. I even like it cold.

Makes 4 Servings:
½ cup cooked pasta and 1½ cup vegetables

45 Minutes to Prepare and Cook

2 tsp olive oil

1 onion, diced

3 garlic cloves, peeled and sliced

2 medium eggplants, peeled and diced (2 cups)

1 small zucchini, diced (do not peel, about 1 cup)

1 red bell pepper, cored, seeded, and diced (1 cup)

Dash sea or kosher salt

Dash black pepper

1 tsp fresh thyme (about 2 sprigs)

1 bay leaf

1½ cups low-sodium petite diced canned tomatoes (with juice)

8 ounces whole-wheat penne

2 tsp shredded fresh basil leaves

1. Add 2 quarts of water to large pot and bring to a boil for the pasta.

2. While the water is heating, place a heavy-bottomed saucepan over medium heat and add the oil. When hot, add the onions and garlic and sauté for 2 minutes. Add the eggplant, zucchini, and red bell pepper; continue to sauté for 3 minutes. Add the salt, pepper, thyme, and bay leaf. Stir and add tomatoes. Continue to cook uncovered for 20 minutes, stirring occasionally.

3. Once the water boils, add the pasta and cook according to package directions. Once the vegetables are tender, remove the bay leaf and stir in the fresh basil. Serve over pasta.

Per Serving: 209.5 calories, 3.1 g total fat, 0 mg cholesterol, 234 mg sodium, 41.8 total carbs, 9.1 g dietary fiber, 7.9 g protein

Make It a Meal:
Add a serving of Turkey Meatballs (page 205) (370 calories) • Serve with baked chicken (359 calories)

Slow-Cooker Lasagna

What a great dish for one of those nights when your kids have a late soccer game! Brown the meat, layer in the ingredients, set your slow cooker on low, and go! Please note that the cooking time should not exceed 4 hours. This is not an "all day" slow-cooker meal.

Makes 8 Servings:
  1 heaping cup per serving

25 Minutes to Prepare; 4 Hours to Cook

1 pound ground beef, 96% lean

¼ tsp red pepper flakes

2 tsp dried thyme

One 24-ounce jar low-sodium marinara sauce

One ¾-pound eggplant, unpeeled, diced (2 cups)

15 ounces part-skim ricotta cheese

1 cup shredded Italian five-cheese blend (see Note)

¼ cup egg substitute (or 1 egg white)

1 tbsp chopped fresh parsley

6 no-boil lasagna noodles

1. In a skillet over moderate heat, brown the ground beef and drain any excess fat. Stir in red pepper flakes, thyme, tomato sauce, eggplant, and 1¼ cup water.

2. In a mixing bowl, combine the ricotta, shredded cheese blend, egg substitute, and parsley.

3. Coat the inside of the slow cooker with non-stick cooking spray. Place enough meat sauce in the slow cooker to cover the bottom. Top with 2 or 3 lasagna noodles (break them up as needed) to cover the meat sauce. Repeat layer.

4. Top the second layer with all of the cheese mixture and finish with a top layer of the remaining meat sauce.

5. Cover and set the slow cooker on low. Cook for 3½ to 4 hours.

Note: If you can't find the Italian five-cheese blend, shredded part-skim mozzarella will work just fine.

Per Serving: 271 calories, 10.2 g total fat, 56.6 mg cholesterol, 283.8 mg sodium, 18 g total carbs, 1.6 g dietary fiber, 24.8 g protein

Vegetable Lasagna

SLIM IT DOWN: Leave out the noodles (23 calories).

Lasagna is a dish that's great for a crowd, but having an entire pan of a rich dish can be too tempting when you're trying to control portions and eat right. This version serves four. We added vegetables to bulk up this family favorite, used whole-wheat noodles, and slashed the fat by skipping the meat. We cut back slightly on the cheese, but we kept a layer on top so you'll really taste it.

Makes 4 Servings:
¼ lasagna per serving

1 Hour to Prepare and Cook

For the Sauce:

2 tsp olive oil

1 medium onion, finely diced (1 cup)

3 garlic cloves, smashed and chopped

1 tsp dried thyme

1 tsp dried basil

¼ tsp red pepper flakes

2 tsp tomato paste (see Note)

One 14.5-ounce can low-sodium petite diced tomatoes

3 whole-wheat lasagna noodles

1 tsp olive oil

8 ounces baby portobello mushrooms, sliced

One 1-pound eggplant, peeled and chopped (about 3 cups)

3 cups baby spinach

1 tbsp lemon juice

½ cup reduced-fat ricotta cheese

½ cup part-skim shredded mozzarella cheese

1. Preheat the oven to 350° F. Prepare a 7" x 10" baking dish with nonstick cooking spray.

2. Make the tomato sauce. Heat olive oil in a sauté pan until warm. Add the onions and garlic and sauté over moderate heat until the onions are soft, about 4 minutes. Rub the thyme, basil, and crushed pepper between your hands to sprinkle them over the pan, then add the tomato paste and tomatoes. Simmer until the sauce thickens, about 15 minutes.

3. Cook the lasagna noodles according to package directions. Do not salt the water.

4. Heat another sauté pan with 1 teaspoon olive oil. Once the oil is hot, add the mushrooms and eggplant, and then spinach. Allow the spinach to wilt before stirring the pan. Sauté until the eggplant is tender, 5 to 7 minutes.

5. While the vegetables are cooking, use a fork to whisk the lemon juice and ricotta together in a bowl. Cut the cooked lasagna noodles in thirds.

6. Assemble the lasagna: place one third of the tomato sauce in the bottom of the baking dish. Layer on a third of the noodles, then half of the vegetable mixture and half the ricotta cheese. Repeat those steps for the second layer. Top with the remaining pasta and sauce, then cover the dish with foil and bake for 15 minutes. Spritz the underside of the foil with nonstick cooking spray so it doesn't stick to the cheese.

7. Remove the foil, sprinkle on the mozzarella, and bake another 15 minutes, until the cheese has melted and the top is slightly browned. Allow to set for 5 minutes before cutting and serving.

Note: To freeze leftover tomato paste, open both ends of the can and push out the remaining paste. Place in a zip-top plastic bag and store in the freezer for up to 3 months. You can also look for double-concentrated tomato paste that comes in a tube. You squeeze out what you need and the rest is stored indefinitely in the refrigerator.

_____

Per Serving: 177.1 calories, 7.3 g total fat, 15.6 mg cholesterol, 341.7 mg sodium, 18.9 g total carbs, 4.7 g dietary fiber, 9.9 g protein

> **Make It a Meal:**
> Just add fruit and a cup of milk.

CHEF MEG'S TIPS:

- Make the sauce ahead of time or use your favorite low-sodium jarred sauce.

- To release the flavor of dried herbs, rub them together between your hands over the pan.

- Swap no-cook lasagna noodles to save time.

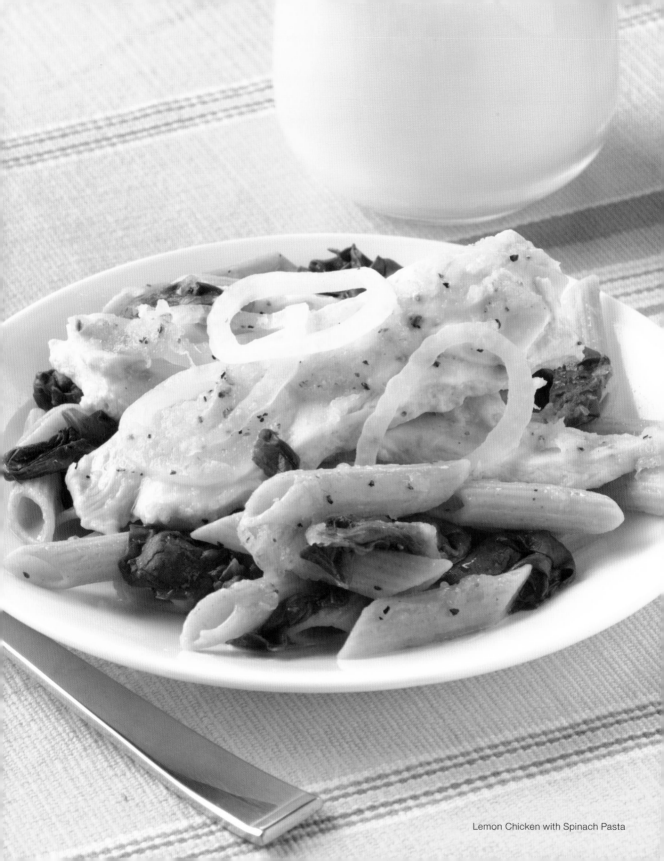

Lemon Chicken with Spinach Pasta

Lemon Chicken with Spinach Pasta

SLIM IT DOWN: Skip the pasta (180 calories).

You can mix up the sauce and marinade for this tasty dish before work, then cook the chicken and pasta when you get home. Thirty minutes and about 350 calories later, you have a filling, healthy meal. Add a serving of steamed broccoli and a cup of milk for a full meal. To make this dish vegetarian, replace the chicken with firm tofu that has been drained and sliced, or seitan (wheat gluten).

Makes 4 Servings:
3–4 ounces chicken and 1 cup pasta per serving

1 Hour 15 Minutes to Prepare and Cook

1 pound boneless, skinless chicken breasts

1 small onion, sliced thin

1 lemon, zested and juiced

3 tbsp white wine or rice-wine vinegar

1 tbsp olive oil

¼ tsp salt

¼ tsp white or black pepper

8 ounces whole-wheat penne

4 cups spinach, washed and trimmed

1. Prepare a glass baking dish with nonstick cooking spray. Trim the chicken of any remaining fat. Place chicken between two sheets of plastic wrap or parchment paper and use a meat mallet, rolling pin, or the bottom of a heavy pan to pound the meat until it is ½- to ¾-inch thick. Slice each breast into four strips and place into the prepared baking dish. Sprinkle the sliced onions over the chicken.

2. Prepare the marinade. In a mixing bowl, whisk together the lemon zest, lemon juice, vinegar, oil, salt, and pepper. Pour half the mixture over the chicken and onions and reserve the second half for the sauce. Marinate in the refrigerator for 30 minutes or up to 8 hours.

3. Preheat oven to 350° F. Cover with foil and bake chicken and onions for 30 minutes.

4. While the chicken is cooking, cook the pasta according to package directions until al dente (firm to the bite). Reserve ¼ cup of the pasta water before draining the pasta. Return the pasta and the reserved pasta water to the pan. Add the spinach, cooking until it wilts. Add the reserved marinade mixture and heat just until warm. Serve with cooked chicken.

Per Serving: 353.6 calories, 6 g total fat, 65.7 mg cholesterol, 238.3 mg sodium, 47 g total carbs, 8.1 g dietary fiber, 34.4 protein

Make It a Meal:
Just add a cup of milk and a piece of fruit!

CHEF MEG'S TIPS:

- Use green beans, broccoli, or asparagus in this recipe instead of spinach. Chop the vegetables into bite-size pieces.

- Add a few chopped sun-dried tomatoes or olives for another layer of flavor.

- Add ½ teaspoon of dried tarragon, dill, or oregano to the marinade and sauce.

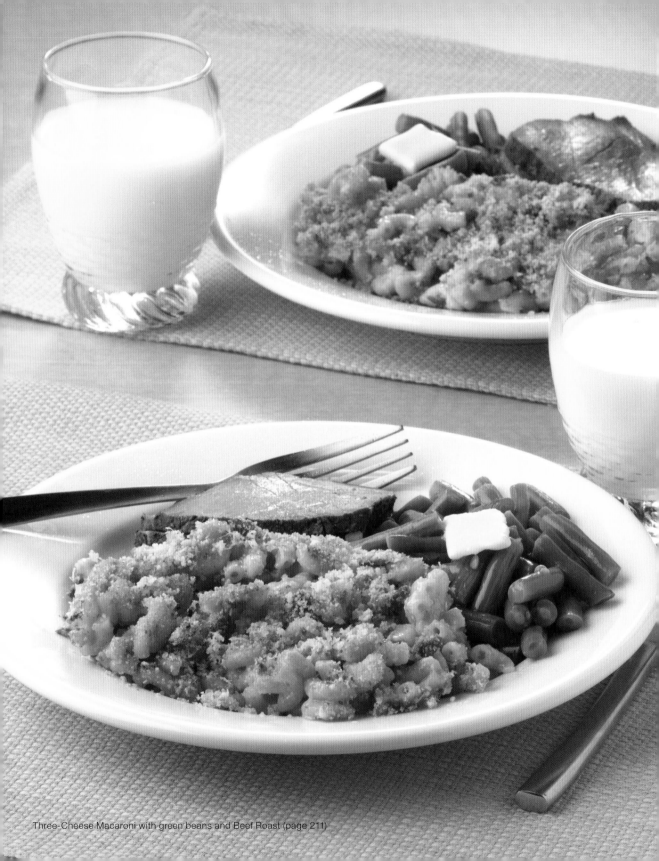

Three-Cheese Macaroni with green beans and Beef Roast (page 211)

Three-Cheese Macaroni

SLIM IT DOWN:
Nix the bacon (35 calories) or the Parmesan and breadcrumbs (16 calories).

In my house, macaroni and cheese never comes from a box or the freezer—it's always home-made. If there is a food more comforting and satisfying than homemade macaroni and cheese, we haven't found it. But a typical homemade recipe—made with cream, butter, and full-fat cheese—has about 400 calories and 25 grams of fat per serving; our version has a third of the fat and about 250 calories per cup. We slightly reduced the amount of cheese, used whole-wheat pasta, and chose flavorful ingredients to create a version that tastes good while cutting extra calories.

This recipe still keeps some fat, which is what adds flavor to this dish. You could make macaroni and cheese with fat-free cheese and no butter, but would you want to eat it?

Though it seems counterintuitive, eating a smaller quantity of a rich dish can be more satisfying than a larger quantity of a dish made with "filler" foods, those that have little flavor and nutritional value. This is a comfort food that you can feel good about eating.

My three boys love this dish. We usually serve it as a side dish rather than an entrée—it goes great with Spicy Turkey Mini Meatloaves (page 201) or just grilled chicken breasts. You can leave out the turkey bacon to make this dish vegetarian; add a pinch of dry mustard to the sauce for a sharper flavor.

Makes 6 Servings:
⅔ cup pasta per serving

45 Minutes to Prepare and Cook

For the Sauce:

2 tbsp light butter

2 tbsp all-purpose flour

1½ cups skim milk

1 bay leaf

⅛ onion, cut in a wedge

2 cloves

¼ cup shredded reduced-fat Swiss cheese

¼ cup shredded cheddar cheese

¼ tsp salt

1 pinch cayenne

8 ounces whole-wheat elbow pasta, dry (see Note)

6 slices turkey bacon, cooked and chopped

1 slice whole-wheat bread, processed into crumbs

2 tbsp grated Parmesan cheese

1. Preheat the oven to 375° F. Prepare a 9" x 13" casserole dish with nonstick cooking spray.

2. Place the butter in a medium saucepan, melt over medium-low heat, and cook until foaming. Add the flour and stir well with a wooden spoon for 1 to 2 minutes. Slowly pour in the milk, whisking to incorporate.

3. Attach the bay leaf to the onion wedge using the cloves. Drop the studded onion into the milk mixture with the clove/bay leaf side down. Cook, stirring occasionally, until the mixture thickens, about 15 minutes.

4. Meanwhile, cook the pasta according to package directions, but don't salt the cooking water.

5. Remove the studded onion from the sauce and discard. Add the Swiss and cheddar cheeses. Stir to combine and heat the sauce until the cheese is just melted. Season with salt and cayenne.

6. In a large mixing bowl, combine the sauce, bacon, and cooked macaroni; toss to coat. Combine the breadcrumbs and Parmesan in a small bowl.

7. Pour the pasta mixture into the prepared baking dish and top with the breadcrumbs and Parmesan. Bake uncovered until bubbly and golden, about 15 minutes.

Note: You can swap half the pasta for 3 cups of blanched broccoli or cauliflower to add fiber and make this dish even healthier.

Per Serving: 259.6 calories, 7.9 g total fat, 12.9 g total fat, 12.9 mg cholesterol, 425.3 mg sodium, 39.5 g total carbs, 4.1 g dietary fiber, 12.6 g protein

Make It a Meal:
Add on steamed broccoli and lean roast beef (450 calories) • Serve with mixed greens salad with vinaigrette and grilled chicken (443 calories)

A PERFECT PIZZA

Who doesn't love the taste of a warm and chewy pizza? I can name pizza joints in cities from here to Europe and back, and each one is different but still delicious. Though a slice of meat-lover's pizza can have up to 400 calories a slice (and you don't even want to know how much fat), don't fret. Pizza can still be a part of your life! Choose whole-wheat doughs and flavorful sauces, limit fatty and processed meats, and sprinkle on small amounts of flavor-packed cheeses and good-for-you vegetables.

Whether you pre-make batches of our healthy pizza dough to keep on hand in the freezer, or purchase dough from the supermarket or your local pizza parlor, you'll find that pizza made at home can be just as quick as the delivery kind.

Pizza toppings, like most foods, can change with the seasons. In the summer when herbs are in abundance, a grilled shrimp pizza with pesto and a crumbly cheese is on the menu. In early fall when the garden is going wild, I gravitate to the Grilled Vegetable Pizza (page 275). Winter brings a Barbecue Chicken Pizza (page 272) because we are looking for some warmth from our food. Then when spring rolls around, I take advantage of the spring greens with a pizza of herb oil, wilted lettuce, lean ham, and shavings of Parmesan.

Whether pizza is on the menu at home or at a restaurant, you can make healthy choices.

- Start with a green salad with vinaigrette to settle down your appetite. Your brain will start to feel full before the pie arrives.

- Opt for a thin-crust pizza rather than a thick crust or a deep dish to save hundreds of calories per slice. (Better yet, order or make whole-wheat or blended wheat dough.)

- Choose healthy toppings such as artichoke hearts, turkey bacon, grilled peppers, roasted tomatoes, mushrooms, spinach, and loads of herbs.

- If the pizza is shining with oil from the cheese, take a disposable napkin and blot away some of the excess to remove up to 100 calories a slice.

- At a restaurant, ask your server for a take-home box right away and put aside what goes home. When you get home wrap each slice and freeze them to avoid temptation in the wee hours or the next morning. When you want another slice, you'll have to plan ahead and thaw it out.

- At home, with your family and with guests, serve pizza with healthy sides. One slice looks lonely on a plate, but if you pair it with some veggies or cut fruit, it starts to look like a real meal.

- If you are a guest at a party, have your slice and then move away from the pizza. Everyone ends up in the kitchen at my parties, so when all the guests have been served, I put the pizza back into a warm oven and let everyone know where it is. This serves two purposes: the pizza stays warm, but it also moves it out of sight, so we're not mindlessly eating.

- Eat your slice with a knife and fork. Not only is it the Italian way, but it keeps your hands clean and reminds you to slow down and savor your slice as well. Pizza is one of those foods that's easy to inhale, so take your time and think before you have a second or third.

- Use pizza night as a teaching moment. Kids love pizza, and as you'll read in our Afterword, Raising Kids to be Healthy Eaters (page 389), making pies at home is a great way to get children involved in what goes on in the kitchen.

Favorite Pizza Combinations

A few tips about toppings. Less is more. Though I'm a fan of piling on the veggies, play around with the quantity. Too many toppings and you'll end up with a soggy pie.

You only need an ounce of cheese or less per slice. For a whole pie, you don't want any more than a cup—and usually ½ cup will suffice. Sure, all that gooey cheese is delicious, but it can easily overpower other ingredients.

Beyond pepperoni and cheese—a combo we rarely have at home—there's an entire world of pizza toppings. Be creative! Here are some of my favorites. Some are familiar and others exotic, but there's no recipe needed. Just pile the toppings on a crust, bake it up, and you're all set.

- Spicy black bean and roasted corn with cilantro

- Baked eggplant parmesan

- Spinach and mushroom

- Tomato and basil

- Lean ham and pineapple

- Roasted red onion, grilled peppers, turkey bacon, and goat cheese, with a drizzle of balsamic vinegar

- Smoked salmon with wilted arugula

- Turkey meatballs with a thick vegetable tomato sauce

- Roasted asparagus, parsley-walnut pesto with shaved Parmesan cheese

- Artichoke hearts, olives, grape tomatoes, and herb oil

- Turkey bacon, wilted lettuce, and tomatoes

- Shrimp with roasted tomatoes

SparkPeople Cooking Challenge:
The next time you make a pizza at home, try something new. Abandon your beloved sausage and mushroom for a more daring combination. Pizza night is a great chance to use up leftovers!

Basic Pizza Dough

Once you make the switch to whole-wheat flours and bread products, you won't want to go back to white versions, but adjusting to the change in texture and taste can take some time. Baked goods made with 100 percent whole-wheat flour tend to be tougher and denser than those made with all-purpose or white flours. To retain some lightness in texture but add the nutrition of whole wheat, I like to mix the two. This is a good basic recipe to use for whole pizzas, mini pizzas, calzones, or my favorite—Grilled Vegetable Pizza (page 275).

Chef Meg's Tip: If you don't have a food processor, mix the flours, salt, and yeast together in a large bowl. Make a well in the center. Pour the honey and water into the well, and, using a fork, slowly incorporate the flour into the water until thoroughly mixed. Then proceed with the recipe starting with Step 3.

Makes 8 Servings:
    1 slice per serving

1 Hour, 20 Minutes to Prepare and Rise

1⅓ cups all-purpose flour

⅔ cup whole-wheat flour

¾ tsp salt

1 package instant yeast (2¼ tsp)

2 tsp honey, warmed

⅔ cup water (heated to 100° to 110° F, see Note)

1 tbsp flour, for dusting

1. Place the flours, salt, and yeast in a food processor and pulse three or four times.

2. Combine the warm water and honey, turn on the machine, and pour the liquid through the feed tube. Process until the dough forms a ball.

3. Turn the dough out onto a counter and use the heel of your hands to knead until the dough is smooth, about 5 minutes. If the dough sticks to your hands, add a little bit more flour.

4. Prepare a bowl with nonstick cooking spray. Add the dough and turn it to coat on all sides. Cover with plastic wrap and place in a warm, draft-free area until the dough doubles in size, about 1 hour. If you are freezing the dough, wrap the ball tightly in plastic wrap and place in the freezer. It will keep for up to 3 months. When ready to use, thaw the dough overnight in the refrigerator and proceed to the next step.

5. Remove the dough to a floured surface, then roll out with a rolling pin. Roll out to a 16-inch circle and top with sauce and your favorite toppings.

Note: Be careful your water isn't too hot or it will kill the yeast and your dough won't rise. The water should feel like bath water—not so hot you can't dip a finger into it.

Per Serving: 117.8 calories, 0.4 g total fat, 0 mg cholesterol, 218.6 mg sodium, 25.3 g total carbs, 1.8 g dietary fiber, 3.6 g protein

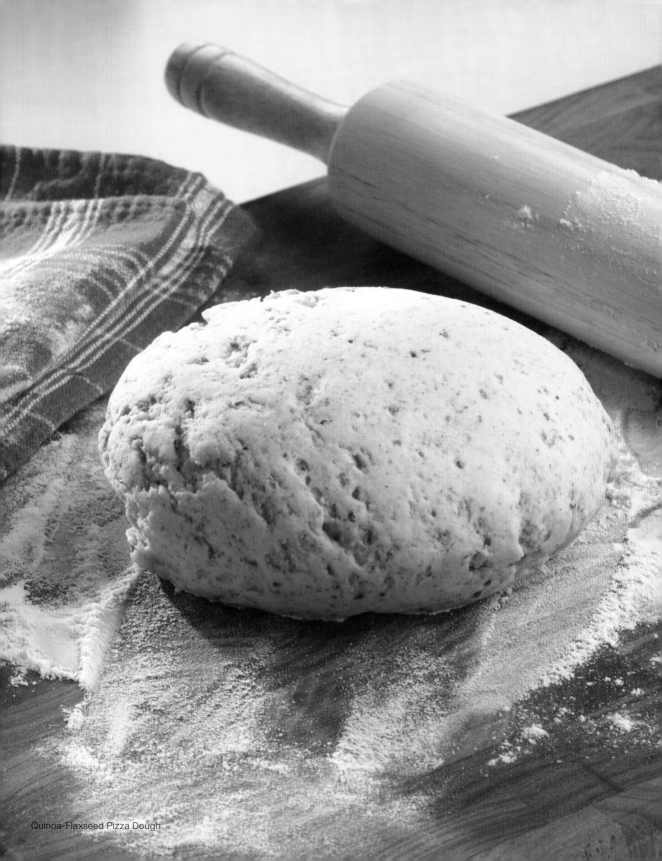

Quinoa-Flaxseed Pizza Dough

Quinoa-Flaxseed Pizza Dough

When choosing a pizza dough, it's often a battle of nutrition versus taste. White-flour varieties lack fiber, but whole-wheat versions lack texture. The solution is a hybrid dough. In this recipe, I experimented with quinoa, a seed that's eaten like a grain. High in fiber and full of protein, I wanted to see whether it could be ground up and used to boost the nutrition of our pizza dough. Combined with some ground flaxseeds, this dough is tasty and more nutritious than a standard pizza dough. Use all quinoa flour and you'll have a gluten-free dough. (For more on quinoa, see Chew on This on page 296.)

If you can't find quinoa flour, make your own by grinding whole quinoa in a clean coffee grinder. One-third cup whole quinoa yields ½ cup quinoa flour.

. . . .

Chef Meg's Tip: If you don't have a food processor, place the flours, flaxseeds, salt, and yeast in a bowl and stir to combine. Make a well in the center of the dry ingredients. Combine the honey and water, and then pour them into the well. Using a fork, slowly incorporate the dry ingredients into the wet until thoroughly mixed. Then proceed with the recipe starting with Step 3.

. . . .

Makes 8 Servings:
　　1 slice per serving

1 Hour, 20 Minutes to Prepare and Rise

1½ cups all-purpose flour

½ cup quinoa flour

2 tbsp ground flaxseeds

½ tsp salt

1 package instant dry yeast (2¼ tsp)

1 tsp honey

⅔ cup water (heated to 100° to 110° F)

1 to 2 tbsp all-purpose flour, for dusting

1. Place the flours, flaxseeds, salt, and yeast in a food processor and pulse to combine.

2. Combine honey and water, then pour into the feed tube of the food processor. Process until the dough forms a ball.

3. Turn the dough out onto a counter and use the heel of your hands to knead until it is smooth, about 5 minutes. If the dough sticks to your hands, add a little more flour.

4. Prepare a bowl with nonstick cooking spray. Add the dough and turn it to coat on all sides. Cover with plastic wrap and place in a warm, draft-free area until the dough doubles in size, about 1 hour. If you are freezing the dough, wrap the ball tightly in plastic wrap at this point and place in the freezer. It will keep for up to 3 months. When ready to use, thaw the dough overnight in the refrigerator and proceed to the next step.

5. Remove the dough to a floured surface, then roll into a 16-inch circle with a rolling pin and top as desired.

Per Serving: 130.8 calories, 1.3 g total fat, 0 mg cholesterol, 147.9 mg sodium, 25.8 g total carbs, 2.1 g dietary fiber, 3.8 g protein

Barbecue Chicken Pizza

My boys love this, and so do their friends! For easy single-serve portions, cut eight rounds from the dough to make mini pizzas—and don't tell them that the sauce is full of vegetables: they'll never know. To make this recipe mom-friendly too, make the chicken and the sauce ahead of time.

This recipe will make 2 cups of tomato sauce; if you have any left over, let it cool, and then freeze for future use. You can also substitute the Sweet and Spicy Barbecue Sauce (page 383) for the tomato sauce.

Makes 8 Servings:
    1 slice per serving (see Note page 273)

For the dough: 20 Minutes to Prepare, 1 Hour to Rise. For the pizza: 45 Minutes to Prepare and Cook.

1 recipe Basic Pizza Dough (page 269)

10 ounces boneless, skinless chicken breasts (2 breasts)

1 tsp Low-Sodium Barbecue Rub (page 384)

For the Sauce:

2 tsp olive oil

½ cup chopped onion

2 cloves garlic, minced

½ tsp Low-Sodium Barbecue Rub

One 14.5-ounce can low-sodium petite diced tomatoes

1 small eggplant (¾ pound), peeled and chopped (2½ cups)

2 tbsp no-salt-added tomato paste

1 cup shredded part-skim mozzarella cheese

1. Make the dough according to the instructions on page 269. If using frozen dough, allow the dough to thaw 1 hour at room temperature (or overnight in the fridge) before shaping. Raise the oven rack to the highest level, then preheat the oven to 400° F.

2. Pat the chicken dry with a paper towel. Place in small dish, then sprinkle with the rub. Prepare a sauté pan with nonstick cooking spray and sauté the chicken until cooked through and no longer pink, about 5 minutes. Remove the chicken from the pan and, once cool, chop into ¼-inch cubes and set aside.

3. To make the sauce, place a sauté pan over moderate heat and add the oil. Once hot, add the onion and garlic. Sauté until onions are tender, about 3 minutes. Stir in the rub. Add the tomatoes, eggplant, and tomato paste and stir to combine. Reduce the heat and simmer for 15 minutes to thicken.

4. Sprinkle 1 tablespoon of flour onto a flat surface. Using a rolling pin, shape the dough into a 16-inch circle. Place the rolling pin in the center of the dough, then fold the dough over the rolling pin to help transfer it to a baking stone or sheet pan.

5. Spread the sauce over the dough, then layer on the chicken and cheese. Bake 18 to 20 minutes, until the cheese is bubbly and the crust is light brown. Cut into 8 wedges to serve.

Per Serving: 227.9 calories, 4.4 g total fat, 28.8 mg cholesterol, 390 mg sodium, 31.5 g total carbs, 3.3 g dietary fiber, 16.1 g protein

Make It a Meal:
Add on Romaine, tomato, and cucumber salad with Homemade Ranch Dressing (page 367) (328 calories) • Eat with carrot and celery sticks with hummus (320 calories)

Meg-herita Pizza

You've probably heard of Pizza Margherita, the traditional Italian pizza with tomato, sliced mozzarella, basil, and olive oil. The story goes that it was created to honor the queen and includes all three colors of the Italian flag.

This pizza includes those same colors but bumps up the nutrition a bit. Instead of white-flour dough, we're using our dough made partly with quinoa and flaxseeds; tangy, creamy goat cheese instead of mozzarella; grape tomatoes; and a puree of basil and spinach instead of plain basil. The result is a pizza that's light enough to fit into a well-balanced meal and tasty enough to fulfill the craving for a really great pie.

Makes 8 Servings:
1 slice per serving (see Note)

For the dough: 20 Minutes to Prepare, 1 Hour to Rise. For the pizza: 25 Minutes to Prepare and Cook.

1 recipe Quinoa-Flaxseed Pizza Dough (page 271)

1 recipe Better-than-Pesto Puree (page 377)

1 cup grape tomatoes, halved lengthwise

4 ounces soft goat cheese, crumbled

1. Raise the oven rack to the highest level, then preheat oven to 400° F. If using a pizza stone, place it in the oven to preheat.

2. Place the dough on a pizza screen or preheated stone, spread with the pesto, then scatter the tomatoes and cheese across the top.

3. Bake until the dough is nicely browned and crispy, 18 to 20 minutes.

Note: Pizza pans vary in size. We base our recipes on a 16-inch pan with eight slices per pie.

Per Serving: 219.9 calories, 9.7 g total fat, 3.3 mg cholesterol, 181.6 mg sodium, 28 g total carbs, 2.7 g dietary fiber, 5.7 g protein

Make It a Meal:
Mix up a tomato and cucumber salad with Tomato-Basil Vinaigrette (page 387) (345 calories) • Enjoy with spinach and carrot salad with Honey-Mustard Dressing (page 382) (294 calories).

CHEF MEG'S TIPS:

- Use provolone or mozzarella instead of goat cheese or feta, which can be strong in flavor.

- Swap halved grape tomatoes for cherry or plum (Roma) tomatoes—whatever's fresh in the market or the garden.

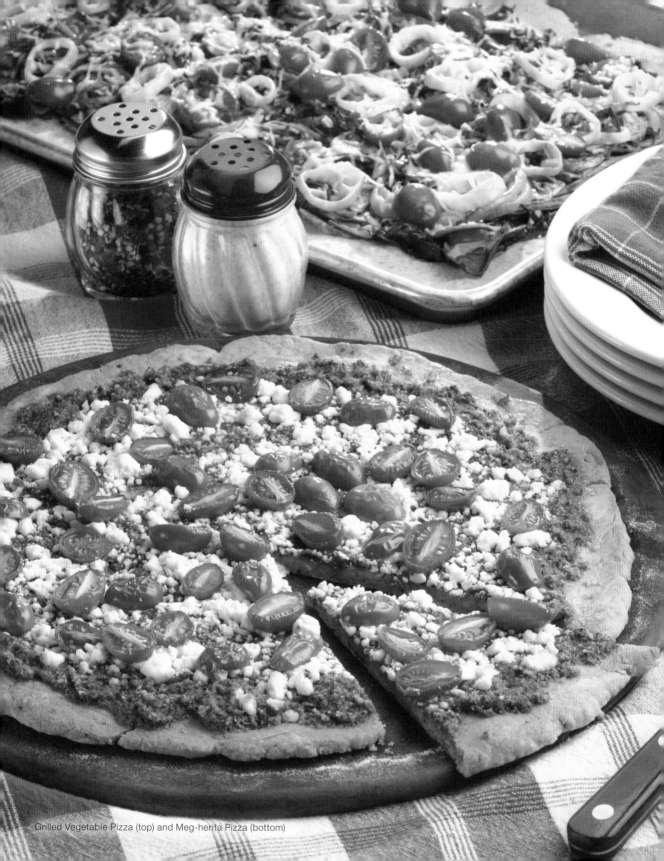

Grilled Vegetable Pizza (top) and Meg-herita Pizza (bottom)

Grilled Vegetable Pizza

When it's too hot to turn on the oven, make pizza on the grill—it's just an outdoor oven with a bigger flame. We raided the garden and loaded up our grilled pizza with veggies. Use whatever you have on hand, but remember to thinly slice or chop your vegetables so they'll cook evenly. Try fresh mozzarella, feta, or goat cheese on this pizza.

Makes 8 Servings:
1 slice per serving (see Note)

For the dough: 20 Minutes to Prepare, 1 Hour to Rise. For the pizza: 30 Minutes to Prepare and Cook.

1 recipe Basic Pizza Dough (page 269)

1 recipe Spicy Garlic Oil (page 384)

To Top the Pizza:

1 red onion, thinly sliced (about 1½ cups)

8 ounces mushrooms, sliced (about 2½ cups)

6 cups fresh spinach, tough stems removed

2 banana peppers, sliced, seeds removed

½ head radicchio, thinly sliced (about 1½ cups)

1 cup grape tomatoes, halved

½ cup shredded part-skim mozzarella

1. Preheat the grill to high. Use a grill brush to clean the grates.

2. Place the onions and mushrooms on a sheet of aluminum foil and wrap to form a parcel. Place on the grill to steam for 10 minutes. Remove from the grill and set aside.

3. Roll out the pizza dough to a large circle. Place the dough on a pizza screen or flat sheet pan to slide the dough onto the grill. Grill for three to four minutes, or until the dough becomes marked from the grill.

4. Using metal tongs or a pizza peel, turn the dough over and brush with 1 tablespoon of the garlic oil. Flip the dough and brush the other side with a second tablespoon of oil.

5. Layer on the vegetables: onions, mushrooms, spinach, peppers, and radicchio. Top with the tomatoes and cheese. Drizzle the final tablespoon of oil over the dough, close the grill lid, and cook for 15 minutes.

Note: Pizza pans vary in size. We base our recipe on a 16-inch pan.

Per Serving: 256.8 calories, 10.6 g total fat, 8.2 mg cholesterol, 308.3 mg sodium, 29.5 g total carbs, 3.7 g dietary fiber, 9.1 g protein

Make It a Meal:
Serve with chickpeas and chopped bell peppers with vinaigrette (450 calories) • Enjoy with cottage cheese and sliced tomatoes (360 calories)

WHOLE GRAINS

I don't buy into that low-carb hype. Breads and grains really are part of the foundation of a healthy diet and, according to the food pyramid, we need 6 to 11 servings of them each day. They provide vitamins, complex carbohydrates, minerals, and, most important, fiber. When I train for marathons, I count on carbs to fuel me through the long runs. Beyond the nutritional significance, bread has a symbolic presence in our lives. After all, it is the "staff of life."

Despite its importance to our diet and culture, not all breads are created equal. Place a slice of white bread and a slice of whole wheat side by side and take a close look. What do you see? The white bread is, well, white, with a dark crust. The whole wheat is a nutty brown color throughout. Now touch it. The white bread is spongy and moist, with a downy soft crust and smooth bottom. The wheat bread: it's slightly rougher all over, but it feels firmer.

Now take a bite. The white bread sticks to your teeth, your tongue, the roof of your mouth. As you chew it falls apart, it gets slimy, and it tastes sweet. Bits cling to your teeth and there's a sweet aftertaste. The wheat bread is firm to the tooth, takes longer to chew, and tastes nutty. It doesn't feel sticky, and there's less of an aftertaste. Which bread do you want to eat?

Compare the nutrition facts:

	Whole-wheat bread (1 slice)	White Bread (1 slice)
Calories	69	66
Protein (g)	3.6	1.9
Fiber (g)	1.9	0.6

That additional protein and fiber, in addition to the nutty taste and hearty texture, will keep you satisfied longer than the white bread, which has virtually no staying power.

Bread is the king of the grain group, but there are plenty of others out there. Rice, pasta, crackers, and cereals are all grains, too, and the same rules apply: whole grain is better. White rice, white pasta, and sugary refined cereals aren't welcome in my shopping cart. They are lacking in trace vitamins and minerals, and have little protein and fiber, which leaves us feeling hungry soon after eating them.

Whole grains have incredible health benefits, too: a 2006 study by Tufts University showed that people who consumed the most whole grains were 42 percent less likely to develop diabetes.[1] Researchers from the Harvard School of Public Health found that people with a diet high in whole grains showed a lower risk of both diabetes and heart disease.[2] In 1997, the FDA authorized the claim that the soluble fiber in oats reduced the risk of coronary heart disease; this approval was extended in 2005 to include the fiber in barley as well.

This chapter will not only show you how to use whole-grain versions of foods you already know and love, like bread and rice (see Chapter 8 for recipes using whole-wheat pasta and our homemade pizza dough), but we will introduce you to other whole grains you might not have tried yet: bulgur, quinoa, wheat berries, even farro.

If you're apprehensive about the taste of whole grains, don't be. We think you'll find the added flavor and chewy texture to be a welcome change. SparkPeople members do. JULIEIRENE said "the switch to (whole) wheat was pretty easy for us. It seems more substantial and filling, which especially helped as I was learning to reduce portion sizes." As for the taste, it's not strong or unpleasant. TRICIAN13 finds grains to be bland on their own, so she uses chicken or vegetable broth when cooking whole grains such as rice or barley to impart an added layer of flavor.

Whole Grains 101

Every grain starts as a whole grain. This whole grain (actually the seed or kernel of the plant) has three parts: the bran, the germ, and the endosperm. A whole grain is one that contains all three parts of the kernel.

The bran is the outer skin of the seed that contains antioxidants, B vitamins, and fiber. (Wheat bran or oat bran can be purchased individually and are also common ingredients in certain cereals.)

The germ is the "baby" of the seed, which grows into a new plant when germinated. It contains many vitamins, along with protein, minerals, and healthy fats. (You can purchase toasted wheat germ in most supermarkets; it can be added to a variety of foods to boost nutritional content.)

The endosperm is the seed's food supply; it provides the energy needed for the young plant to grow. The largest portion of the seed, it contains carbohydrates and smaller amounts of protein, vitamins, and minerals.

SparkPeople Cooking Challenge:
Swap brown rice for white the next time you make dinner. If you're nervous, cook a batch of white and a batch of brown and mix the two. Slowly work your way up to all brown rice.

COUNT ON CARBS

Carbohydrates are the main calorie-providing nutrients in grains. Carbohydrates are broken down by digestion into the "blood sugar" called glucose, which is the body's most important fuel and the primary source of energy for the body, brain, and nervous system. Carbohydrates also spare protein from being used as energy, therefore freeing protein for its important functions of building, repairing, and maintaining body tissues. Carbohydrates aid in fat utilization and promote the growth of beneficial bacteria, which synthesize certain vitamins in the intestinal tract. The indigestible carbohydrate called fiber helps prevent constipation and lowers the risk for certain diseases such as cancer, heart disease, and diabetes.

It's a "Complex" Issue

The type of carbohydrates in grain-group foods are classified as complex carbohydrates—also called starches. Starches are found in grain products, such as bread, crackers, cereals, pasta, and rice. Starchy vegetables, like potatoes, corn, sweet peas, lima beans, dry beans, dry peas, and lentils, also contain complex carbohydrates. Some foods containing complex carbohydrates are better choices than others. Food products using unrefined grains, called whole grains, contain all three parts of the kernel of grain and therefore retain their original vitamins, minerals, protein, and fiber. When one or more of the kernel parts are removed, the result is a refined grain. This refining process removes some of the vitamins, minerals, protein, and most of the fiber from the grain. Therefore, unrefined grain products are more nutritious and higher in fiber, which is very beneficial when trying to achieve and maintain a healthy weight. High-fiber foods take longer to chew, slow down your

eating speed, and add bulk to your diet. These may help you to feel fuller longer, and you will be less likely to overeat. The digestion and absorption process is also slowed down, the result being healthier blood-sugar levels. While both unrefined and refined grain foods can be a part of a healthy diet, the food pyramid recommends that half of your grain food selections be from whole-grain foods.

Breaking Down Bread

When looking for good-for-you breads, become a detective. Look for clues on the package and within the nutritional analysis.

- Purchase 100% whole-wheat breads for optimal fiber and staying power. Double-check the label: whole grain is not 100% whole wheat. Manufacturers sometimes like to trick us with this one.

- Avoid bad oils like hydrogenated or partially hydrogenated oils (trans fats).

- Personally, I look for breads that have added nuts or seeds (like flaxseeds) as a crunchy finish.

LESS IS MORE

All you really need to make bread is flour, water, yeast, salt, and a little bit of sugar (to activate the yeast). But breads these days have long and complicated ingredients lists. These extra ingredients are usually added to help improve the taste, texture, shelf life, or nutritional profile of the bread so that consumers will find it more appealing. Some fiber-rich additions (like processed oat, cottonseed, pea, or wheat fibers) boost the fiber content. Other manufacturers use additional sweeteners (like sugar, corn syrup, or honey) to make their bread—especially whole-wheat ones—taste sweeter. Often, high-fructose corn syrup replaces sugar in many breads to reduce cost and prolong shelf life. And many breads are enriched with vitamins and minerals so that they'll appear to be more nutritious.

It's up to every individual consumer to decide whether they want a bread that contains corn syrup, preservatives, or other additives. But one thing we could all do is look for breads that have shorter ingredients lists and recognizable ingredients in general.

At the supermarket. To make sure you are getting 100% whole-wheat bread, look at the ingredients list, not the front of the package. "Whole-wheat flour" or "100% whole-wheat flour" should be the first ingredient—and the only flour listed. Don't fall for deceitful terms like "wheat flour," "unbleached wheat flour," "multi-grain," "enriched," or "stone-ground wheat flour." These are just sneaky ways of saying refined white flour.

Besides ingredients, here are some guidelines from Becky, our SparkPeople Head Dietitian, for picking a loaf that is healthy and nutritious. Look for these Nutrition Facts:

- Calories: 100 or fewer per slice

- Fiber: 2 grams or more per slice

- Sodium: 225 mg or less per slice

At the bakery. Search out a bakery in your area that makes artisanal whole-grain breads and support their hard work. Be sure to ask questions about what goes into each loaf, as bakery bread doesn't often have a nutrition facts label. Most artisan bakers offer at least one whole-grain option. For optimal taste, eat the day it is baked, but don't feel the need to eat the entire loaf. Day-old bread is good for breadcrumbs, French toast, or croutons.

Once you get the loaf home keep it tightly wrapped in a dry area. Never put breads in the refrigerator, as they will go stale quickly. If you purchase extra bread, wrap it in plastic wrap, place it in the freezer, and allow it to come to room temperature before using.

BUYING AND STORING GRAINS

Whole grains are found prepackaged near the pasta and in bulk bins. Prices will be lower when you buy in bulk, but be sure to label your purchases. Many whole grains can look alike to the novice healthy cook.

Grains should always smell fresh, not musty or stale. Always buy from a source with good turnover on the shelves to ensure a fresh supply. Store your grains in a tightly sealed bag or lidded container—in a cool, dark cabinet or the refrigerator. It varies from grain to grain, but most will remain fresh for at least two months with proper storage.

BULK UP YOUR MEALS IN NO TIME

Whole grains take longer to cook than refined grains because they still contain their tough outer layer, called the bran; but it's that bran that provides the bulk of the nutrition of the grain.

We recommend making one or even two whole-grain side dishes on nights when you have some extra time. Many require very little prep time, and take just a bit longer to cook than refined grains. Pull leftovers out of the fridge and serve hot or cold alongside simple meals like grilled chicken, lean roast beef, or steamed fish. Heat up your favorite frozen vegetable or sauté a fresh one, add a cup of skim milk, and dinner is ready!

LOVE YOUR LEFTOVERS

When life gives you leftovers, you have three options: 1. You can eat seconds at dinner. 2. You can throw them away or leave them in the fridge to rot. 3. You can transform them into a healthy lunch. Successful SparkPeople members choose option 3. They tell us that packing their lunch helps them save money and avoid temptation at work.

If you say you don't like to eat the same thing over and over, that's fine. Here are some easy ways to transform leftovers into a new meal:

1. Place Wild Rice with Roasted Shallots and Garlic (page 291) on your favorite salad.

2. Add Grilled Fish with Mango Salsa (page 223) to a whole-wheat wrap, along with some chopped lettuce.

3. Put Mushroom-Cheese Frittata (page 91) on a toasted English muffin for a quick sandwich.

4. Break up a Black-Bean Burger with Lime Cream (page 139) over brown rice or a serving of pasta, then top with salsa.

5. Mix Slow-Cooker Salsa Chicken (page 181) into your favorite vegetable soup.

Bruschetta with Cilantro Pesto and White Beans

Cocktail hours and dinner parties are two of a healthy eater's biggest challenges. Platters of food—often fried—are within reach, and it's hard to keep track of what you've eaten. Take a platter of this bruschetta to your next party, and you'll be able to ward off hunger before the meal without going overboard.

Bruschetta (pronounced broos-KET-uh), meaning "grilled bread," takes its name from a verb in the Roman dialect of Italian. Though the grilled or toasted bread was traditionally topped with olive oil and rubbed with garlic, today bruschetta refers to any topped, toasted bread.

In this version, the cannellini beans offer protein and fiber, which will help fill you up with few calories. One of these will set you back just 52 calories.

If you don't have beans on hand, just top your bread with the pesto and Parmesan. Try the Better-than-Pesto Puree (page 377) or Tomato Jam (page 378) with the beans and Parmesan. You can mash the beans slightly to get them to stay on the toast better.

Makes 12 Servings:
1 bruschetta per serving

20 Minutes to Prepare and Cook

12 ounces whole-wheat baguette, about ⅔ loaf, cut into 12 slices

2 tbsp Coconut-Cilantro Pesto (page 376)

¾ cup canned cannellini beans, drained and rinsed

2 tbsp Parmesan cheese, shaved with a vegetable peeler

1. Preheat oven to 250° F. Place the bread slices on a baking sheet and toast until light brown, about 7 minutes. Remove the bread from the oven, raise the oven rack to its highest settings, and turn on the broiler.

2. Top each slice of bread with ½ teaspoon of pesto, 1 tablespoon of beans, and 1 teaspoon of Parmesan; return the baking sheet to the oven. Broil just until the cheese is melted, leaving the door ajar, and keeping a close eye on the broiler the entire time. Serve warm.

Per Serving: 52.5 calories, 0.8 g total fat, 1 mg cholesterol, 88.4 mg sodium, 8.9g total carbs, 1.3 g dietary fiber, 2.6 g protein

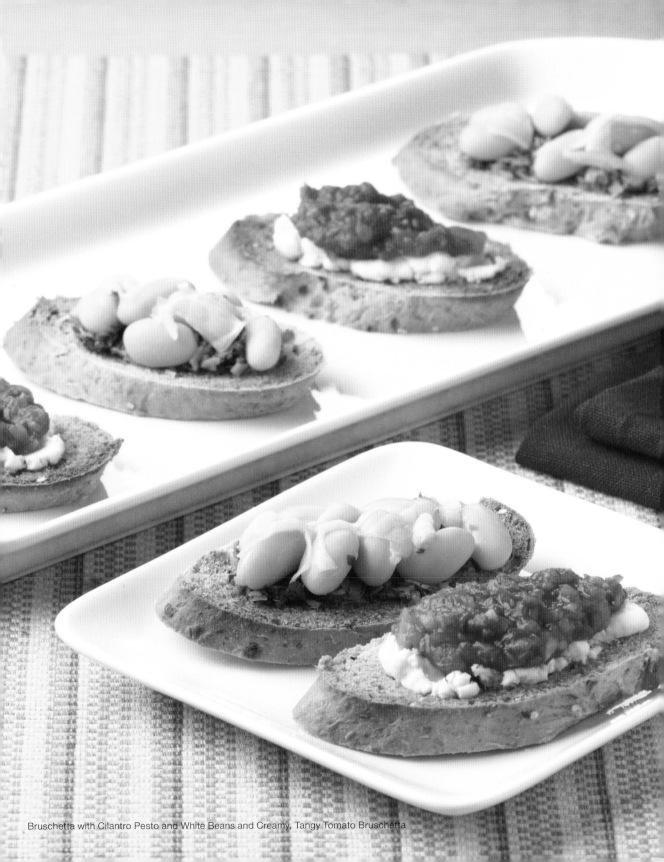

Bruschetta with Cilantro Pesto and White Beans and Creamy, Tangy Tomato Bruschetta

Creamy, Tangy Tomato Bruschetta

SLIM IT DOWN: Nix the goat cheese (38 calories).

This is a prime example of how a little bit of a rich ingredient, like goat cheese, can go a long way. By pairing it with the tangy contrasting flavor of the tomato jam, it cuts the richness and invigorates your taste buds. If you want to add a bit of green, finish the bruschetta with a sprinkle of chopped parsley.

This jam is incredibly versatile, but I really like it best on bruschetta. (See the recipe on page 378 for more uses.) To turn this into a lunch, use whole-wheat sandwich bread, spread on 1 ounce of goat cheese, 2 tablespoons of the jam, and a handful of arugula. You could also add some roasted chicken.

Makes 4 Servings:
2 bruschetta per serving

20 Minutes to Prepare and Cook

8 ounces whole-wheat baguette (about half a loaf), cut into 8 slices

2 ounces goat cheese, softened

½ cup Tomato Jam (page 378)

1. Preheat oven to 250° F. Place the bread slices on a baking sheet and toast until light brown, about 7 minutes. Remove the bread from the oven, raise the oven rack to its highest settings, and turn on the broiler.

2. Spread about 1 teaspoon of goat cheese on each slice of bread, then layer on 1 tablespoon of jam. Return the baking sheet to the oven and broil with the oven door ajar just until the cheese starts to melt. Keep a close eye on the broiler the entire time. Serve warm.

Per Serving: 140.9 calories, 4.7 g total fat, 6.5 mg cholesterol, 281.8 mg sodium, 20.2 total carbs, 2.5 g dietary fiber, 5.9 g protein

HOW TO COOK RICE

Of all the cooking woes that I hear about from students, friends, and fellow shoppers in aisle four at the supermarket, the one I hear the most is, "I cannot cook rice! It either turns out mushy, dry, or burned." You *can* make perfect rice every time. All it takes is a little practice and a few practical tips.

Know Your Varieties

- *Enriched rice* is rice that has been coated with vitamins.

- *Short- and medium-grain rice* have small round kernels that become sticky when cooked. Used for sushi.

- *Long-grain rice* has long and slender grains that fluff when cooked.

- *Parboiled rice* is long-grain rice that has been partially cooked then redried. It cooks quickly and doesn't stick together when cooked.

- *Brown rice* still has the bran of the kernel, which gives it a brown color and a chewy texture. This is the best choice nutritionally.

- *Wild rice* is really not a rice but the seed of a grass. It adds both color and flavor to rice dishes and is delicious on its own as well.

- *Aromatic rices* are varieties of rice that have a nutty flavor and aroma. Popular varieties include jasmine and basmati. Frequently used in Asian and Indian cooking, they are light and fluffy when cooked. Available in brown and white varieties.

- *Arborio rice* is a shorter-grain rice that is high in starch, traditionally used in risotto. Available in white and brown varieties.

Cooking Methods

There are three methods used to cook rice and grains: simmer, pilaf, and risotto. If you are just starting out in the kitchen and don't have a rice steamer, I would suggest the pilaf method. To me, it is the most foolproof. (**Note:** These cooking techniques can be used for all whole grains, not just rice.) The general rule of thumb is 2 parts of water to 1 part rice.

Simmer. This is the most common method and yet it's the trickiest to master. Basically you just simmer the rice in water or broth on the stovetop until it is cooked to your desired tenderness. The grains are stirred into boiling water, the heat is reduced, the pot is covered, and the grain slowly cooks. Sounds easy, right?

The problem is that it is hard to control your heat. If the heat is too high, the water evaporates and the starch burns on the bottom of the pan—what a mess to clean up! When in doubt add a bit of water and lower the heat. You can always drain a bit of excess water at the end, but one bit of burned rice will ruin the whole pot.

Just a note: Most package directions will say that oil and salt should be added for flavor—this is not necessary. I prefer to add flavor by cooking my rice in homemade broth, adding garlic, shallots, citrus zest, or a bay leaf.

Pilaf. This is my favorite method. The grain is coated in a small amount of fat, cooked for a few minutes, and then liquid is added. The mixture is brought to a boil, reduced to a simmer, covered with a tight-fitting lid, then placed in the oven to finish cooking. No problem controlling the heat, no constant stirring, just easy and tasty rice.

Risotto. The Italian root of this word, "riso," means rice. It's the perfect example of the Italian kitchen. The process is slow. The rice is cooked in a small amount of fat then stock or water is slowly added to it until all the liquid is absorbed. This is a "needy" method. The liquid has to be added a small amount at a time with pretty constant stirring, but it can also be a relaxing process—just you and the rice, stirring for up to an hour. Try this method with grains like farro or barley.

Most risotto recipes call for massive quantities of butter and cheese, but they're not necessary. You'll achieve a creamy consistency with constant stirring as the starch leaves the rice grains. If you do add a bit of butter or cheese, do so at the end, when you'll really be able to taste it.

So while making rice can often take awhile—brown rice can take an hour to cook—you can make it in large batches that last for several meals. You can keep it in the fridge until you need it later in the week. Rice, particularly the long-grain varieties, also freezes well. Let the rice cool, then pack in zip-top plastic bags. Reheat in the microwave; the length of time depends on the amount of rice: one cup takes about 2 minutes on high.

Spanish Rice

Spanish rice is a dish that's part of the curriculum at my cooking school. I have the pleasure of tasting 32 Spanish rice dishes every 9 weeks! I had come to hate Spanish rice—until now. Changing the white rice to brown, cooking the tomato paste, and adding sweet peas makes all the difference in the world.

If you don't have 40 minutes, feel free to use instant brown rice—I do on busy nights! Follow the recipe but reduce cooking time according to package directions.

Makes 6 Servings:
¾ cup per serving

45 Minutes to Prepare and Cook

1 tbsp canola oil

½ onion, finely diced (½ cup)

2 tbsp tomato paste

1 tsp cumin

1 tsp sweet or hot paprika

1 tsp chili powder

¼ tsp salt

1 cup brown rice

2 bell peppers (red, yellow, or orange), cored, seeded, and chopped (2 cups)

1 cup peas, frozen

1. Prepare a large, heavy, lidded saucepan with nonstick cooking spray. Warm the pan over moderate heat, then add the oil to warm. Add the onions and cook until soft, about 4 minutes. Do not let them brown.

2. Add the tomato paste, cumin, paprika, chili powder, and salt to the saucepan. Stir and cook for 1 minute; a crust will form on the bottom of the pan. Slowly pour 1 cup of water into the pan and scrape the bottom of the pan with a wooden spoon to remove the crust. Add the rice and pour in an additional 1½ cups of water. Bring to a simmer, cover, and cook over low heat for 20 minutes.

3. Add the peppers and peas to the rice, replace the cover, and cook until the rice is tender, about 10 minutes more. Remove from the heat and serve warm.

Per Serving: 180.2 calories, 3.6 g total fat, 0 mg cholesterol, 131.1 mg sodium, 35.5 g total carbs, 5.3 g dietary fiber, 2.1 g protein

Baked Lemon-Spiced Rice

A lot of people have trouble cooking rice. It's a simple process, but one that's easy to mess up. That's why I encourage people to try the pilaf method: it adds more flavor than traditional simmering methods and is fairly error-free. (See How to Cook Rice, page 285.)

I also know that people tend to avoid cooking brown rice because it takes so long. It does, but the nutritional benefits leave white rice in the dust—and we think you'll find this rice is so delicious that it's worth the extra cooking time. Coriander, the fruit of the cilantro plant, provides a spicy, citrus flavor. If you don't have shallots, substitute two cloves of minced garlic or an equal amount of minced onion.

Makes 4 Servings:
¾ cup per serving

1 Hour to Prepare and Cook

1 tbsp olive oil

2 tbsp finely diced shallot

1 cup brown rice

1 tsp salt

1 tsp coriander seeds, crushed

1 lemon, zested into large strips

1 bay leaf

Pinch of white pepper

1. Preheat the oven to 350° F. Heat the oil in an ovenproof saucepan with lid over moderate heat; add the shallots and sauté, uncovered, until soft, about 2 minutes. Do not let them brown. Add the rice and stir to coat in the oil.

2. Add 2 cups of water to the saucepan, stir, then add the salt, coriander, lemon zest, bay leaf, and pepper. Bring to a simmer, cover with a tight-fitting lid, and place in the preheated oven. Bake for 50 minutes, remove from the oven, and discard the bay leaf. Fluff the rice with a fork before serving.

Per Serving: 88.3 calories, 3.8 g total fat, 0 mg cholesterol, 584.5 mg sodium, 12.3 g total carbs, 1 g dietary fiber, 1.4 g protein

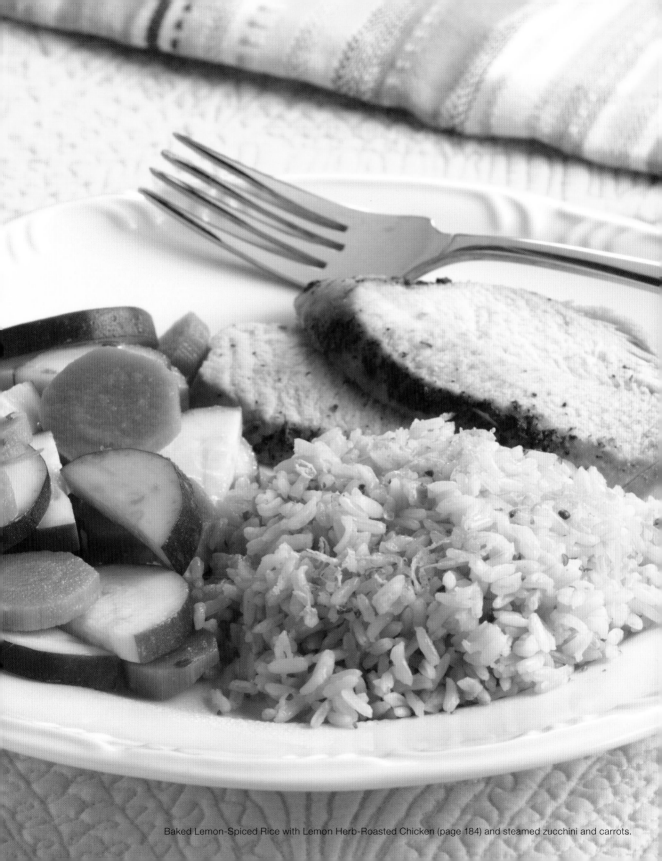

Baked Lemon-Spiced Rice with Lemon Herb-Roasted Chicken (page 184) and steamed zucchini and carrots.

Ten Easy Ways to Get More Fiber into Your Diet

Why do we put so much emphasis on eating fiber? Because fiber keeps your digestive system healthy and running smoothly, and a diet rich in fiber has been shown to reduce cholesterol levels and play a part in the battle against heart disease and diabetes. While the recommended daily amount of fiber is 25 to 35 grams, knowing which foods are fiber-rich is easier than counting numbers.

Fiber comes in two forms, *soluble* and *insoluble.* Soluble fiber, found in foods such as whole grains and beans, mixes with water and coats the intestinal tract. This gummy substance binds to cholesterol, reduces its absorption, and delays absorption of glucose. Insoluble fiber is found in the "bran" of whole grains and the skins of fruits and vegetables. It absorbs water and helps keep the digestive system running smoothly.

Eating too much fiber too quickly may cause constipation or stomach discomfort. Increase fiber amounts in your diet slowly, and boost your fluid consumption by drinking at least 8 cups of water daily.

Not sure where to start? Here are some easy ways to integrate more fiber each day. In addition, we've included this symbol 🌾 to note recipes that are high in fiber!

1. Start the day with a bowl of oatmeal. It's filling enough to get you through the morning.

2. Add bran flakes or flax meal to oatmeal or cereal. Start with a teaspoon, and work your way up to 2 tablespoons as your system adjusts to the added fiber.

3. Eat a piece of fruit instead of drinking fruit juice, which has had most of the fiber removed.

4. Enjoy 1 to 1½ ounces (about a handful) of mixed nuts and seeds as a snack or in salads.

5. Eat brown rice instead of white.

6. Read the labels carefully and buy only whole-grain breads, wraps, crackers, and whole-wheat pasta.

7. Eat your fruits and vegetables! Adding even a handful of veggies to a cup of a soup and a sandwich can help. Berries are an especially good source of fiber.

8. Add a can of rinsed and drained beans—black, white, pinto, red—to salads, soups, and casseroles. (Rinsing the beans removes sodium and the starch that can cause gas.)

9. Start your meal with a salad full of dark, leafy greens—arugula, escarole, spinach, and kale

10. Eat the skins of fruits (apples, pears, peaches) and vegetables (potatoes, sweet potatoes, squash). Be sure to wash them well first.

Wild Rice with Roasted Shallots and Garlic

Wild rice is actually not a rice but the seed of an unrelated grass. The grains are long, slender, and dark brown or even black. You will notice that wild rice is much chewier, with a stronger flavor than brown or white rice.

Why do people add butter or salt to their rice? Because rice doesn't have much flavor on its own. If you're serving rice as a side dish rather than a component of an entrée where it will soak up sauce, it's important to flavor the rice. Who wants to eat plain rice? Not me.

The strong flavor of the wild rice with the shallots and garlic make this a great pairing with beef dishes. Our Caramelized Onions (page 310) could be added instead of the shallots.

Makes 8 Servings:
½ cup per serving

1 Hour 15 Minutes to Prepare and Cook

3 cloves garlic

4 whole shallots, peeled, sliced in half

2 cups homemade or low-sodium chicken stock

1 cup wild rice, rinsed well

½ tsp salt

1 tsp dried thyme

1. Preheat oven to 375° F. Place the garlic and shallots on a roasting pan and roast until softened and golden brown, 20 minutes, stirring occasionally. Remove from the oven, set aside until cool enough to handle, and then roughly chop.

2. In an ovenproof saucepan with a lid, bring the stock to a boil. Add the rice, salt, and thyme. Bring the mixture back to a boil, cover, and transfer the pan to the oven. Cook until rice begins to split and is tender, 45 to 50 minutes. Drain any excess liquid.

3. Stir the roasted shallot mixture together with the rice. Serve warm.

Per Serving: 96.6 calories, 0.3 g total fat, 0 mg cholesterol, 80.1 mg sodium, 19.8 g total carbs, 1.7 g dietary fiber, 3.6 g protein

CHEF MEG'S TIPS:

- Freeze any leftovers or add to vegetable soups.

- Use vegetable stock to make this dish vegetarian.

- Rework the dish for a second meal by adding Roasted Root Vegetables (page 315).

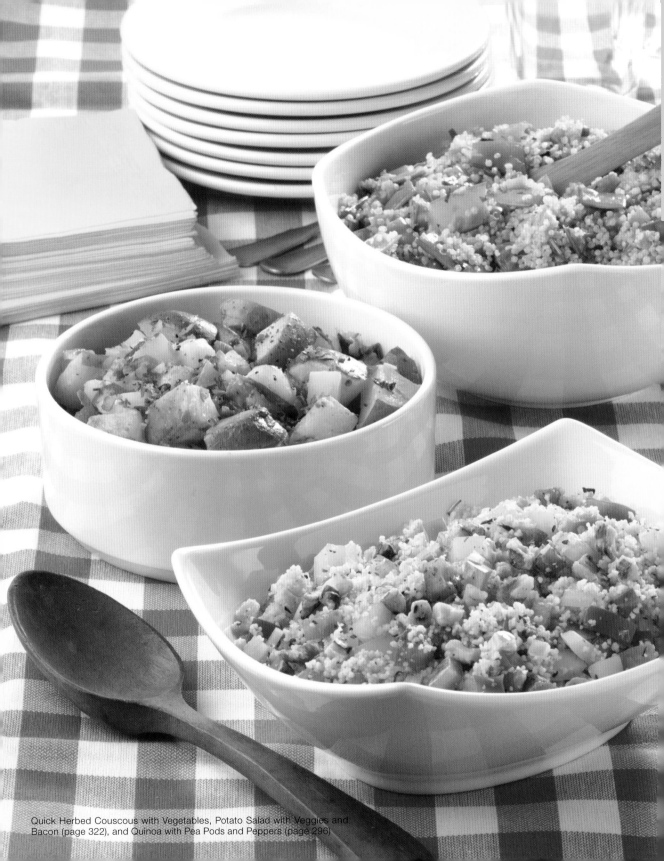

Quick Herbed Couscous with Vegetables, Potato Salad with Veggies and Bacon (page 322), and Quinoa with Pea Pods and Peppers (page 296)

Quick Herbed Couscous with Vegetables

Couscous is one of the quickest and easiest side dishes to make: Just place in a bowl, cover with an equal amount of boiling water, then cover and let sit for 15 minutes. Fluff with a fork and serve! This dish is great warm or cold. If you have any leftovers, serve as part of a salad. (See Chew on This for more on cooking and serving couscous.)

Beware of the flavored couscous on store shelves. We all love the little boxes that scream, "I am easy and quick to fix!" Those little boxes are loaded with sodium and dried vegetables. This dish might take an extra five minutes to cook, but you're adding about two servings of fresh vegetables!

Whole-wheat couscous can be a bit hard to track down, but it's affordable and nutritious. You might need to ask your grocery store to order it. I found it in the bulk bins at my local health-food store.

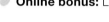 **Online bonus:** Learn how to toast nuts. Visit SparkRecipes.com for Chef Meg's video.

Makes 4 Servings:
1¼ cups per serving

25 Minutes to Prepare and Cook

1 cup whole-wheat couscous

1 cup boiling water

1 tbsp Italian Herb Seasoning (page 369)

1 tsp olive oil

1 lemon, zested and juiced

1 large or 2 small shallots, finely chopped (¼ cup)

2 bell peppers, cored, seeded, and chopped (2 cups)

3 plum (Roma) tomatoes, chopped (1½ cups)

2 tbsp walnuts, toasted and chopped

1. Place the couscous in a large mixing bowl, cover with boiling water, stir, and allow to sit covered for 7 to 8 minutes. Fluff with a fork.

2. In a small bowl, combine the herb seasoning, oil, lemon zest and juice, shallots, peppers, and tomatoes; toss into the couscous and stir to combine. Garnish with the walnuts before serving.

Per Serving: 142.7 calories, 5.8 g total fat, 0 mg cholesterol, 10.6 mg sodium, 22.4 g total carbs, 4.2 g dietary fiber, 4.1 g protein

Chew on This: Couscous

Couscous is a tiny pasta traditionally made from semolina flour that's been coated with wheat flour. The whole-wheat version is made from whole-wheat flour. It hails from northern Africa, where it is steamed and served at most meals. You might also see Israeli couscous at the market. That is a low-fiber version of couscous that is much larger—it's sometimes referred to as "pearl pasta." It's tasty but not made from whole grains. Most couscous in Western supermarkets has been pre-cooked and dried, which makes it a breeze to cook. When you're short on time and need a whole-grain side dish, whole-wheat couscous is your best friend.

Tabbouleh

Whether you spell it tabbouleh, tabouli, or tabuli, this Middle Eastern salad is fresh and easy to make. A mix of bulgur, parsley, tomatoes, green onions, lemon, and olive oil, tabbouleh is about as versatile as a side dish can be, and it's ready in no time flat.

Try it with Lemon Herb-Roasted Chicken (page 184), Chicken Kebob Pitas with Creamy Cucumber Sauce (page 140), or Black-Bean Burgers with Lime Cream (page 139). (Tabbouleh is pictured on page 141, served with Chicken Kebob Pitas.)

· ·

Chef Meg's Tip: Chopping parsley into "dust" is a rite of passage for all culinary-school students. They chop and chop and chop some more, then come to me for approval. "Is this enough, Chef?" they ask, their eyes eagerly widening. "Nope, not yet," I reply as they return to the chopping block.

Before chopping parsley for any recipe, be sure to wash it and dry it well. For most dishes, you'll want to chop it until it is as small as granulated sugar. (It's a great way to improve your knife skills.) If the parsley is wet, it will clump together, making it impossible to sprinkle.

When making tabbouleh, your knife can take a break. Since there is so much parsley in the recipe, I would suggest using the food processor on pulse mode. I prefer flat-leaf, or Italian, parsley to the curly varieties. It has a darker color and looks prettier on the plate.

· ·

Chew on This: Fresh Herbs vs. Dried Herbs

I always prefer to use fresh herbs and they're the standard in our recipes. Whether right out of the garden or snipped from a small pot on the kitchen windowsill, fresh herbs add an incomparable brightness of flavor to any dish. But what if it's the dead of winter, or you just don't happen to be growing a particular fresh herb that's called for in a recipe? That's what dried herbs are for! Feel free to substitute dried for fresh, just remember that drying intensifies the flavor of the herb, so use half as much as you would if using fresh.

Makes 4 Servings:
    1 cup per serving

30 Minutes to Prepare and Cook

1 cup bulgur

1 large bunch flat-leaf parsley, chopped
    (about 3 cups)

4 green onions, white and green parts,
    chopped (about 1 cup)

2 tomatoes, diced

1 lemon, zested and juiced

⅛ tsp salt

½ tsp black pepper

1 tbsp olive oil

1. Place the bulgur and 2 cups water in a medium-size saucepan with lid. Bring to a boil, cover, and reduce to a simmer. Cook until the bulgur is tender, about 12 minutes.

2. Spread the bulgur on a plate to cool. In a large mixing bowl, combine the parsley, green onions, tomatoes, lemon zest and juice, salt, pepper, and oil. Add the cooled bulgur and toss to combine. Cover and chill for 15 minutes before serving.

Per Serving: 179 calories, 4.3 g total fat, 0 mg cholesterol, 112.1 mg sodium, 32.5 g total carbs, 8.7 g dietary fiber, 6.2 g protein

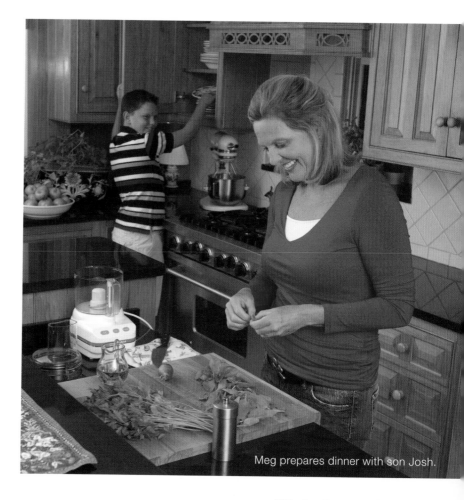

Meg prepares dinner with son Josh.

Quinoa with Pea Pods and Peppers

Quinoa is perfect for a busy night. A good source of protein and fiber, this whole grain (actually a seed) is ready in about 15 minutes. You could eat it plain, but like any grain, it benefits from added flavors. Sautéing garlic, shallots, and other vegetables in a bit of olive oil adds a layer of flavor to the dish, then lemon and parsley add freshness.

Quinoa is more calorie- and nutrient-dense than rice or couscous. If you prefer a lighter side dish, cook half as much quinoa or cut the serving size in half. It can also be a light vegetarian entrée. Instead of snow peas, try frozen peas, chopped asparagus, broccoli, or cauliflower.

Makes 4 Servings:
    1 cup per serving

30 Minutes to Prepare and Cook

1 cup quinoa

1½ cups vegetable stock or water

2 tsp olive oil

4 small shallots, chopped (¼ cup)

3 cloves garlic, chopped

6 ounces snow peas, sliced (about
    2 cups)

1 yellow or orange bell pepper, cored,
    seeded, and chopped (about 1 cup)

1½ tbsp lemon juice

¼ cup parsley, chopped

1. Rinse the quinoa in a fine-mesh strainer under cold water until the water runs clear. Place the quinoa into a medium-size saucepan with lid and add the stock. Bring to a boil, cover, and reduce to a simmer. Cook until the quinoa is tender, 15 to 18 minutes.

2. While the quinoa is simmering, heat a sauté pan over moderate heat. Once hot, add the oil. When the oil is hot, add the shallots and garlic to the pan. Sauté until the shallots become tender, 3 to 4 minutes. Add the snow peas and peppers and sauté for 3 minutes more.

3. Drain any remaining stock from the quinoa; add the quinoa to the vegetables and stir to combine. Remove from heat and add the lemon juice and parsley. Serve warm or cold.

Per Serving: 228.6 calories, 5.3 g total fat, 0 mg cholesterol, 4.5 mg sodium, 39.1 g total carbs, 4.5 g dietary fiber, 7.9 g protein

Chew on This: Quinoa

Quinoa is an ancient seed that has been harvested and used as a grain in South America for more than 5,000 years. The Incas considered it a sacred food and called it the "mother grain." Quinoa is a nutritional powerhouse: it's high in protein (up to 18 percent) and because it also contains all nine essential amino acids, it's a complete protein as well. It is naturally gluten-free and an excellent source of dietary fiber.

Although most of the quinoa available today is pre-rinsed, it's always a good idea to rinse quinoa before cooking to remove any trace of saponin, a coating on the grain that can leave a bitter taste.

When cooked, quinoa has a light and nutty taste; try it hot or cold for a protein-packed breakfast. Look for red and black varieties as well; they have the same excellent flavor and look pretty on the plate.

Farro-Arugula Salad with Walnut Vinaigrette

Tangy, nutty, bitter, peppery, and sweet all wrapped up into one. Regardless of what you're craving, this salad will hit the spot. Adding whole grains to a salad is a great way to increase satiety. We also added a serving of goat cheese for some protein and texture.

This recipe is easy to adapt. It's a good basic cold grain salad recipe—if you want to have some fun or don't feel like running to the market, you can change it up. Spinach and escarole make a great substitute for the arugula, and brown or wild rice will work in place of the farro. Cook the grains ahead of time to save time on prep—or make this salad when you have leftover grains. Top with three ounces of grilled chicken or low-sodium turkey deli meat to boost the protein and make it a meal.

Makes 4 Servings:
    2 cups per serving

1 Hour to Prepare and Cook

1 cup farro

½ tsp salt

4 cups arugula, stems removed

2 tbsp coarsely chopped walnuts

2 tsp brown sugar

½ tsp black pepper

1 tbsp sherry vinegar

1 tbsp canola oil

2 Granny Smith apples, unpeeled, cored, and sliced

4 ounces goat cheese, crumbled

1. Place the farro in a bowl and cover with water to soak for 25 minutes, then drain and rinse in a fine-mesh strainer.

2. Place the soaked farro into a lidded saucepan with 3 cups of water and the salt. Bring to a boil, cover, and simmer on moderate to low heat for 25 minutes. Don't overcook, the farro should be firm to the bite, like al dente pasta. Remove from heat and drain before placing into a serving bowl. Immediately add the arugula and toss to wilt.

3. Place the walnuts in a small saucepan over low heat. Cook, shaking the pan, until the walnuts are toasted. Add the sugar, stir to combine, and remove from heat.

4. Mix the pepper and vinegar together in a bowl, then slowly add the oil, whisking to emulsify.

5. Combine the farro mixture, vinaigrette, walnuts, apples, and cheese. Toss to combine. Serve at room temperature.

Per Serving: 240.6 calories, 12.8 g total fat, 13.1 mg cholesterol, 395.7 mg sodium, 27.7 g total carbs, 5.3 g dietary fiber, 10.8 g protein

Chew on This: Farro

Farro (pronounced FAH-ro) is a variety of wheat popular in Italy. Sold dried, it is often soaked before simmering and usually served al dente (with a bite to the texture). If you can't find farro (sometimes called emmer wheat), substitute wheat berries, barley, spelt, or your favorite whole grain.

Wheat Berry and Broccoli Salad

Have you ever had broccoli salad at a picnic or a salad bar? Between the mayo, the bacon, and the cheese, a half cup can have 300 calories and 30 grams of fat. Sure, broccoli is a superfood, but even it can't save that salad.

I kept the crunch of the salad but decided to start from scratch with this recipe. Most of the fat is gone, and in its place is a salad that's full of interesting, healthy ingredients. Slivered, toasted almonds replace the bacon but retain a slight smokiness to the dish. A vinaigrette replaces the mayo, while tomatoes bulk up the salad.

You can leave the broccoli raw or slightly steam it in the microwave. Don't overcook it, though—it should still be crunchy. If you have any salad left, pack it for lunch the next day. I love it on a bed of spinach. (For more on wheat berries, see Chew on This.)

Makes 6 Servings:
    1 cup per serving

1 hour 15 Minutes to Prepare and Cook (plus overnight soaking, see Note)

¾ cup wheat berries, washed, soaked in 3 cups cool water for 12 hours or overnight (see Note)

3 cups broccoli, chopped (1½ pounds)

1 cup grape tomatoes, sliced in half

1½ tbsp lemon juice

2 tbsp slivered almonds, toasted

For the Dressing:

2 tsp Dijon mustard

1 tbsp white-wine vinegar

¼ tsp black pepper

4 tsp olive oil

2 tbsp finely diced shallots

1. Drain the wheat berries, discard the soaking liquid, and place the wheat berries in a medium-size saucepan with 2½ cups of water. Bring to a boil, reduce to a simmer, cover, and cook until berries are tender but still have a slight crunch, 50 minutes to 1 hour. If you hear the wheat berries popping in the pan, quickly add more water.

2. Steam the broccoli in a microwave for 2 minutes. Transfer the broccoli to a large mixing bowl, add the tomatoes and the hot wheat berries, and stir to combine. Pour lemon juice over the mixture.

3. Make the dressing. Combine the mustard, vinegar, and pepper in a blender or food processor (or in a bowl if using an immersion blender). Process and slowly pour in the oil to emulsify. Stir in shallots. Pour the dressing over the wheat-berry mixture and stir to combine. Garnish with the almonds.

Note: Forget to soak your wheat berries? Boil them for 1 hour 15 minutes to 1½ hours, until they reach the desired chewy texture.

Per Serving: 138.2 calories, 4.6 g total fat, 0 mg cholesterol, 55.1 mg sodium, 21.1 g total carbs, 4.9 g dietary fiber, 5.1 g protein

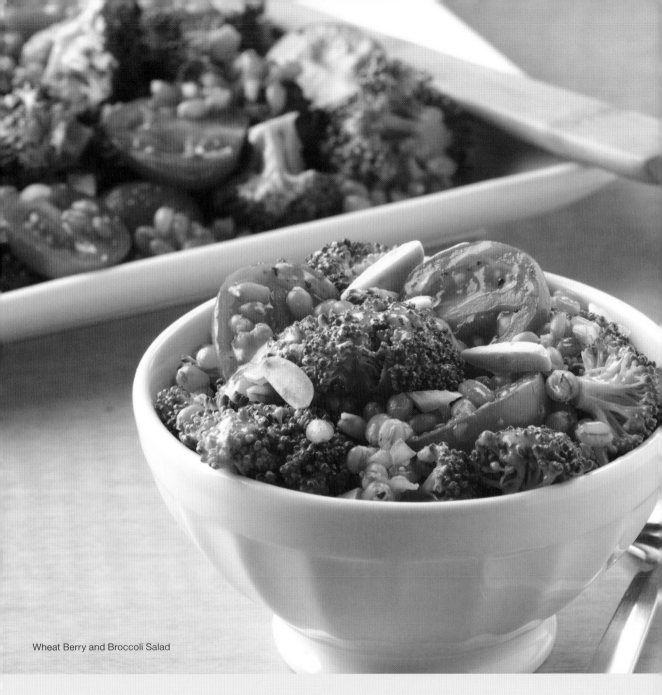

Wheat Berry and Broccoli Salad

Chew on This: Wheat Berries

Wheat berries are a trendy food right now. What are they? Just wheat kernels. You can find them in the whole-grain section of the supermarket. They do require some soaking time, but their nutty and slightly sweet taste is worth the extra effort. I soak grains on Saturday nights, then cook up a big batch on Sundays so I have them on hand to add to salads and soups throughout the week. Per half-cup cooked, they have 5 grams of fiber and 6 grams of protein—more than twice as much of both as brown rice.

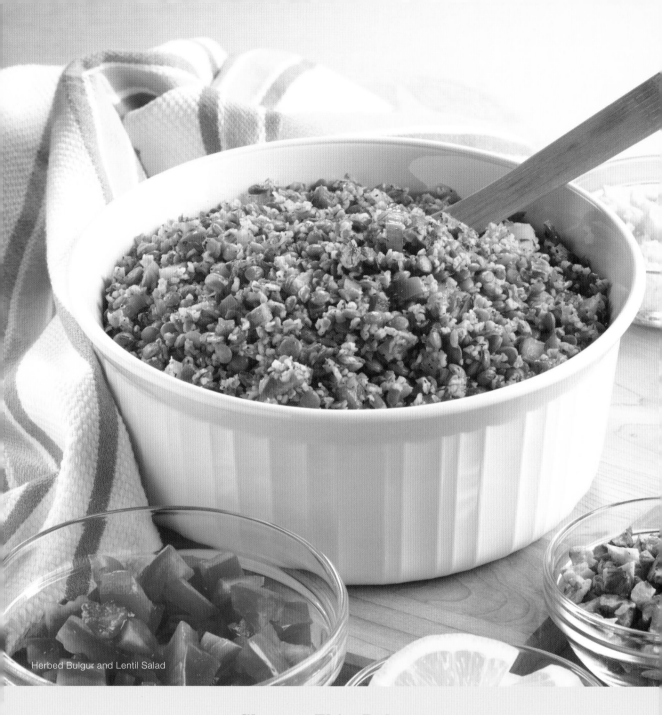

Herbed Bulgur and Lentil Salad

Chew on This: Bulgur

A quick-cooking whole grain, bulgur is wheat that has been parboiled, steamed, and crushed to remove the bran. It's not the same as cracked wheat, which is just crushed wheat kernels. Bulgur is a staple of Mediterranean and Middle Eastern cooking and adds its nutty flavor to pilafs, salads, and stews, and is often mixed with meat. Look for bulgur in the same supermarket aisle as other grains and baking items.

Herbed Bulgur and Lentil Salad

SLIM IT DOWN: Swap chicken broth for the oil (57 calories).

I love how easy and delicious this salad is. The longer it sits in the fridge, the better it tastes, so I make a big batch and eat it throughout the week. This hearty salad provides a filling and fiber-rich base for Lemon Herb-Roasted Chicken (page 184).

Makes 4 Servings (1 cup per serving) or 8 Servings (½ cup per serving)

30 Minutes to Prepare and Cook

1 cup lentils, preferably French or yellow (see Note)

1 cup bulgur

¼ cup olive oil

¼ cup lemon juice (1 to 2 lemons)

2 cloves garlic, crushed

1 tsp salt

2 tbsp chopped mint

2 to 3 tbsp chopped dill

Black pepper, to taste

¼ cup chopped flat-leaf parsley

⅓ cup finely minced red onion

1 red or yellow bell pepper, cored, seeded, and diced

1 stalk celery, finely chopped

1. Place the lentils in a fine-mesh strainer, rinse, and pick out any stones. Place in a medium-size saucepan with lid, add 2 cups water, and bring just to the boiling point. Turn the heat down, partially cover, and simmer without stirring until tender but not mushy, about 20 minutes (see Note). Drain well, and then transfer to a large bowl.

2. While the lentils are cooking, place the bulgur in a small bowl. Add 1 cup boiling water, cover with a plate, and let stand 10 to 15 minutes.

3. Add the olive oil, lemon juice, garlic, salt, mint, dill, black pepper, parsley, onion, bell pepper, celery, and the bulgur to the lentils. Mix gently but thoroughly, cover tightly, and refrigerate for 30 minutes before serving.

Note: If using yellow or pink lentils, adjust cooking time to 15 minutes.

Per 1-Cup Serving: 159.2 calories, 7.1 g total fat, 0 mg cholesterol, 300.4 mg sodium, 21 g total carbs, 5.7 g dietary fiber, 4.8 g protein

CHEF MEG'S TIPS: SALAD ADDITIONS

- ½ cup crumbled feta cheese (add 25 calories, 2 g fat per ½-cup serving)

- ½ cup Niçoise or other black olives (add 10 calories, 1 g fat per ½-cup serving)

- 1 tomato, diced (add 19 calories, 0 g fat per ½-cup serving)

- ½ cup walnuts, toasted and chopped (add 50 calories, 5 g fat per ½-cup serving)

Multigrain Rolls

When I started to track my recipes and daily meals on SparkPeople, I felt reassured that I was eating a well-balanced diet. One thing did surprise me: I seemed to be consuming more sodium than I had thought. I cook with as little salt as possible, so I knew it wasn't coming from my recipes. I eat very little processed foods and no fast food, so those weren't to blame. The culprit: bread!

Homemade bread contains much less sodium than supermarket bread, so if sodium is a concern for you, you should be making your own bread at home. It's easier than you think. You can make hearty, healthy, homemade bread in just a couple of hours.

Rolls are easier to bake than a whole loaf of bread, and they're instantly portion controlled. There's no guessing about how much you're really eating, and these are portable and versatile. The recipe yields two dozen rolls, but if you want to use them for sandwiches, shape them into 12 rolls and bake an additional 10 minutes or until lightly browned.

Makes 24 side or 12 sandwich rolls

3 Hours to Prepare and Bake

1 packet active dry yeast

1 tsp sugar

2 cups white whole-wheat bread flour

1 cup whole-wheat flour

1 tbsp flaxseed meal

1 tsp kosher salt

½ tsp olive oil to coat bowl

For the Topping:

1 tbsp sunflower seeds

1 tbsp flaxseeds

2 tbsp rolled or old-fashioned oats

1 tbsp sesame seeds

1. In a glass, mix together the yeast, sugar, and 2 ounces of 110° F water. Let the mixture sit in a warm location for 5 minutes; it should double in size according to package directions.

2. In the bowl of an electric stand mixer fitted with a dough hook, combine the flours, flax meal, and salt. Slowly pour in the yeast water, then an additional 1 cup of water. Mix together until a well-developed dough forms, about 10 minutes. The dough should be smooth, moist, and slightly sticky. Additional water may be necessary depending on the humidity.

3. Coat a large bowl with the olive oil. Smooth the dough into a ball and place it in the prepared bowl. Cover the bowl with plastic wrap and place it in a warm spot. Allow dough to rise until double in size, about 1 hour 15 minutes.

4. In a flat dish, combine the sunflower seeds, flaxseeds, oats, and sesame seeds.

5. Remove dough from bowl and press down to expel the gases that have built up in the dough. Divide the dough into 24 balls, each slightly smaller than a golf ball. Roll just until smooth, then coat in the topping. Place the rolls

2 inches apart on a parchment-lined sheet pan. Cover with plastic wrap, or a damp towel, and allow to rise in a warm place until double in size, about 40 minutes.

6. Preheat the oven to 375° F. Brush each roll with water, then place in the oven and bake until golden brown, about 15 minutes. The rolls should firm and sound hollow when tapped. The rolls can be kept frozen for up to 2 months, thawed and reheated before serving.

Per Side Roll Serving: 65.8 calories, 1 g total fat, 0 mg cholesterol, 77.4 mg sodium, 12.4 g total carbs, 2.3 g dietary fiber, 2.4 g protein (Double this info for bun-size rolls)

Chew on This: Flaxseeds

Packed with fiber, antioxidants, and omega-3 fatty acids (the good kind of fats that fight inflammation), flaxseeds are a great addition to your diet. Your body can't break down whole flaxseeds, and they pass through undigested, so grind them in a coffee or spice mill before using—or buy flax meal, which is simply ground flaxseeds. Whichever form you buy it in, store flaxseeds in the refrigerator, away from light and use it by the expiration date. Because flaxseeds are so high in unsaturated fat, they can quickly go rancid. (In the Multigrain Rolls, we left them whole for crunch.)

VEGETABLES

On menus and in kitchens across the country, vegetables play second fiddle. Some of us have relegated them to understudy, only eaten when every other option has been exhausted. Proteins always get first billing: Poached Salmon with Broccoli and Brown Rice. Pot Roast with Mashed Sweet Potatoes. Grilled Chicken with Mushrooms and Green Beans.

In my kitchen, vegetables are not the supporting players, they are the stars. You can really take any vegetable-based side dish and turn it into a meal. Take, for example, grilled vegetables like eggplant, peppers, and zucchini. Alone, they're not much, but add Tomato-Basil Vinaigrette (page 387) and low-fat cheese, place on top of whole-wheat bread and—presto!—you have a healthy meal ready to go.

And even if vegetables do stay on the side, there's no reason for them to be boring. As we learned in our Debunk the Diet taste test, bland and boring vegetables just don't satisfy. We can only stomach plain steamed carrots for so long, but when we eat Sautéed Cumin Carrots, we're much more likely to eat them again. Three

fourths of participants knew that steamed carrots were "healthy," but more than half wouldn't eat them again. They wanted the more flavorful sautéed variety. At least three people asked for the recipe when they left, and one woman said those were the first carrots she'd ever liked—take that, ranch dressing!

Holly was 29 years old before she learned to eat any vegetables, and when she came to the taste test, she was apprehensive. She stared down the carrots, but bravely tried them. What she tasted was sweet and citrusy, with a familiar smoky, savory note—cumin, a spice that her Mexican-American mother used in almost every meal growing up. She gobbled down the entire portion—and voted to eat them again. Since then, she has been working to overcome her aversion to vegetables, even enlisting Stepfanie to guide her through the maze of produce at the supermarket. She reached a goal of liking ten vegetables by her 30th birthday! Next up: increasing the number of servings.

While we need two to four servings of protein per day (for most of us, that's two to three ounces of meat per serving), we should be eating more than twice as many vegetables: five to nine servings.

According to the 2009 annual report from the nonprofit Trust for America's Health, "Consumption of fruits and vegetables in the United States increased by 19 percent from 1970 to 2005; however, Americans still are not meeting the Dietary Guidelines' recommendations of two cups of fruit and two and a half cups of vegetables per day."

The Spark's Secrets of Success survey supports that. Among those surveyed who reached their weight-loss goals or lost 100 pounds or more, the No. 1 nutritional strategy was to eat more fruits and vegetables. Ninety percent of those who met their goals and reached their ideal weight now eat more fruits and veggies.

Now 55 pounds lighter and a spinning instructor, ARCHIMEDESII surprised even herself. "I crave vegetables more than chocolate. I never thought that something like that would happen. I love eating a leafy green salad."

When she joined SparkPeople, JANEY2010 admittedly ate few vegetables. She has dropped 115 pounds and hasn't missed her five-a-day servings of fruits and vegetables in more than a year. "Amazing," she says of her transformation from veggie ambivalence to love.

SATISFACTION, NOT GUILT

At our house, raw veggies rule. The boys prefer them as nature intended, often with a low-fat dip or hummus, and that's fine by me. We encourage the boys to eat their fruits and vegetables first. They do it, mostly because I tend to serve them what they like. They have to try every dish I serve, but if they would rather eat raw broccoli, carrots, and celery than a cooked version, I'm okay with that.

Ideally, they would love every dish I set in front of them, but in reality, I'm happy that they have at least a half-dozen vegetables they'll willingly and regularly eat. You shouldn't worry that you hate asparagus, as long as there are other green veggies you like. I'll confess—you'll never see me eat a green pepper. They're too strong and bitter. But you will see me eat orange, red, and yellow ones. Eating your vegetables isn't about perfection or guilt. It's about finding what you like, eating a range of colors, and experimenting with new cooking techniques and vegetables.

MONEY WELL SPENT

No doubt about it, fruits and vegetables are more expensive than ramen noodles and potato chips. But if you look beyond the sticker cost to see the real value, you'll find that you can work produce into your diet on any budget, whether it's fresh or frozen. (And frozen is just as nutritious as fresh—and sometimes more so.)

Once you start giving up the frozen dinners, prepackaged snacks, and canned meals, you'll have more money for "real" food—like fruits and vegetables. And how do you put a dollar amount on these benefits?

Eating a diet full of fruits and vegetables may help:

- Lower blood pressure

- Reduce your risk of heart disease, stroke, and some cancers

- Lower your risk for digestive issues

The next time you think twice about the cost of fresh fruits and vegetables, do what ~INDYGIRL did. After losing 141 pounds (and she's still going), she stopped feeling guilty about treating her body well. Her tip: "Buy yourself or your family a fruit or vegetable tray. They are already made, taste great, and make you feel pampered. Personally, I used to feel they cost too much, but wouldn't think twice about spending that same amount on something unhealthy like a fast-food meal."

No matter what your excuse for not eating them, we can counter it. Vegetables and fruit are a crucial part of a healthy diet. In this chapter you'll learn that you don't have to eat like a rabbit and gobble down pounds of raw vegetables to meet your quota. Even broccoli can satisfy you.

Pop quiz time: how many servings of fruits and vegetables did you eat yesterday? Don't count the pickles on your sandwich or the fries you ate alongside it. No need to be exact—was it over or under five?

SparkPeople Cooking Challenge:

Increase the servings of vegetables you eat each day until you finish a week with five per day. After just a couple of weeks, your glowing skin and hair and newfound energy will be proof enough of the health benefits of vegetables.

On SparkPeople.com, we have a feature called "SparkStreaks" that allows members to challenge themselves to see how many consecutive days they can reach a goal. Eating fruits and vegetables is one of the most common goals people set!

A serving of fruit or vegetables is not as large as you think, and one large salad a day can knock out several of your servings, which are:

- 1 small piece of fruit

- ½ cup raw or cooked vegetables

- ½ cup fruit

- 1 cup leafy greens

Still overwhelmed? Measure out your vegetables. It only takes four to six broccoli florets to equal a half-cup serving. That doesn't seem overwhelming, does it?

So why aren't vegetables at the center of the plate? You might notice that in this book, they kind of are. We packed at least one serving into every dish we possibly could. Half of your plate should be filled with nonstarchy vegetables, and the other half should be equally filled with whole grains or a starchy vegetable and lean protein. Our recipes are meant to reflect that.

Vegetables shouldn't be an afterthought to the meal, though heating up a bag of frozen broccoli or a can of low-sodium green beans is a fine addition to any meal. That attitude is why many of us don't like vegetables to begin with.

If you're tempted to skip this chapter because no way, no how, will you eat your vegetables, we offer you a dare. We bet that you will find at least one recipe that will get you to learn to like vegetables. In fact, there is one recipe that started as a dare, a challenge by Stepfanie for our members who said they couldn't stomach any vegetables. And guess what? It worked. Check out Roasted Root Vegetables on page 315 if you don't believe me.

Frances, whose story is featured on page 66, came running up to Stepfanie at a SparkPeople

Convention in 2009. She "had to meet" the woman responsible for a blog post titled "The Magical Cooking Technique That Will Get You to Eat Your Veggies." Frances wasn't a vegetable lover when she joined SparkPeople, but she recently e-mailed Stepfanie to tell her she had roasted and frozen 25 pounds of tomatoes from her garden to keep on hand for winter. (Find the recipe for Oven-Roasted Tomatoes on page 311.)

From veggie loather to veggie lover, in less than a year!

Now let's go back to those excuses. Stepfanie, who has never met a vegetable she dislikes, considers it her personal mission to make everyone a vegetable lover. Here, she debunks common excuses.

I Can't Afford to Buy Them

- *Buy what's in season.* When you buy asparagus in winter, it has to be shipped in from somewhere else and you pay a premium price. In spring, when the crop is plentiful, the price will be lower—and its flavor at its peak.

- *Be flexible.* If your recipe calls for broccoli but cauliflower is on sale, make the swap. Once you are familiar with vegetables, you'll instinctively know which vegetable can be substituted with another.

- *Weigh the costs.* Consider that you are getting nutrient-dense foods that your body craves, full of vitamins and minerals. They are certainly better buys than chips, cookies, and soda, which we

normally buy regardless of cost. Healthy food now or medical bills later—it's a choice we can all make.

- *Keep an eye on them.* Store fruits and ready-to-eat vegetables on the top shelf of the fridge, or on the kitchen counter or table. If you see them several times in a day, you will be more likely to eat them before they spoil.

- *Sacrifice for them.* If you're having trouble fitting fruits and veggies into your budget, cut back in another area. Two-liter bottles of soda are on sale at my supermarket for $3 each—that's the price of two bags of frozen broccoli. Buy one fewer bottle of soda—or none—and you'll have more money for healthy foods.

I Don't Have Time to Make Vegetables

- *Use shortcuts.* Take advantage of your grocery salad bar, which provides already sliced varieties. Eat them in snack form or toss in a salad with less prep time. Buy shredded carrots, washed lettuce, and chopped stir-fry vegetables. If spending a little more means you'll cook instead of picking up fast food on the way home, those extra dollars were well spent.

- *Stock up.* Always keep frozen and canned fruits and vegetables on hand. These are simple to prepare in the microwave and offer similar nutritional value to the fresh variety. Sometimes frozen vegetables lock in nutrients better than "fresh" ones that have sat on shelves and in trucks for a few days or weeks. If buying canned food, look for the low-sodium varieties—and always rinse and drain your canned vegetables to remove excess salt.

- *Prep in advance.* Wash, slice, and dice them ahead of time. Store in a clear container in the front of your fridge where you can see and reach for them on a daily basis for immediate use. (Only prep a few days' worth at a time to avoid wasted food, and wash delicate salad greens just before use.)

I Don't Like the Taste

- *Buy in season.* Your taste buds as well as your pocketbook appreciate in-season foods. Taste a strawberry in November, then taste one in June. When food is in season and allowed to ripen in the field, it tastes infinitely better.

- *Try, try again.* According to research, it can take up to ten times for our taste buds to adjust to a new food. If you tried peppers once and couldn't stomach them, try them again, prepared in another

way. If you don't like steamed carrots, try them roasted or raw and dipped in hummus. Raw broccoli turns your stomach? Steam it and top it with your favorite spice blend, add it to an omelet, or toss it with a vinaigrette. Did you like to exercise when you started? Probably not, but you kept it up because you knew it was good for you. Take the same approach with vegetables.

- *Say No to "No, thank you."* Trying new foods is terrifying for some people. Be patient with yourself, but don't give up. If you just can't stomach an entire portion of a new food, institute a new rule: If someone offers you a food, instead of saying "No, thank you," take one bite. Accepting a "no, thank you helping" was the required response at my house growing up.

- *Be Sneaky.* If you don't like vegetables, start by tricking yourself. Puree spinach into your pesto (as we do with Better-than-Pesto Puree on page 377), shred them and add them to casseroles or one-pot meals (like Slow-Cooker Salsa Chicken on page 181) or grate them and cover them with another flavor (like the Dark Chocolate Cake on page 360).

I Don't Know How to Cook Them

Keep reading, and by the end of this chapter, that will no longer be an excuse.

Caramelized Onions

Make a batch of these sweet and tangy onions in advance and keep them in a container in the refrigerator to use all week. They're great on a sandwich, grilled bread, pizza, or on the side with pork or beef. You can even make a "skinny" French onion soup by adding beef broth to them. Serve these flavorful onions atop our Beef Roast (page 211) and Chef Meg's Beef and Blue Sandwich (page 135). (Caramelized Onions are pictured on page 137, served atop a Beef and Blue Sandwich.)

Makes 8 Servings:
  2 tbsp per serving

35 Minutes to Prepare and Cook

1 tsp unsalted butter

4 to 5 medium white or yellow onions,
    sliced thin (4 cups)

½ tsp black pepper

1. Place a large sauté pan over moderate heat. Once the pan is warm, add the butter. When the butter begins to foam, add the onions. Cook, stirring the onions occasionally, for 10 minutes.

2. When the onions start to turn light brown, add 2 tablespoons of warm water to the sauté pan and use a wooden spoon to scrape up the browned bits from the bottom of the pan. Continue cooking and repeat two more times, every 10 minutes. Season with pepper.

Per Serving: 26.4 calories, 0.6 g total fat, 1.3 mg cholesterol, 1.8 mg sodium, 5 g total carbs, 1.1 g dietary fiber, 0.7 g protein

Oven-Roasted Tomatoes

This is a great basic to always have on hand! Instead of spending money on expensive, oil-packed, sun-dried tomatoes, make your own. Make large batches when tomatoes are in season, then freeze them for winter use. Serve them in a sauce over whole-wheat pasta, on a sandwich, or in a green salad. They're quite versatile and affordable—especially if you're using tomatoes from your own garden. Some people even eat them like candy.

Makes 12 Servings:
¼ cup per serving

2 Hours 5 Minutes to Prepare and Cook

3 pounds plum (Roma) tomatoes

2 tbsp extra-virgin olive oil

3 cloves garlic, minced

1 tsp dried basil

2 tsp Italian Herb Seasoning (page 369)

½ tsp cracked black pepper

1. Preheat the oven to 275° F. Cut off the top and bottom of the tomatoes and then cut in half lengthwise. Scoop out the seeds and inner flesh and discard. Cut the slices into 2-inch strips.

2. In a bowl, combine the oil, garlic, basil, herb seasoning, and pepper. Add the tomato strips and toss to coat.

3. Lay a roasting rack or a cooling rack over a baking sheet and lay the tomato strips on top in a single layer. Roast the tomatoes for 2 hours (1½ hours if using a convection oven). Remove from oven and allow to cool. To freeze, place ½-cup servings into freezer bags, press out any excess air, and date and label before storing in the freezer. These will keep for up to 6 months.

Per Serving: 28.9 calories, 2.4 g total fat, 0 mg cholesterol, 3.4 mg sodium, 2 g total carbs, 0.4 g dietary fiber, 0.4 g protein

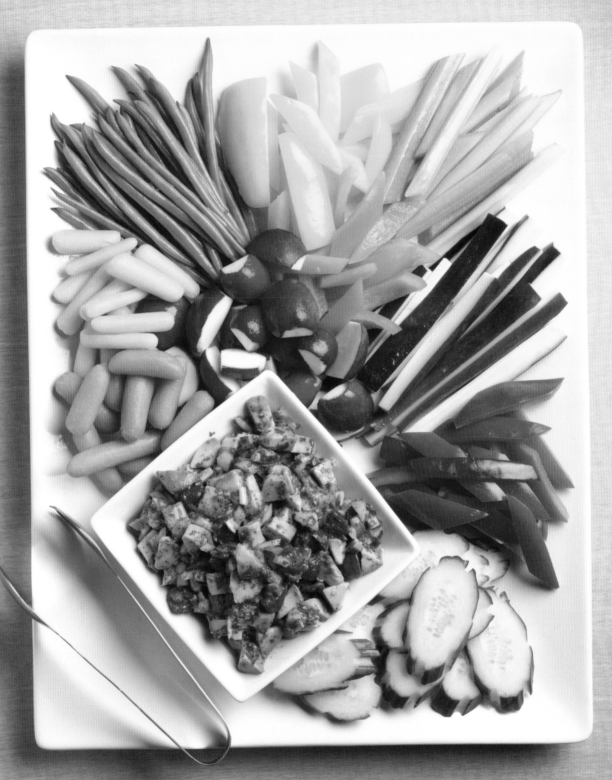

Avocado Cherry-Tomato Salsa, served with a variety of veggie dippers

Avocado Cherry-Tomato Salsa

SLIM IT DOWN:
Halve the avocado (35 calories).

Decades of bland diets have maligned the avocado. Full of fiber and flavor, avocados are a fruit that we happily include on our shopping list. While the fat they contain is primarily the heart-healthy variety, a little avocado goes a long way. That's why, instead of a traditional guacamole in which the avocado is the headliner, this recipe casts it as a co-star with tomatoes. If you like a spicier mix, add a chopped jalapeño pepper. Serve this salsa over a simple green salad alongside Grilled Southwest Flat-Iron Steak (page 220).

Makes 4 Servings:
½ cup per serving

15 Minutes to Prepare and Cook

1 avocado, diced

¼ red onion, diced (¼ cup)

8 cherry tomatoes, quartered (see Note)

1 lime, zested and juiced

2 tbsp chopped cilantro

½ tsp salt

½ tsp black pepper

In a large mixing bowl, stir together the avocado, onion, tomatoes, lime zest and juice, cilantro, and salt and pepper. Serve immediately at room temperature.

Note: Instead of cherry tomatoes, you can substitute 2 chopped plum (Roma) tomatoes or 16 halved grape tomatoes.

Per Serving: 88.9 calories, 6.8 g total fat, 0 mg cholesterol, 298 mg sodium, 7.7 g total carbs, 3.8 g dietary fiber, 1.4 g protein

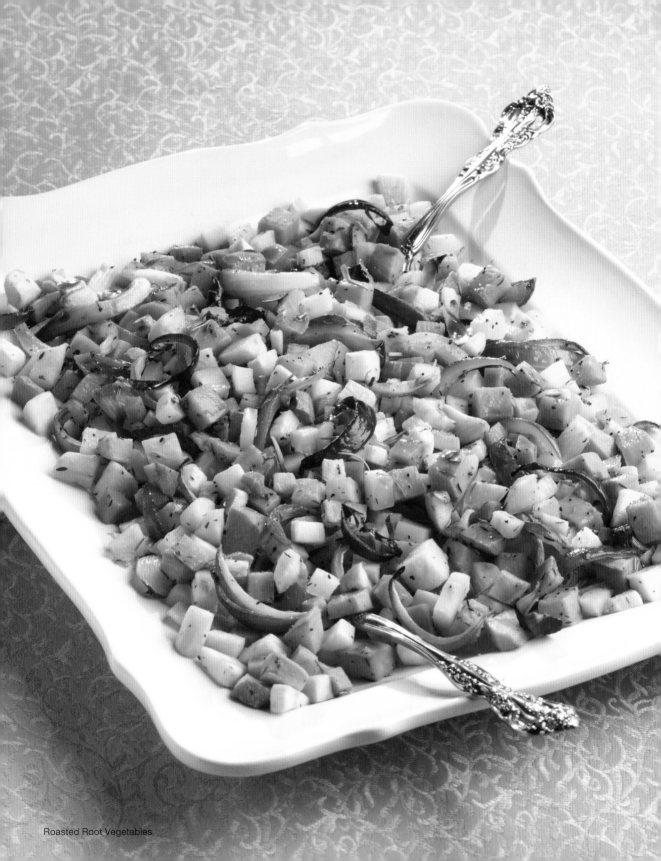

Roasted Root Vegetables

Roasted Root Vegetables

Frances credits this recipe for helping her learn to love veggies. She's such a fan of roasted vegetables that she will even eat them cold as a snack!

She says, "Mix a variety of firm and root vegetables with a little chili powder, lots of cumin, and a drizzle of olive oil and roast them to get a rainbow of tasty, sweet goodness. The taste compares to candy but the nutrition is phenomenal. Just watch it disappear at dinnertime."

This recipe sings of the fall and early-winter harvest. Take advantage of the local farmers' market and buy whatever root vegetables they have. I add a bit of extra richness by drizzling a small amount of balsamic vinegar over the vegetables while they are still hot.

This roasting technique works with almost any vegetable, fresh or frozen, so use whatever vegetables you have on hand and adjust the portion sizes accordingly—just make sure the pieces are about the same size. Try roasted artichoke hearts, broccoli, asparagus, or cauliflower.

Feel free to double up on this recipe—or any veggie recipe—and pack in two tasty servings of vegetables!

Makes 8 Servings:
 ½ cup per serving

45 Minutes to Prepare and Cook

1 tbsp olive oil

1 red onion, sliced

4 cloves garlic, peeled and cut in half

2 carrots, peeled and diced

1 turnip, peeled and diced

1 yam or sweet potato, peeled and diced

2 parsnips, peeled and diced

1 tsp dried rosemary

1 tsp dried thyme

Pinch of salt

½ tsp black pepper

1 tbsp balsamic vinegar (optional)

1. Preheat the oven to 375° F. Prepare a baking sheet with nonstick cooking spray.

2. Combine the oil, onion, garlic, carrots, turnip, yam, parsnips, rosemary, thyme, salt, and pepper in a mixing bowl; toss to combine.

3. Spread the mixture on the prepared baking sheet in a single layer. Bake for 30 minutes, turning the vegetables every 10 minutes until they are tender and slightly browned. Drizzle with balsamic vinegar, if you like, before serving.

Per Serving: 82.1 calories, 1.9 g total fat, 0 mg cholesterol, 36.6 mg sodium, 15.8 g total carbs, 3.2 g dietary fiber, 1.3 g protein

Roasted Red Potatoes with Garlic Herb Oil

The days of potatoes being banished from the plate are over. Potatoes contain vitamin C, potassium, and fiber (especially if you eat the skin) and there are plenty of ways to prepare them without all the added fat and salt of mashed and fried versions. Small potatoes are great for roasting, which is healthier than frying but still produces a crispy skin and tender flesh.

Makes 8 Servings:
½ cup per serving

50 Minutes to Prepare and Cook

1½ pounds red or new potatoes

2 tbsp olive oil

3 cloves garlic, smashed and sliced

1 tbsp fresh thyme

1 tsp chopped rosemary

½ tsp kosher or sea salt

1. Preheat the oven to 400° F. Prepare a baking sheet with nonstick cooking spray.

2. Scrub the potatoes, but do not peel; cut them into quarters. In a large mixing bowl, toss together the potatoes, oil, garlic, thyme, rosemary, and salt.

3. Spread the potatoes in a single layer on the prepared baking sheet. Roast for 20 minutes, stir, and roast an additional 25 minutes or until the potatoes are tender and light brown. Serve warm.

Per Serving: 93.8 calories, 3.5 g total fat, 0 mg cholesterol, 150.8 mg sodium, 14.1 g total carbs, 1.6 g dietary fiber, 1.7 g protein

Steamed Asparagus with Citrus Vinaigrette

SLIM IT DOWN: Use half the dressing (55 calories).

In springtime, asparagus is delicious on its own—just steamed, perhaps with a drizzle of olive oil and a pinch of salt and pepper. But if you want to serve asparagus as a starter for a meal or as an alternative to a green salad, pair it with a citrus fruit and this sweet and tangy vinaigrette. The Dijon mustard in the dressing acts as an emulsifier, which keeps the oil and vinegar from separating.

Asparagus can quickly go from vibrant green and crisp to off-color and stringy, so to prevent that, we blanch it. Immediately after removing the asparagus from the steamer, place it in a bowl of ice water to "shock" it. This will keep it crisp and bright green.

Makes 4 Servings:
 4 stalks asparagus and
 ½ orange per serving

30 Minutes to Prepare and Cook

2 oranges

1 tsp Dijon mustard

1 tbsp orange juice

2 tbsp rice- or white-wine vinegar

2 tbsp olive oil

1 tbsp finely diced shallot

16 stalks asparagus, tough ends snapped and thicker stems peeled

1 bowl of ice water

1. Zest the oranges, then, with a sharp knife, peel away the remaining pith. Segment the fruit while holding it each over a bowl to catch the juice by cutting away the sections in a V, leaving behind the membrane. Set aside the orange zest, juice, and segmented fruit.

2. Prepare the dressing by placing the Dijon mustard, orange juice, and vinegar in a small bowl or blender. While whisking, or with the motor running, slowly add the oil in a steady stream.

3. To cook the asparagus, use a steamer or place a large sauté pan over medium-high heat along with 2 tablespoons of water. Add the asparagus to the pan in a single layer and cover. Steam the asparagus until just tender, about 5 minutes. Remove from heat and immediately place in a bowl of ice water.

4. Drain the asparagus and place in a mixing bowl. Pour the vinaigrette over the asparagus and toss with segmented oranges, shallot, and orange zest.

Per Serving: 121.7 calories, 7 g total fat, 0 mg cholesterol, 31.7 mg sodium, 14.6 g total carbs, 3.6 g dietary fiber, 2.4 g protein

Roasted Asparagus

Asparagus is a harbinger of spring. When those first tender green stalks appear in the market, you know that winter is over. And while you've probably steamed or sautéed asparagus, have you ever roasted it? Roasting tempers any bitterness in out-of-season asparagus and adds great caramelization and a layer of flavor any time of year.

Serve this with Light Lemon Sauce (page 379); it's great for pouring or dunking. Asparagus is low in calories, so load up on it while it's in season!

Makes 8 Servings:
about 8 stalks per serving

15 Minutes to Prepare and Cook

2 bunches asparagus (see Note)

Pinch of salt

Pinch of pepper

1. Preheat the oven to 400° F. Prepare a baking sheet with nonstick cooking spray.

2. To trim the woody ends, hold one end of the asparagus stalk in each hand. Snap the asparagus; the stalk will naturally break at end of the thick, woody end. Trim any remaining tough flesh away with a paring knife or vegetable peeler.

3. Place the asparagus on the prepared sheet pan in a single layer. Spritz the asparagus with additional cooking spray and season with the salt and pepper. Roast for 10 minutes, turning the stalks over halfway through.

Note: When you buy the asparagus, make sure the tips are tight and compact. Cut off just the ends of the stalks and store upright in the refrigerator in a small dish of water, just like you would flowers.

Per Serving: 29.6 calories, 0.2 g total fat, 0 mg cholesterol, 41.4 mg sodium, 5.8 g total carbs, 2.6 g dietary fiber, 3 g protein

Baked Sunburst Fries

Who doesn't like fries? They're crispy, they're crunchy, and you can eat them with your fingers. In our house, fries aren't fried, and they aren't made from just potatoes. You can turn just about any root vegetable into a fry, but carrots, parsnips, and sweet potatoes are tops at our house. We call these sunburst fries because of their lovely pale yellow and bright orange colors.

Fries are traditionally made by squaring off a potato and cutting it into sticks. That's fine with a large sweet potato, as there's not much waste, but for carrots and parsnips, I recommend that you cut them in half lengthwise, then into wedges. Instead of plain ketchup, offer our Spicy Yogurt Sauce (page 380) or Honey-Mustard Dipping Sauce (page 382). (Baked Sunburst Fries are pictured on page 143, served with our Crunchy Cod Sandwich, page 142.)

Makes 4 Servings:
 1 cup per serving

40 Minutes to Prepare and Cook

1 sweet potato or yam, peeled and cut into ½-inch sticks

1 large parsnip, peeled and cut into ½-inch wedges

1 carrot, peeled and cut into ½-inch wedges

1 tbsp olive oil

½ tsp kosher or sea salt

½ tsp black pepper

1. Preheat oven to 400° F. Coat a sheet pan with nonstick cooking spray.

2. Place the potato, parsnip, and carrot in a bowl; toss with the oil, salt, and pepper (see Note).

3. Spread the vegetables on the sheet pan in a single layer. Bake for 15 minutes, then stir to ensure even cooking. Return the pan to the oven and bake an additional 15 minutes. Don't overcook the vegetables, they should still be crunchy.

Note: If you don't want to dirty a bowl, drizzle the olive oil directly on the baking sheet, spread the vegetables on top in a single layer, and then sprinkle on the seasonings. Mix well using your hands.

Per Serving: 152.9 calories, 3.8 g total fat, 0 mg cholesterol, 341.3 mg sodium, 29.2 g total carbs, 4.4 g dietary fiber, 1.9 g protein

Trio of Grilled Vegetables with Balsamic Glaze

This is as much a method as it is a recipe. As with roasting, grilling will bring out the natural sweetness of the vegetables, but it adds another layer of flavor as well: that great, smoky char. You can grill almost any vegetable, from eggplant to potatoes, to corn, to even lettuce. Green vegetables such as broccoli or asparagus should be blanched (briefly boiled then plunged into ice water to stop the cooking process) before grilling. When grilling root vegetables such as carrots, potatoes, or sweet potatoes, boil them until almost tender before grilling. Use a grill basket to prevent vegetables such as asparagus from slipping through the grates on the grill.

Makes 4 Servings:
1 cup per serving

30 Minutes to Prepare and Cook

For the Herb Oil:

¼ tsp kosher or sea salt

¼ tsp black pepper

1 tbsp dried basil

1 tbsp olive oil

1 small red onion, peeled, quartered, and layers separated

2 small yellow squash (about 4 ounces), sliced lengthwise, ¼-inch thick

2 small zucchini (8 ounces), sliced lengthwise, ¼-inch thick

For the Glaze:

¼ cup balsamic vinegar

1. Preheat the grill to 375° F or moderate heat (see Note).

2. In a large bowl, whisk together the salt, pepper, basil, and oil. Add the onion and squash to herbed oil, and toss to coat.

3. Place the onions on the grill and cook for 4 to 5 minutes. Add the squash to the grill in single layers, and cook for 3 minutes. Turn the squash over and cook for 2 minutes more.

4. Meanwhile, place the vinegar into a small saucepan. On the stovetop, bring the vinegar to a simmer and cook until it is reduced by half. (This step can be done ahead of time if you are planning an outdoor event.)

5. Remove the vegetables from the grill and place them on a platter, then drizzle them with the vinegar glaze. For a nice effect, you can drizzle the glaze on the plate instead.

Note: Never spray the grill with nonstick cooking spray: it's flammable. If the grill's surface is clean and hot, your food will not stick. Clean the grill grates with a metal brush before use and always preheat before placing food on the grill surface.

Per Serving: 60.2 calories, 3.6 g total fat, 0 mg cholesterol, 153 mg sodium, 6.5 total carbs, 1.3 g dietary fiber, 1.7 g protein

Herbed Mushrooms with Bacon

SLIM IT DOWN: Leave out the bacon (35 calories).

There are so many mushrooms on the market that have great flavor. Button or white mushrooms are fine for most recipes, but for this dish, try a mixture of mushroom varieties for boosted flavor. This would be a good side dish for pork, chicken, or beef; you could also serve it over toasted whole-grain bread, polenta, or whole-wheat pasta.

Fresh spinach is much easier to clean these days, thanks to the triple-washed bags available at most supermarkets.

Makes 4 Servings:
½ cup per serving

30 Minutes to Prepare and Cook

4 slices turkey bacon, diced

3 cups mixed mushrooms (shiitake, baby bellas, cremini, or white), sliced into ½-inch slices

2 cloves garlic, finely chopped

1 packed cup baby spinach, stems removed

¼ cup white wine or 1 lemon, juiced

1 tsp dried thyme

¼ tsp salt

¼ tsp black pepper

¼ cup shredded Parmesan cheese

1. Place a nonstick skillet over moderate heat. Add the bacon and cook until just crisp. Remove from the pan and set aside on a paper towel.

2. Add the mushrooms and garlic to the warmed pan and sauté for 3 to 4 minutes. Add the spinach and cook until just wilted.

3. Add the wine or lemon juice, and stir with a wooden spoon to scrape up any brown bits from the bottom of the pan.

4. Season with the thyme, salt, and pepper, and add the Parmesan and cooked bacon. Toss to combine. Serve warm.

Per Serving: 101.4 calories, 4.7 g total fat, 4.9 mg cholesterol, 451.7 mg sodium, 10.4 g total carbs, 2.8 g dietary fiber, 6.9 g protein

Potato Salad with Veggies and Bacon

Who needs mayo? Not potato salad! The traditional recipe has 360 calories, 21 grams of fat, and a staggering 1,300 milligrams of sodium—and much of that damage comes from the mayonnaise. This smoky potato salad has a not-so-secret ingredient (bacon) that will make you forget the creamy version of this picnic staple. Serve it warm or at room temperature—it's terrific either way. (Potato Salad with Veggies and Bacon is pictured on page 292.)

Makes 4 Servings:
1 cup per serving

30 Minutes to Prepare and Cook

1½ pounds red potatoes

2 slices bacon, chopped

1 medium red onion, chopped (1 cup)

1 red bell pepper, cored, seeded, and chopped

1 yellow or orange bell pepper, cored, seeded, and chopped

1 tbsp white-wine vinegar

½ tsp black pepper

1 tbsp chopped parsley

1. Scrub the potatoes, but do not peel them; cut each potato into 8 pieces. Place in a saucepan and cover with water. Bring to a boil and cook until the potatoes are just tender, 6 to 8 minutes, then strain.

2. Cook the bacon in a large sauté pan over moderate to low heat until the fat melts and the meat starts to brown. Remove the bacon from the pan and increase the heat to high. Add the onion and potatoes, then sauté until they just start to brown, 4 to 5 minutes.

3. Add the peppers to the pan and continue to cook for 2 to 3 minutes. Add the vinegar to the pan and stir to combine. Remove from heat, then add the black pepper, the cooked bacon, and chopped parsley. Serve hot or at room temperature.

Per Serving: 161.5 calories, 2.1 g total fat, 2.7 mg cholesterol, 63 mg sodium, 32.1 g total carbs, 5.1 g dietary fiber, 5.1 g protein

Chew on This: Bacon Is Back

Bacon is often thought of as being forbidden in a healthy diet. Instead of banning its smoky, rich, and, yes, fatty deliciousness from your plate, reclassify it. Stop thinking of bacon as a protein source, and think of it as a condiment instead. (Becky tells us that nutritionally it has always been in the fat group.) For example, our potato salad has just two slices of bacon—a half-slice per person. We even kept the bacon fat, and each serving still has just two grams of fat.

To keep your fat and cholesterol in check, you do have to limit your intake of fatty or cured meats like bacon, sausage, or ham. But with these "rarely eaten" foods, just remember that a little goes a long way. Crumble a slice of bacon or a tablespoon of sausage meat or finely chopped ham on a salad or in an omelet, and be sure to blot the grease unless you're using it to flavor a dish.

Easy Steamed Vegetable Packets

Cooking in parchment paper packets is a technique known as *en papillote*. That might sound complicated, but it's oh-so-easy and, because everything is cooked in the parchment, cleanup is a breeze! The food stays moist without any added fat, and the herbs lend flavor to the vegetables. Be sure to slice your vegetables thinly to ensure even cooking. We used peppers, mushrooms, and leeks here, but you can choose your favorites: peppers, asparagus, carrots, onions, zucchini, and green beans are all good choices. Switch up the herbs and spices, too: try adding garlic, basil, or oregano to mix the flavors. (Easy Steamed Vegetable Packets are pictured on page 225, served with Easy Steamed Fish Packets, page 224.)

Makes 4 Servings:
    ¾ cup per serving

30 Minutes to Prepare and Cook

2 leeks, thinly sliced

2 red or yellow bell peppers, cored,
    seeded, and thinly sliced

1 cup button mushrooms, caps only,
    sliced

2 lemons, zested and cut in half

1 tbsp chopped parsley

1 tsp chopped thyme

1. Preheat oven to 450° F. Fold four sheets of 15" x 15" parchment paper in half (see Note). Coat one half with nonstick cooking spray and place it—with the coated side up—on a sheet pan.

2. On the coated side of the parchment, layer one fourth of the leeks, peppers, and mushrooms; sprinkle the lemon zest, parsley, and thyme on top; followed by the juice of half a lemon. Fold over the uncoated half of the parchment and crimp the edges to form a packet. Repeat with the remaining sheets of parchment paper.

3. Bake 12 to 15 minutes, depending on the thickness of the vegetables. Serve the vegetables in the packets, allowing everyone to open their own packet at the table. (Remember the escaping steam can be quite hot.)

Note: To make two servings of 1½ cups of vegetables, use only two sheets of parchment.

Per Serving: 107.8 calories, 0.7 g total fat, 0 mg cholesterol, 22.4 mg sodium, 25.9 total carbs, 4.8 g dietary fiber, 3.7 g protein

Braised Swiss Chard with Beans

This dish is more of an entrée than a side dish—it's that filling. The creamy white beans add fiber and staying power to the Swiss chard and mushrooms. Serve this dish with Lemon Herb-Roasted Chicken (page 184) and Wild Rice with Roasted Shallots and Garlic (page 291) for a special dinner. We also like it over plain brown rice as a vegetarian supper. For a side dish, feel free to cut the portions in half.

Swap escarole or spinach for the chard if you want, and use chicken stock if that's what you have on hand.

Makes 4 Servings:
    1 cup per serving

30 Minutes to Prepare and Cook

2 tsp olive oil

1 small red onion, thinly sliced into strips
    (about 1 cup)

4 portobello mushrooms, gills removed,
    sliced into ½-inch strips

1 can (15.5 ounces) cannellini beans,
    drained and rinsed

¼ tsp red pepper flakes

½ tsp chopped fresh rosemary

½ tsp black pepper

4 cups thinly sliced Swiss chard leaves

½ cup homemade or low-sodium
    vegetable stock

1 tbsp plus 1 tsp balsamic vinegar

1. Place a large sauté pan with lid over moderate heat; when the pan is hot, add the oil. When the oil is hot, add the red onion and sauté until softened, 4 to 5 minutes. Add the mushrooms and sauté 1 to 2 minutes more.

2. Add the beans, red pepper, rosemary, black pepper, and Swiss chard; sauté 1 to 2 minutes. Pour the stock over the vegetables, cover, and cook for 8 to 10 minutes. Stir in the vinegar before serving.

Per Serving: 167.7 calories, 2.4 g total fat, 0 mg cholesterol, 326.2 mg sodium, 34 g total carbs, 13.1 g dietary fiber, 13.5 protein

Sautéed Cumin Carrots

Even the pickiest of children usually will eat carrots, although they usually like them best when dunked in ranch dressing. And plenty of cooked dishes accentuate carrots' natural sweetness with honey, brown sugar, or maple syrup, but does anyone really need more sugar? This dish, which won over cooked-carrot haters in our taste test, uses whole and ground cumin to add a smoky, savory element to the carrots.

You'll get two servings of vegetables for the whole family with this recipe, which makes a great side for chicken, pork, or beef.

Makes 4 Servings:
   1 cup per serving

30 Minutes to Prepare and Cook

¼ tsp whole cumin seeds

1 tbsp butter

3 large carrots, peeled and sliced into
   1-inch disks (about 4 cups)

¼ cup orange juice

¼ tsp ground cumin

¼ tsp salt

¼ tsp white pepper

1 lime, zested and juiced

1. Place the cumin seeds in a medium saucepan with a tight-fitting lid, then warm the pan over medium heat to toast the seeds. Once the seeds start to pop, add the butter and melt until foamy.

2. Add the carrots, orange juice, ground cumin, salt, white pepper, and ¼ cup of water. Cover and simmer for 10 minutes. Remove the lid, add the lime zest, and continue to simmer the carrots until they are just firm to the bite, about 5 minutes. Sprinkle the lime juice over the carrots before serving.

Per Serving: 74.5 calories, 3.2 g total fat, 7.8 mg cholesterol, 214.6 mg sodium, 11.4 g total cars, 2.9 g dietary fiber, 1.1 g protein

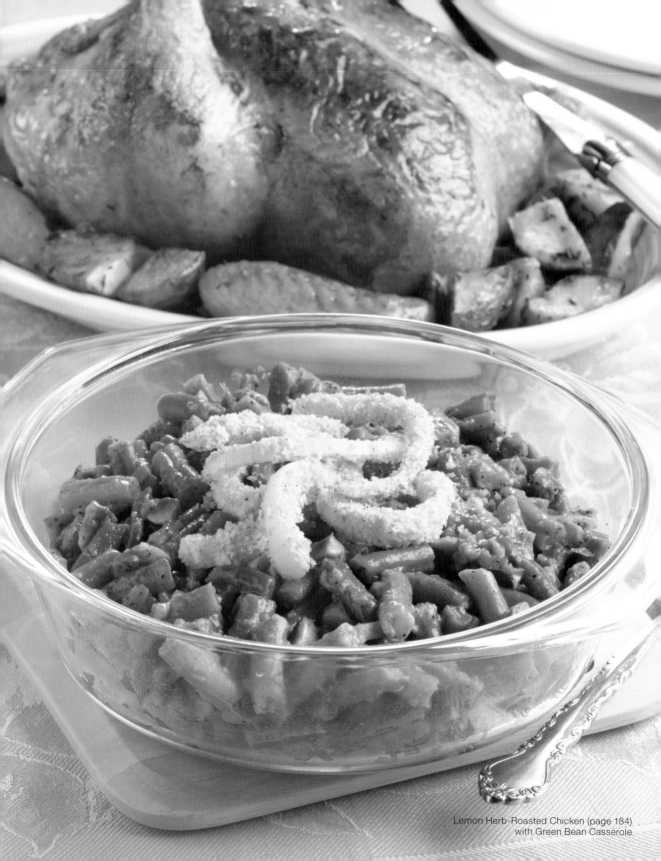

Lemon Herb-Roasted Chicken (page 184)
with Green Bean Casserole

Green Bean Casserole

SLIM IT DOWN: Omit the onions (40 calories).

When did the green bean casserole earn a place at the holiday dining table? That this back-of-the-soup-can recipe quickly became a favorite is no surprise: green beans are coated in a rich, creamy sauce, then topped with fried onions. You get fat, salt, crunch, and cream—all in one bite. You also get 120 calories, 8 grams of fat, and more sodium than a large order of McDonald's French fries in a scant half cup.

We kept those same four components but lightened them up. Gone is the condensed soup, and in its place is a quick broth-based sauce. The onions are still crunchy, but they're baked. We added fresh mushrooms and frozen green beans to boost the veggies and the nutrition. Our serving size is doubled with far fewer calories—so go ahead and make room at the Thanksgiving Day buffet for this one!

For your next Sunday supper, serve Green Bean Casserole with Lemon Herb-Roasted Chicken and Baked Lemon-Spiced Rice (360 calories, 8.6 g fat, 293 mg sodium). You'll even have room for dessert!

. . . .

Chef Meg's Tip: Try these crispy baked onions atop the Tuna Noodle Casserole (page 231), atop a salad, or in a sandwich for a bit of crunch.

. . . .

Makes 6 Servings:
1 cup per serving

45 Minutes to Prepare and Cook

For the Sauce:

1 tsp unsalted butter

1 tsp all-purpose flour

1 cup homemade, low-sodium, or no-salt-added chicken or vegetable stock

For the Onions:

1 tbsp cornstarch

1 egg white

¾ cup panko (Japanese breadcrumbs)

¼ tsp paprika

¼ onion, sliced into thin strips

For the Casserole:

2 cups small button mushrooms, cut in half

4 cups frozen green beans

½ tsp black pepper

1. Preheat the oven to 350° F.

2. Make the sauce. Place the butter into a small saucepan over moderate heat. When the butter has melted, add the flour and cook, stirring constantly, until the flour turns a light brown color, 2 to 3 minutes. Slowly pour the stock into the saucepan and whisk to combine. Turn up the heat to bring to a boil, then reduce to a simmer and cook for 10 to 15 minutes.

3. Meanwhile, make the onions. Lay out two pie plates or flat-bottomed bowls; place the cornstarch in one, place the egg white in the other

and whisk. Place the panko and paprika in a plastic bag. Toss the onions in the cornstarch, dip them into the egg white, and then place them in the plastic bag. Shake to coat. Place in a single layer on a baking sheet and bake until golden, about 8 to 10 minutes. Remove from the oven and set aside. Do not turn off the oven.

4. Coat a saucepan with nonstick cooking spray and place over high heat. Add the mushrooms and sauté until golden, 4 to 5 minutes. Add the beans, season with pepper, and pour in the sauce. Stir to coat and cook for 1 to 2 minutes.

5. Transfer to an ovenproof casserole dish prepared with nonstick cooking spray and bake for 10 minutes. Sprinkle the breaded onions over the beans and bake for 5 minutes more.

Per Serving: 95.5 calories, 0.8 g total fat, 1.8 mg cholesterol, 24.2 mg sodium, 16.0 g total carbs, 3.6 g dietary fiber, 4.3 g protein

Braised Spinach with Pine Nuts

SLIM IT DOWN: Skip the pine nuts (15 calories).

Spinach is a superfood, but I often hear people say they don't like it when cooked. Raw spinach is wonderful in salads, but with the proper cooking techniques, cooked spinach can be just as delicious.

Spinach cooks quickly, and overcooking it yields a slimy, brownish-green mess. The trick here is to add enough water to cook it but not so much as to leave it soggy. What we're doing here is braising—a technique we usually think of for slow cooking meat. But you can also braise vegetables: it doesn't take long, and it adds great flavor that simply steaming could not. You'll be surprised at how much spinach shrinks during cooking. Two cups of raw spinach—two servings—yields just about ½ cup when cooked.

If you don't have pine nuts on hand, substitute an equal amount of your favorite chopped nut.

. . . .

Chef Meg's Tip: Although it takes some time, I recommend removing the stems of fresh spinach, which are fibrous and don't soften during cooking. Turn the spinach upside down, grasp the stem, and rip it out. Of course, if you want some added fiber in your diet, you can leave them! To save time, leave the stems!

. . . .

Makes 4 Servings:
½ cup per serving

20 Minutes to Prepare and Cook

1 small shallot, chopped (about 1 tbsp)

8 cups spinach (about 10 ounces), large stems removed

1 lemon, zested and juiced

¼ tsp black pepper

2 tbsp pine nuts

1. Coat a large lidded sauté pan with nonstick cooking spray and place over moderate heat. Add the shallot and cook until softened, about 2 minutes. Do not let the shallot brown.

2. Add ½ cup of water to the pan and bring to a boil. Add the spinach, toss, and cover the pan. Reduce the heat to low and cook for 2 to 3 minutes.

3. Uncover and remove the pan from the heat. Add the lemon zest, juice, and pepper to season. Garnish with the pine nuts.

Per Serving: 33.2 calories, 1.7 g total fat, 0 mg cholesterol, 56 mg sodium, 3.5 g total carbs, 1.7 g dietary fiber, 2.4 g protein

SNACKS & DESSERTS

SNACKS

Confession: I am the poster child for snacking, and in my boys, I have created three clones. We are all snackers. For me, it is because of my profession and my health. It seems like I am constantly eating, whether it's for taste analysis and grading or to keep me from seeing stars from low blood sugar. For my boys, it's because they're always on the go, with sporting events or practices almost daily. They can't exercise with a full belly, so they eat two small meals, one before and one after a game or practice.

So how do my pants—from my skinniest jeans to my baggy checkered chef's trousers—still fit? I'm smart about snacking, follow the SparkPeople experts' guidance, and use snacks to my advantage: they don't replace meals, they're spread out from meals by at least an hour or two, and they total a couple hundred calories or less. I make sure most of my snacks contain 5 to 10 grams of protein to sustain me until my next meal. And I don't wait until

I'm hungry to search for a snack; I think about snacks in advance and make sure I have some on hand so I don't end up eating the cake scraps left in the kitchens at school or candy out of a bowl on someone's desk!

In recent years, dietitians, doctors, and researchers have rethought the "no eating between meals" rule. Snacks are important, especially when you live an active life or are trying to lose weight. If you go hours on end without eating, your blood sugar will drop, your stomach will grumble, and you'll start to get grouchy—and you'll ultimately eat your way through whatever's in the kitchen. Eating every few hours keeps your hunger levels down so you can control your appetite and prevent overeating. Healthy snacks help keep blood-sugar levels in check and keep your energy up.

Just a few well-timed bites have a big impact, says LADYSALUBRIOUS, who is using SparkPeople to "reclaim her body" after two babies in as many years. "I usually go no more than 2 or 3 hours without eating and feel great! I eat only healthy things and typically go as unprocessed as I can. I like to couple fruit or veggies with some type of protein (nuts, cheese, peanut butter), and this usually staves off cravings.

"If I don't eat a snack, then by the time lunch or dinner comes I am ready to eat a continent! Not good 'cause by that time I'm craving greasy burgers and other comfort foods."

Integrating snacks and desserts into your life is an important part of learning to eat right. Snacks are not a chance to load up on empty calories. They are an opportunity to add more heart-healthy fats, whole-grain carbs, and protein—or an extra serving of fruits and vegetables—to your daily intake. Snacks help fuel your body to give you a boost of energy in the afternoon or tide you over until your next meal.

Treating yourself occasionally can help prevent binges later on. Instead of heading to the vending machine when afternoon munchies set in or fatigue hits, grab a healthful snack—of about 200 calories or less. You'll find suggestions to stave off any craving on our Easy Snacks list (page 333). I always drink at least 8 ounces of water right before I eat a snack to help me fill up. Thirst often masquerades as hunger, so this is a great trick when you feel like snacking for no good reason.

SparkPeople Cooking Challenge:

Skipping snacks to save calories for later in the day often leads to extreme hunger and overeating. Add an afternoon snack tomorrow, and note any differences in your hunger levels at dinnertime.

We promote healthy snacking, but it's easy to understand how snacks have earned their bad reputation. Since 1977, America's consumption of salty snacks has increased dramatically, with kids aged two to eight eating 132 percent more in 1996 than they did 19 years prior. Adults aged 19 to 39 ate 133 percent more, according to a 2009 report. That same report found that 85 percent of snacks in school vending machines are of poor nutritional quality, and I believe it.[1] When I see the food my kids have access to at school, I am shocked. And it doesn't stop there.

I love that my boys are active and learning new skills through sports, but I will say that I hate "snack time" for sporting events. (I know this just made me a very unpopular mom.) Why do kids need a cupcake as a reward after every one-hour game? The reward is that they were able to spend time competing in a sport they love. My son Josh's lacrosse coach is a refreshing change: after every practice, he talks to the kids about nutrition and exercise and there's no pushing of sugary snacks or sports drinks after games—it's all about water, water, water.

A healthy snack can save you from making food decisions that you'll regret later. Without hunger pangs gnawing at your belly, you'll be able to drive past the fast-food restaurant after work, resist the cake in the office kitchen in the afternoon, and say no to the cookies the size of your face at the mall. Here are some strategies for healthy snacking no matter where you are.

HEALTHY SNACKS ON THE GO

- *In the car.* SparkGuy stashes healthy snacks in his glovebox or console.

Energy bars, nuts, dried fruit, and even baggies of whole-grain crackers are great on-the-go snacks.

- *In the bag.* Keep small containers of granola, trail mix, or an apple in your gym bag or purse.

- *At the office.* Store a few portion-controlled snacks in your desk drawer so you can fight the urge to hit the vending machines. Keep a fruit bowl on your desk as a reminder to eat right all day long.

HEALTHY SNACKS AT HOME

- Designate a shelf in your pantry and in your fridge for healthy snacks. If you have kids, place it at their eye level. By keeping snacks within reach in one place, you'll be less tempted to search for less-healthy options.

- Fill a small plate with your snack and leave the kitchen. Just walk away. When your plate is empty, snack time is over.

- Limit yourself to a single serving. Never bring the entire container with you to eat in front of the television or computer.

- Enjoy your snack without distraction and you won't be tempted to reach for more.

- Plan out your snacks just like you would a meal. Is one cookie worth the calorie cost, when you could eat a plate of fresh fruit instead?

SparkPeople Cooking Challenge: Make a game plan. The next time hunger strikes at home, measure out your snack, put the box or bag away, then eat with as few distractions as possible. Ideally, snacks should be consumed sitting down at the dining table.

EASY SNACKS

At SparkPeople, we love snacks. The majority of our members can't imagine staying on an eating plan that didn't allow them to snack between meals, and the latest research shows that that's a good thing! If too much time passes between meals, hunger and cravings set in. If you are prepared to answer that call with a healthy delicious snack, you'll keep your metabolism high, satisfy your craving, and support your healthy lifestyle.

Here are some of our favorite healthy snacks.

- 2 rice cakes spread with 1 tablespoon peanut butter

- 1 ounce low-fat cheese cubes

- 1 hardboiled egg

- 6 ounces low-fat yogurt with fresh fruit, ¼ cup nuts, or trail mix

- ½ cup cut vegetables with 2 table-spoons low-fat dip (packets of low-fat salad dressing from salad bars work as easy-to-pack dip)

- 1 cup cucumber slices or other raw vegetables with ¼ cup hummus

- 3 ounces leftover chicken or turkey slices (great to eat cold)

- ½ cup healthy, fiber-rich or whole-grain cereal (easy to eat dry from a plastic bag)

- Half a large whole-wheat bagel with 1 tablespoon light cream cheese

- 1 medium apple with 1 tablespoon peanut butter

- 1 cup fresh berries with ½ cup low-fat vanilla yogurt

- 1 ounce whole-wheat crackers and 1 piece of low-fat string cheese

- 1 cup frozen grapes with ½ ounce mixed nuts

- Tuna or cottage cheese in 4-ounce mini-containers

- 1 medium piece of fruit and a 6-ounce container of low-fat yogurt

- 1 packet of oatmeal made with skim milk

- ¼ cup of trail mix with nuts and dried fruit

- 4 ounces low-fat cottage cheese and ½ cup of fruit

- Half a peanut butter or turkey/chicken sandwich on whole-grain bread

- 1 ounce whole-grain crackers with 1 tablespoon nut butter or 1 ounce cheese

- 2 whole-grain fig (or fruit) Newton cookies

- 8 ounces low-fat milk (especially low-fat chocolate milk)

- 8-ounce yogurt smoothie (with added protein powder, if desired)

- 2 celery sticks with 1 tablespoon peanut butter and several raisins on top

- A protein or energy bar

Sweet and Spicy Pecans

Nuts are a great snack. They're portable and full of protein, fiber, and heart-healthy fats.

I like to set out dishes of these nuts at parties; I also give them away as hostess gifts. These are a much better option than anything I'll find at the concession stand at the boys' games. I also like to chop these nuts and add them to a simple green salad. It's a great way to add some staying power. Experiment with other kinds of nuts, if you like, but be sure to portion them out. They are quite addictive!

Makes 16 Servings:
    2 tbsp per serving

15 Minutes to Prepare and Cook

2 cups raw pecan halves or walnuts

1 tbsp sugar

1 tsp cinnamon

¼ tsp cayenne

1 tbsp egg white

1. Preheat the oven to 300° F. Prepare a baking sheet with nonstick cooking spray.

2. In a mixing bowl, combine the nuts, sugar, cinnamon, and cayenne. Stir in the egg white.

3. Spread the nuts in an even layer on the sheet pan. Bake for 3 minutes, shake the pan, then continue to bake for 3 to 4 minutes more. Cool in the pan on a wire rack. When completely cooled, store in an airtight container. They'll keep for a week.

Per Serving: 97.9 calories, 9.7 g total fat, 0 mg cholesterol, 3.5 mg sodium, 2.8 g total carbs, 1.4 g dietary fiber, 1.6 g protein

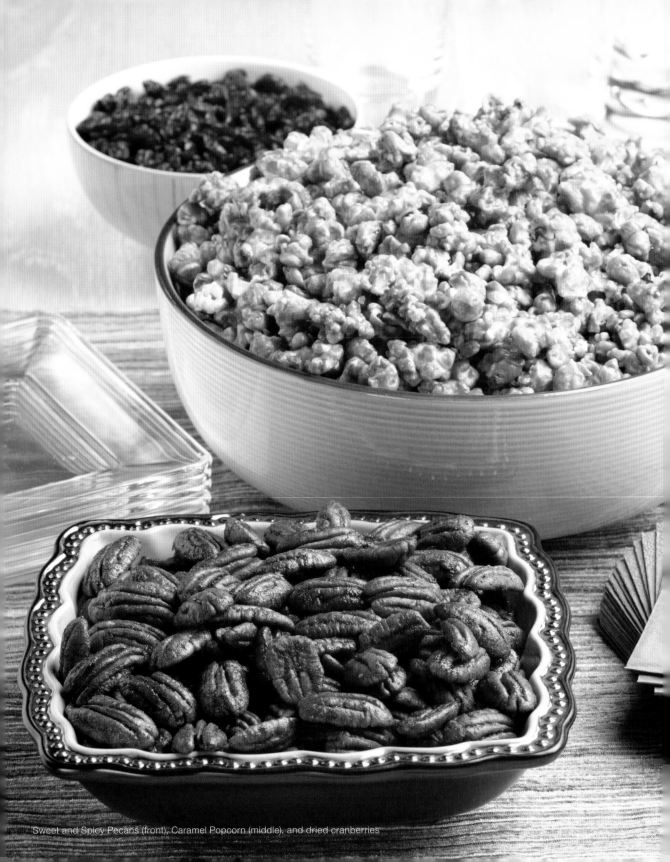

Sweet and Spicy Pecans (front), Caramel Popcorn (middle), and dried cranberries

Caramel Popcorn

SLIM IT DOWN:
Use half the caramel (40 calories).

A number of our members have submitted recipes for this popular treat. I held onto the best parts of all of them, then reduced the sodium and fat. The popcorn glaze doubles as a tasty caramel sauce. Serve it with low-fat frozen yogurt or with apple slices as a treat.

Makes 18 Servings:
about ⅔ cup per serving

1 Hour to Prepare and Cook

1 cup packed dark brown sugar

½ cup light-colored corn syrup

¼ cup butter

1½ tsp vanilla extract

½ tsp baking soda

½ tsp salt

12 cups air-popped popcorn (6 tbsp kernels)

1. Preheat the oven to 250° F. Prepare a large jelly-roll pan or baking sheet with nonstick cooking spray.

2. Combine the sugar, corn syrup, and butter in a medium or large heavy-bottomed saucepan; bring to a boil over medium heat. Cook 4 to 5 minutes, stirring 3 to 4 times to scrape down the sides of the pan and keep the mixture from bubbling up. Be careful; the mixture will burn you if it boils over. If you have a pastry brush, dip it in cool water and use it to brush down the sides of the pan.

3. Remove the pan from the heat; stir in the vanilla, baking soda, and salt. Place the popped popcorn in a large bowl and pour the caramel mixture over in a steady stream, stirring to coat evenly.

4. Spread the popcorn mixture into the prepared pan. Bake for 45 minutes, stirring every 15 minutes.

5. Remove the pan from the oven; stir with a spoon to break up any large clumps. Let cool for 15 minutes before serving at room temperature. To store: let the popcorn cool completely before placing in an airtight container. It will keep for up to a week.

Per Serving: 116.6 calories, 2.8 g total fat, 6.9 mg cholesterol, 115.9 mg sodium, 23.3 g total carbs, 0.8 g dietary fiber, 0.7 g protein

SparkGuy's Best Trail Mix

With a balance of carbs, fat, and protein, trail mix is a great snack. Plus, it eliminates one of life's toughest decisions by mixing salty and sweet. Trail mix doesn't need to be refrigerated, travels well, and is easy to eat.

Our tasty version contains just the right blend of whole-grain cereal, nuts, seeds, natural dried fruit, and even a bit of candy to fulfill your need for a healthy snack. By following the measurements provided, your customized trail mix will provide just the right combination of calories, carbohydrates, protein, and fat to boost energy and satisfy hunger. It's perfect for a pre-workout snack, a mid-morning pick-me-up, and an after-hours munchies cure.

Makes 10 Servings:
¾ cup per serving

3 Minutes to Prepare and Cook

5 cups high-fiber, whole-grain cereal

3 ounces nuts

4 ounces dried fruit, cut into bite-size pieces if necessary

⅓ cup chocolate chips

1. Combine the cereal, nuts, fruit, and chocolate chips in a large bowl and toss lightly.

2. Portion ¾ cup of the combined trail mix into 10 snack bags.

Per Serving (estimated): 158.1 calories, 6.7 g total fat, 0 mg cholesterol, 106.7 mg sodium, 24.5 g total carbs, 3.9 g dietary fiber, 3.7 g protein

Berry Oatmeal Bars

Have you ever read the ingredient list on those "fruit and grain bars"? There doesn't seem to be much of either ingredient. This version has twice the fiber, with a much shorter ingredient list. Use any flavor of all-fruit preserves you prefer, and you could even throw in some dried fruit instead of fresh. Experiment with different flavors. These bars make a great morning meal on the go. Just grab one, along with a piece of fruit and a cup of milk, and you're all set!

Makes 16 Servings:
one 2" x 2" bar per serving

45 Minutes to Prepare and Bake

2 cups old-fashioned oats

½ cup all-purpose flour

1½ cups whole-wheat flour

4 tbsp wheat germ

1 tsp cinnamon

¼ tsp salt

3 tbsp canola oil

1 tsp vanilla extract

¼ cup raw sugar

½ cup skim milk

⅓ cup low-sugar strawberry preserves, or strawberry all-fruit spread

1 cup strawberries, chopped

½ cup blueberries

2 tbsp chopped walnuts

1. Preheat the oven to 325° F. Prepare an 8" x 8" baking pan with nonstick cooking spray.

2. Place 1¼ cups of the oats in a food processor and grind to a flourlike consistency.

3. Combine the ground and whole oats, flours, wheat germ, cinnamon, and salt in an electric stand mixer fitted with a paddle attachment. Mix until evenly combined.

4. Add the oil, vanilla extract, and sugar; pour in the skim milk; and mix until the dough comes together and flours are moistened.

5. Press two-thirds of the dough into the bottom of the prepared pan. Spread preserves over the dough, then top with the strawberries and blueberries. Sprinkle over the walnuts, and then remaining oatmeal mixture.

6. Bake until golden brown, about 45 minutes. Let cool before cutting into 2" x 2" squares.

Per Serving: 158.9 calories, 4.3 g total fat, 0.2 mg cholesterol, 41.1 mg sodium, 33.1 g total carbs, 4.1 g dietary fiber, 4.1 g protein

Coach Nicole's Fresh Guacamole

SparkPeople's resident fitness expert, "Coach Nicole," loves guacamole, but she lightens it up by blending in extra vegetables. Cucumbers give a refreshing flavor to this guacamole, which has a smoother texture without the traditional tomatoes and jalapeño pepper. Feel free to add them if you like. Enjoy with your favorite chips or baked tortillas.

Makes 8 Servings:
¼ cup per serving

6 Minutes to Prepare and Cook

2 ripe avocados, peeled and chopped

⅓ medium cucumber, preferably organic (see Note), chopped

⅓ medium onion, chopped

1 garlic clove, minced

1 tsp ground cumin

1 to 2 tbsp lemon juice

Salt to taste (about ½ teaspoon)

Combine the avocado, cucumber, onion, garlic, cumin, and lemon juice in a blender or food processor. Pulse to desired consistency. Add the salt. Serve chilled.

Note: If using conventional (not organic) cucumber, peel the cucumber and discard the skin.

Per Serving: 77.5 calories, 6.8 g total fat, 0 mg cholesterol, 145.8 mg sodium, 4.8 g total carbs, 3.2 g dietary fiber, 1 g protein

Antipasto Kebobs

Antipasto means "before the pasta." In Italy, a platter of olives, cured meats, cheeses, and pickled vegetables is often served as a starter, along with some bread. While packed with flavor, most of those ingredients are also packed with fat, calories, and salt. Because you're eating a bite of this and a bite of that, it's hard to limit your portions.

I created a lighter antipasto platter that's portion controlled by making kebobs. Mushrooms, tomatoes, and artichoke hearts are much lower in fat than olives, and we ditched the cured meats in favor of a bit of cheese. Feel free to adjust this recipe to suit your tastes. I love Manchego cheese, which is a semisoft Spanish cheese, but feel free to switch it up with Swiss or Parmesan. The cheese is your high-calorie food. Swap it out for olives or even a small piece of salami, and use roasted red peppers or sun-dried tomatoes (not packed in oil) instead of grape tomatoes.

Serve these kebobs as a starter to a meal (try it with Weeknight Spaghetti, page 256) or ditch the skewers and add the ingredients to four cups of spinach for a salad.

Makes 8 kebobs, 2 skewers per serving

20 Minutes to Prepare and Cook

4 wooden skewers, broken in half

For the Dressing:

1 tsp Dijon mustard

1 tbsp white-wine vinegar

1 tbsp olive oil

¼ tsp black pepper

1 tbsp chopped fresh basil or thyme

For the Kebobs:

8 baby cremini mushrooms

16 grape tomatoes

4 artichoke hearts, not packed in oil, quartered

4 ounces Manchego or Parmesan cheese, cut into ½-inch cubes

1. Make the Dressing. Place the mustard and vinegar into a food processor, or a bowl if using an immersion blender. Process and slowly add the oil until the mixture emulsifies. Stir in the pepper and chopped herb.

2. Make the Kebobs. Alternate the mushrooms, tomatoes, artichoke hearts, and cheese on the skewers. Place the kebobs in a flat-bottomed bowl.

3. Pour the dressing over the kebobs and marinate for at least 20 minutes in the fridge. Serve at room temperature.

Per Serving: 121.9 calories, 8.7 g total fat, 15 mg cholesterol, 253.6 mg sodium, 5.9 g total carbs, 1.6 g dietary fiber, 5.7 g protein

DESSERTS

Though we've grouped them together in one chapter, snacks and desserts aren't interchangeable. Snacks are nutritious small meals with 200 calories or less that tide over your hunger until your next meal, fuel you through a workout, or replenish your body after a sweat session. Desserts are treats, an occasional sweet that isn't meant to fulfill any nutritional requirements.

That said, our desserts are healthier than most—and even more satisfying than anything you'll find at the bakery or in a 100-calorie pack. Even so, limit these satisfying, healthier desserts to "sometimes" food—meaning twice a week at most.

Oh my gosh, do I like desserts! At school, I am in the baking labs daily. Students are always handing me desserts, fellow teachers are proffering bites of their latest creations, and the cake decorators—they're the most evil of them all! They trim the edges off their beautiful cakes and the discarded pieces are just lying there waiting to be eaten! It's so tempting, but I usually resist. Because of the daily temptation at work, I only bake at home for special events and parties.

Special events can be as simple as good grades on a report card, but I still want my family to be excited about desserts. If you constantly have them around, the excitement fades. For me this has been a life lesson. My mother used to reward us regularly with desserts, and later in life I realized I used desserts not only as a reward but a crutch when life was stressful. I now reward myself with a run, flowers, or just a hug from my family.

I have trained my kids well when it comes to desserts. We are all "snobs." Fake icing, ingredients that we cannot pronounce, and waxy chocolate will not enter our mouths. We want the real flavors! I have learned over the years that there are some tricks with dessert preparation that can sway them to the healthier side of the scale—upping the nutrient density is my favorite. I prefer whole-wheat pastry flours and additions of whole grains, nuts, seeds, and dried fruits. Even though what's inside might be slightly healthier, I always make real buttercream when I bake a cake. A small sliver of cake with a moderate layer of sweet, buttery, melt-in-your-mouth frosting is so supremely satisfying—to me, there's just no substitute!

Low-fat baking might seem like an oxymoron, but it can be done. The trick to it—like so many other areas of life both inside and outside the kitchen—is balance.

In our taste test, we offered up two muffins. The first, an Applesauce Oatmeal Muffin with Walnuts and Raisins, had 94 calories, 3 grams fat, and 2 grams of fiber. The ingredient list: Splenda brown sugar blend, unsweetened applesauce, soy flour, whole-wheat flour, egg whites, plus leavening agents, dried fruit, and spices. While flavorful, the muffin was described as dense, chewy, heavy, clunky, and just plain bad. I think I overheard someone calling it "hippie food."

The other muffin, which we actually call a Spring Cupcake with Citrus Icing (page 348), contains egg and egg whites, brown sugar, canola oil, whole-wheat pastry flour, various spices and leavening agents—and a half serving of zucchini and carrots per cupcake. It was described as "decadent," and almost three quarters of participants wanted to eat it again.

The biggest surprise is that they thought the muffin was healthier than the "cupcake." They were wrong. The light, fluffy Spring Cupcake contained about 45 fewer calories, less fat, and the same amount of sodium. The oatmeal muffin had an extra gram of fiber, but the Spring Cupcake has 2.2 grams per serving—better than most cupcakes!

We chose to test these two recipes to demonstrate the good, bad, and the ugly of nutritional baking. For many of the recipes in this chapter, I recruited a good friend and colleague, Megan Ketover, an award-winning pastry chef who has been featured on the Food Network. An expert in healthy baking, she helped us develop amazing recipes that serve as lessons in how to lighten up your baked goods while retaining great taste—and that light texture we all crave.

Although we encourage you to experiment with different flavors and ingredients in many of our recipes, doing so when baking can lead to mixed results. Baking is much like chemistry: cakes rise and cookies turn crispy because of the way ingredients interact. So feel free to substitute one nut for another, or swap out lemon extract for vanilla, but don't use light margarine when the recipe wants full-fat butter. Having to feed the results of your hard work to the birds is no way to save calories!

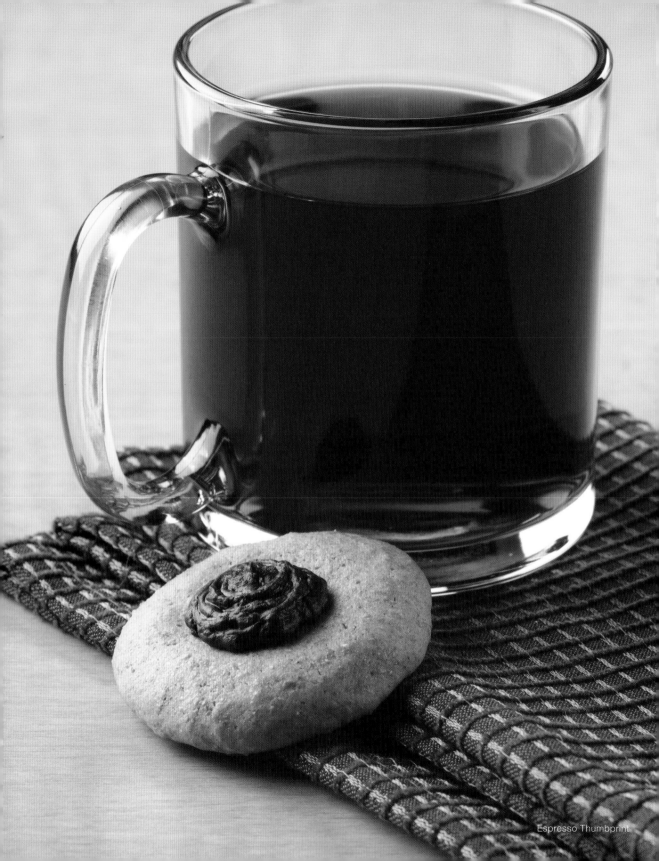

Espresso Thumbprint

Espresso Thumbprints

SLIM IT DOWN:
Skip the frosting (35 calories).

Coffee and chocolate are a great team, each enhancing the flavor of the other. These thumbprint cookies are perfect for a brunch or party.

While you can create glazes or thin icing without using fat, it's virtually impossible to create a thick, creamy frosting without some fat. In this recipe, we decided to use a healthier fat, in the form of almond butter, rather than butter, margarine, or shortening. This is a prime example of making every bite count. You could choose a fat like butter, which adds little nutritionally, or almond butter, which adds small amounts of fiber and protein. We had already used butter in the cookie, so we chose the almond butter for the frosting.

We use a mix of flours here to keep the texture light, but if you don't mind a dense cookie, you can use whole-wheat flour alone.

Makes 24 Servings:
   1 cookie per serving

40 Minutes to Prepare and Bake, plus chilling

½ cup butter, softened

2 tsp instant coffee or espresso powder

1 cup confectioners' sugar

1 egg

1 egg white

¼ tsp salt

1 tsp vanilla extract

½ cup all-purpose flour

⅔ cup whole-wheat flour

½ cup cocoa powder

For the Frosting:

¼ cup almond butter

⅓ cup cocoa powder

¼ cup confectioners' sugar

¼ cup skim milk

1. Preheat the oven to 350° F.

2. In the bowl of an electric stand mixer, cream together the butter, coffee, and confectioners' sugar until well combined. Beat in the egg, egg white, salt, and vanilla.

3. In a separate bowl, sift together the flours and cocoa powder. Slowly add the flour to the mixer bowl, and beat until the flour is moistened and just combined.

4. Chill the dough in the fridge for 1 hour.

5. Roll the chilled dough into 24 balls. Place on the cookie sheet and press the center of each cookie with a moistened thumb to make an indent for frosting. Bake until no longer shiny and slightly crispy on edges, 12 to 15 minutes. Cool on a rack before frosting.

6. Make the Frosting. Combine the almond butter, cocoa powder, and confectioners' sugar in a small bowl. Add the skim milk and stir to combine. Place a dime-sized amount of frosting in the center of each cooled cookie.

Per Serving: 89.3 calories, 5 g total fat, 12 mg cholesterol, 19.2 mg sodium, 10.7 g total carbs, 0.9 g dietary fiber, 1.6 g protein

Fruit Salad with Poppy Seed Dressing

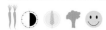

Fruit is Mother Nature's dessert, and by creating a sweet and tangy dressing, you can marry all the flavors of a fruit salad. I especially like to use this dressing in winter, when most fruit isn't at its peak. Any fruit works with this dressing, but try to choose those that are in season. You can use one variety or seven, whatever you have on hand. I like raspberries, peaches, plums, or grapes.

Make sure you smell your poppy seeds. One sniff and you'll know if they're rancid. Always date them when you bring them home, and use them within six months.

Though this makes a great snack, we also like to serve this dish as a breakfast or brunch side dish—or even as a healthy dessert or accompaniment at the dinner table. Leftovers are great in lunches!

Makes 4 Servings:
    1 cup per serving

10 Minutes to Prepare

For the Dressing:

1 lime, zested and juiced

1 tbsp honey

1 tsp poppy seeds

2 cups strawberries, chopped

2 kiwi fruits, peeled and chopped

1 cup blackberries

1. Make the dressing. Combine the lime zest and juice, honey, and poppy seeds in a small bowl and stir to combine.

2. Mix together the strawberries, kiwi, and blackberries in a large bowl. Pour the dressing over the fruit and stir to coat. Serve chilled.

Per Serving: 87.2 calories, 1 g total fat, 0 mg cholesterol, 3.1 mg sodium, 20.8 g total carbs, 5.3 g dietary fiber, 1.3 g protein

Raspberry Streusel Muffins

In baking, streusel usually means a crumb topping of butter, flour, and sugar mixed with nuts. Instead of adding fat and sugar to the top of these sweet raspberry muffins, we took this as a chance to add a bit of fiber—each muffin has 3.6 grams of it, more than a cup of Wheaties.

Have you ever eaten a "light" muffin that was anything but? Cooks often replace all of the oil in recipes with applesauce and all of the eggs with egg whites. The result is a dense, chewy muffin. You can substitute egg whites for one of the eggs if you want, and I have already swapped in applesauce for some of the fat, but for the sake of texture and taste, I prefer to keep some fat in the recipe.

Raspberries are delicate, so fold them in gently at the end. If you use frozen raspberries, thaw them and drain the juice to use in a smoothie. You could also substitute your favorite berry or dried fruit.

Makes 12 Servings:
1 muffin per serving

35 Minutes to Prepare and Bake

4 tbsp low-fat butter baking blend sticks, softened

¼ cup sugar

¼ cup brown sugar

½ cup unsweetened applesauce

2 eggs

1 cup all-purpose flour

½ cup whole-wheat flour

¼ cup plus 2 tbsp wheat germ

2 tsp baking powder

¼ tsp salt

½ cup skim milk

1 tsp vanilla extract

1 pint fresh or 1½ cups frozen raspberries

For the Streusel Topping:

1 tbsp ground flaxseeds

1 tbsp wheat germ

1 tsp olive oil

½ tsp light brown sugar

1 tbsp old-fashioned oatmeal

1. Preheat the oven to 375° F. Prepare a 12-cup muffin tin with paper baking cups or nonstick cooking spray.

2. In the bowl of an electric stand mixer, cream together the butter, sugar, brown sugar, and applesauce until evenly combined, scraping the bottom of the bowl with a rubber spatula halfway through. Add the eggs one at a time and mix well.

3. In a separate bowl, stir together the flours, wheat germ, baking powder, and salt. Add the flour mixture to the butter mixture, and mix until combined, about 1 minute. Add the skim milk and vanilla and beat about 2 minutes. Fold in raspberries.

4. Scoop the batter into the muffin cups, filling each about three-quarters full.

5. In a separate bowl combine the flaxseeds, the remaining wheat germ, oil, brown sugar, and oatmeal; stir with a fork. Sprinkle two teaspoons of the streusel mixture over the muffins. Bake the muffins until they are golden brown and spring back at a touch, 20 to 25 minutes.

Per Serving: 166.4 calories, 5.1 g total fat, 35.6 mg cholesterol, 181.9 mg sodium, 29.1 g total carbs, 3.6 g dietary fiber, 4.2 g protein

Spring Cupcakes with Citrus Icing

SLIM IT DOWN: Axe the icing (20 calories).

Cupcakes are all the rage these days, and for good reason. These diminutive desserts are automatically portion controlled, and they're just darn cute! Instead of traditional vanilla and chocolate, we chose a garden variety: Carrots and zucchini aren't just for salads; they add moisture and texture to desserts as well.

There aren't enough veggies to count for one of your daily servings, but you are getting a tasty treat that has more fiber and less fat than even a slice of traditional carrot cake.

Carrot cake usually has a spicy taste, but we lightened that up by adding a fresh orange flavor. These cupcakes are perfect for an Easter brunch, a children's birthday party (no need to tell them the "confetti" inside comes from vegetables), or a graduation celebration.

These cupcakes were a hit during our taste test!

Makes 18 Servings:
    1 cupcake per serving

45 Minutes to Prepare and Bake

1 egg, at room temperature

1 egg white, at room temperature

¾ cup brown sugar

2 cups grated carrots

2 small zucchini, grated (about 1 cup, excess moisture pressed out with a paper towel)

⅓ cup canola oil

1 tbsp orange zest (see Note)

1 tsp baking powder

½ tsp baking soda

½ tsp cinnamon

¼ tsp salt

2 cups whole-wheat pastry flour

For the Icing:

1 tbsp orange zest (see Note)

2 tbsp orange juice (see Note)

½ cup confectioners' sugar

1. Preheat the oven to 350° F. Fill 18 muffin cups with cupcake liners.

2. Combine the eggs and brown sugar in a bowl, then beat at medium speed with a hand mixer for 2 minutes. Add the carrots, zucchini, oil, and orange zest to the mixture and stir to combine.

3. In a separate bowl, combine the baking powder, baking soda, cinnamon, salt, and flour using a fork; then add to the wet mixture. Using the mixer, blend just until combined.

4. Divide the batter among the muffin cups, and bake until a toothpick inserted in the middle of a cupcake comes out clean, 18 to 20 minutes. (If your oven has hot spots, rotate the pans halfway through cooking.)

5. Allow to cool in the pans for 10 minutes, then remove and cool completely on a wire rack.

6. While the cupcakes are baking, prepare the icing by whisking together the orange zest, the orange juice, and sugar. After the cupcakes have cooled, top each one with 1 teaspoon of icing.

Note: You should be able to get plenty of zest and juice for both the cupcakes and the icing from one large orange.

Per Serving: 145.8 calories, 4.9 g total fat, 11.8 mg cholesterol, 114.7 mg sodium, 24.6 g total carbs, 2.4 g dietary fiber, 2.6 g protein

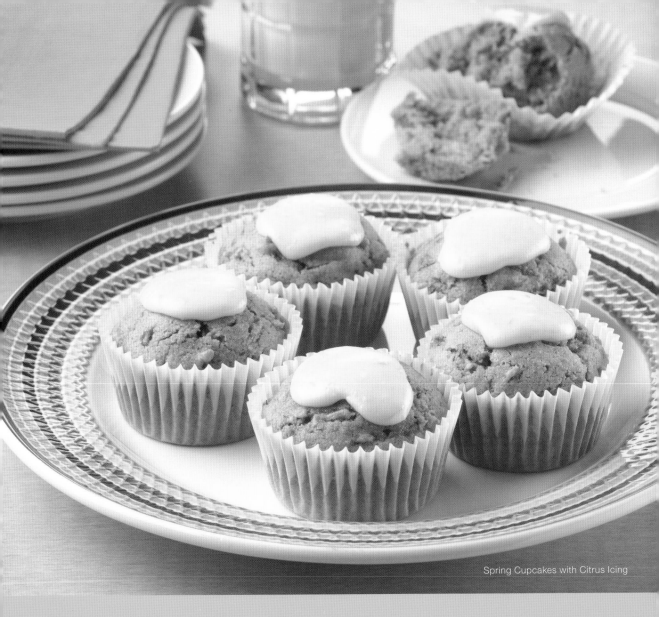

Spring Cupcakes with Citrus Icing

CHEF MEG'S TIPS:

- Use the grating blade on a food processor to shred the carrots and zucchini. If you don't have a food processor, use a box grater and give your arm a workout!

- For even easier prep, buy a 10-ounce bag of shredded carrots, place in the food processor, and pulse 3 to 4 times.

- If you overmix the batter, you'll cause "tunneling," which means that your cupcakes will contain holes and hollow tunnels throughout. Mix just until the wet and dry ingredients are combined.

- If you can't find whole-wheat pastry flour, you can use two parts whole-wheat flour to one part cake flour (available in the baking aisle). You can also use regular whole-wheat flour, but your cupcakes will be much denser.

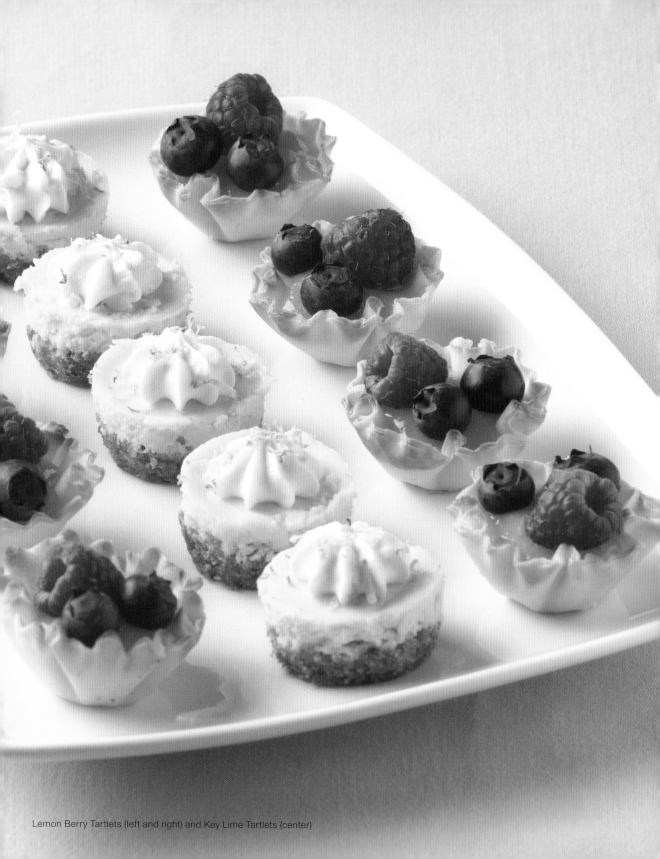

Lemon Berry Tartlets (left and right) and Key Lime Tartlets (center)

Lemon Berry Tartlets

The trend of mini desserts is a healthy eater's salvation. When sweets are pre-portioned, it's harder to cheat. The mini-tarts just say "summertime" to me. I imagine eating them on a patio after a luncheon with my girlfriends while sipping iced mint tea and feeling the warm breeze. They're so refreshing and light.

Phyllo dough is a secret weapon for the healthy baker—it even comes in whole-wheat varieties. The paper-thin layers of dough are often painted in butter for pastries like baklava, but they can also serve as a low-calorie pie crust with minimal added fat.

The "curd" filling is basically a lemon pudding. You can serve it on scones or muffins, as a topping for ice cream or sorbet, or as a pie filling, as you see here.

Makes 12 Servings:
  1 tartlet per serving

25 Minutes to Prepare, 10 Minutes to Bake

For the Lemon Curd:

½ cup lemon juice

2 tsp lemon zest

4 tbsp sugar

Pinch salt

1 egg

½ tsp vanilla extract

For the Tart Shells (see Note):

1 tbsp water

1 tbsp canola oil

6 sheets frozen phyllo dough, thawed

1 cup raspberries and blueberries,
    washed and dried

1. Make the Lemon Curd. In a stainless-steel bowl, whisk together the lemon juice and zest, the sugar, salt, egg, and vanilla. In a saucepan, bring 2 cups of water to a boil, then reduce to a low simmer.

2. Set the bowl over the top of the saucepan and whisk the mixture continuously until it thickens, about 10 minutes. Remove the bowl from the pan, cover the surface of the curd with plastic wrap, and refrigerate the mixture until completely cool. It will thicken further as it cools. The lemon curd can be stored, covered, in the refrigerator for up to 4 days.

3. Preheat the oven to 375° F. Prepare a muffin tin with nonstick cooking spray.

4. Mix together the water and canola oil. On a cutting board, lay out 1 sheet of phyllo dough and brush it with the oil mixture. Layer another sheet of phyllo on top, and brush with oil mixture. Repeat the process until the dough is 6 sheets high. Use a sharp knife or pastry cutter to cut the dough into 12 2-inch squares.

5. Place the squares of dough in the wells of a mini-muffin pan. With water-moistened fingers, press the center of the dough to shape the tartlet shells into place; the dough will overlap and fold into shape.

6. Bake until golden brown, about 10 minutes. Allow to cool completely before filling with lemon curd.

7. Fill each tart shell with about 1 tablespoon of lemon curd, then top with 1 raspberry and 2 blueberries.

Note: To save time, buy premade phyllo dough cups. Look for them in the frozen-food aisle.

Per Serving: 57.6 calories, 1.9 g total fat, 17.7 mg cholesterol, 41.3 mg sodium, 9.6 g total carbs, 0.3 g dietary fiber, 0.9g protein

Key Lime Tartlets

Tartlets are great for portion control—and a great way to serve pie for a crowd. They're easy to serve, everyone gets an equal amount—and they're just plain fun to eat. Serve these at a shower or spring party.

I revamped the crust by swapping Greek yogurt for the melted butter, then added some pecans for flavor and texture, and a bit of olive oil to bind it all together. For the custard, egg whites and fat-free condensed milk keep that thick and rich texture.

Makes 16 Servings:
1 tartlet per serving

1 Hour to Prepare and Bake

For the Crust:

½ cup graham-cracker crumbs

1 tbsp brown sugar

1 tbsp finely chopped pecans

1½ tbsp fat-free Greek yogurt

½ tsp olive oil

For the Filling:

⅓ cup key-lime juice

7 ounces fat-free sweetened condensed milk

1 egg

2 egg whites

For the Topping (Optional, see Note):

¼ cup heavy cream

2 tsp confectioners' sugar

½ tsp vanilla extract

1. Preheat oven to 325° F.

2. Make the Crust. In a mixing bowl, stir together the graham-cracker crumbs, brown sugar, and pecans. In a small bowl, stir together the yogurt and oil. Add the yogurt mixture to the graham-cracker mixture and stir until moistened.

3. Press about ⅓ tablespoon of the mixture into each cup of a nonstick mini-muffin tin. Bake until firm and light golden brown, 9 to 12 minutes. Don't turn off the oven. Let cool completely before filling.

4. Make the Filling. In a saucepan over medium heat, stir together the lime juice and condensed milk. In a separate bowl, whisk together the egg and egg whites. When the lime mixture just begins to simmer, add ¼ cup of the hot mixture to the eggs while whisking constantly. Don't add more than ¼ cup to start, or the eggs will begin to cook. Finish adding the lime mixture to the eggs ¼ cup at a time, and whisk until combined.

5. Fill each tartlet shell with 1 to 1½ tablespoons of the lime mixture. Return the muffin tin to the oven and bake until the filling is set and slightly firm to the touch, 10 to 15 minutes. Allow to cool, but don't try to remove the tartlets from the pan. Place the pan in the refrigerator and, once they have cooled completely, remove the tartlets from the pan by running a paring knife around the edge of the crust.

6. Make the Topping. If you like, beat together the heavy cream, confectioners' sugar, and vanilla to soft peaks. Top each cooled tartlet with a dollop of the whipped cream.

Note: We considered ditching the topping, but ¼ cup of heavy cream yields ½ cup of whipped cream. Divide that among 16 tartlets, and you're only adding 8 calories per tartlet—definitely worth it! If you prefer, the tartlets could be dusted with confectioners' sugar instead.

Per Serving: 73.3 calories, 2.1 g total fat, 17.3 mg cholesterol, 38.3 mg sodium, 11.6 g total carbs, 0.2 g dietary fiber, 2.6 g protein

Banana Honey Cake

Did you know that one slice of cinnamon-walnut coffee cake at a coffee house has about as much fat as a Whopper Jr. from Burger King? To save money and avoid empty calories, I prefer to meet up with friends at home and enjoy our coffee with a home-baked goodie.

This Banana Honey Cake is just as gooey and decadent as coffee cake, but with far less fat. You won't believe there's no butter in this. The cake stays moist thanks to the bananas, tea, and orange juice. Using other low-calorie liquids instead of water is a great way to add flavor to a recipe.

I used a mixture of all-purpose white flour and whole-wheat flour in this recipe to keep the cake lighter. To add more fiber, you could use 1¾ cups of whole-wheat pastry flour if you have that in your kitchen.

Chef Meg's Tip: You might notice that this recipe contains no eggs. That's because it contains flaxseed instead. The same soluble fiber that makes flaxseed useful for helping to lower blood cholesterol levels also makes it a binding agent in baked goods. If you're watching your cholesterol, consider swapping eggs for "flax eggs" in your baked goods. Flaxseed works best in denser baked goods that have flavors that won't be overpowered by their nuttiness. Use them in pancakes, waffles, fruit-based muffins, and quick breads; avoid using them in cakes or any baked goods that you want to be light and fluffy. Simply mix 1 tablespoon of ground flaxseed with 3 tablespoons of water for each egg you want to replace, then stir and let sit until a gelatinous substance forms. Add it as you would eggs.

Makes 16 Servings:
    2" x 2" square per serving

1 Hour to Prepare and Bake

1 tbsp flaxseed meal

1 ripe banana, mashed

¼ cup canola oil

½ cup honey

¼ cup light brown sugar

½ tsp vanilla extract

1 cup all-purpose flour

¾ cup whole-wheat flour

1½ tsp baking powder

½ tsp baking soda

¼ tsp salt

1 tsp cinnamon

¼ tsp ground allspice

⅛ tsp nutmeg

½ cup Earl Grey tea, brewed strong and cooled

¼ cup orange juice

1 tbsp confectioners' sugar (optional)

1. Preheat the oven to 350° F. Prepare an 8" x 8" cake pan with nonstick cooking spray.

2. In a small bowl, mix together the flaxseed meal and 3 tablespoons water; stir until a gelatinous paste forms. Set aside.

3. In the bowl of an electric stand mixer, combine the banana, oil, honey, brown sugar, vanilla, and flaxseed mixture; beat until well combined and slightly lighter in color. In a separate bowl, sift together the flours, baking powder, baking soda, salt, cinnamon, allspice, and nutmeg. Add the flour mixture to the banana mixture and beat for one minute. Slowly pour in the tea and orange juice, and mix the batter for 2 minutes.

4. Pour the batter into the prepared pan and bake until the cake springs back in the center when pressed, about 30 minutes. The cake is best served warm, dusted with confectioners' sugar, if you like.

Per Serving: 136.3 calories, 3.8 g total fat, 0 mg cholesterol, 123.5 mg sodium, 26.4 g total carbs, 1.3 g dietary fiber, 1.8 g protein

Mini Apple Tarts

SLIM IT DOWN:
Skip the caramel sauce (35 calories) or use just the filling (30 calories).

Phyllo dough is not only great for the healthy kitchen, it's incredibly versatile as well. Serve these mini apple pies next Thanksgiving—they offer just enough of a sweet finish to the meal, without being too filling. In a pinch, you can use prepared, frozen tart shells, but we find it's just as easy to make your own—and keep the fat content under control.

Makes 12 Servings:
2 tartlets with 1 tsp caramel sauce each

20 Minutes to Prepare and Bake

9 sheets frozen phyllo dough, thawed

1 lemon, juiced

4 Granny Smith apples, peeled, cored, and diced

2 tbsp unsalted butter

4 tbsp brown sugar

½ cup caramel sauce (optional)

½ cup whipped cream (optional)

1. Preheat oven to 375° F. Prepare a 24-cup mini-muffin tin with nonstick cooking spray.

2. Lay the phyllo dough on a cutting board. With a sharp knife, slice the dough into 1-inch strips, then cut each strip into 2-inch segments. Working with 3 layers of dough at a time, fill the cups, spraying cooking spray between each layer. Repeat process three times then, with water-moistened fingers, press the center of each cup to shape the dough into tart cups.

3. Combine lemon juice and apples in a mixing bowl and set aside. In a cast iron or heavy skillet, heat the butter until frothy. Add the brown sugar and cook until dark in color, 1 to 2 minutes. Add the apples and toss to coat.

4. Fill each tart shell with about 1 tablespoon of the apples. Bake until the shell is golden brown and the apple filling is bubbly, 6 to 7 minutes. Allow the tarts to cool slightly; top with the caramel sauce and the whipped cream, if you like.

Per Serving: 124.2 calories, 4.1 g total fat, 5.2 mg cholesterol, 59 mg sodium, 23.2 g total carbs, 1.6 g dietary fiber, 0.5 g protein

Cocoa Meringue Shells

I shape these meringues to form basketlike bowls; they're a fun treat when served with low-fat vanilla ice cream and fresh fruit. If you don't have parchment paper, try using a brown paper bag from the grocery store.

Egg whites won't stiffen if there is any grease or greasy residue in the bowl or on the beaters of your mixer, so clean them with vinegar and water beforehand to ensure they're grease-free. If you don't have a pastry bag, just snip the corner from a plastic bag and use it instead.

Makes 24 meringues:
    1 meringue per serving

2 Hours, 30 Minutes to Prepare and Bake

12 egg whites at room temperature
    (see Note)

½ tsp cream of tartar

1½ cups granulated sugar

½ cup dark cocoa powder (see Note)

1. Preheat the oven to 275° F. Line three baking sheets with parchment paper.

2. Place the egg whites in the bowl of an electric stand mixer and beat at high speed with a whisk attachment until stiff, about 8 minutes. Add the cream of tartar and continue to beat. Slowly add half the sugar and beat to combine. Remove the whisk attachment and fold in the cocoa powder using a rubber spatula.

3. With the spatula, transfer the mixture to a piping bag fitted with a star tip. Pipe into circles onto the lined trays: pipe one 4-inch base circle, then pipe a second layer on just on the outer top of the circle to create a basketlike bowl.

4. Position the baking sheets in the middle and lower section of the oven and bake for 1 hour. Turn off the oven but do not open the door. Allow the meringues to sit in the warmed oven for 1 hour more. Remove from oven to cool. Store in an airtight container for up to 3 days.

Note: Separate the eggs when the eggs are cold and then let them come to room temperature.

This recipe makes a very richly flavored cocoa meringue. If you prefer a lighter cocoa taste, reduce the cocoa to ⅓ cup.

Per Serving: 55 calories, 0.4 g total fat, 0 mg cholesterol, 28.1 mg sodium, 12 g total carbs, 0.9 g dietary fiber, 3 g protein

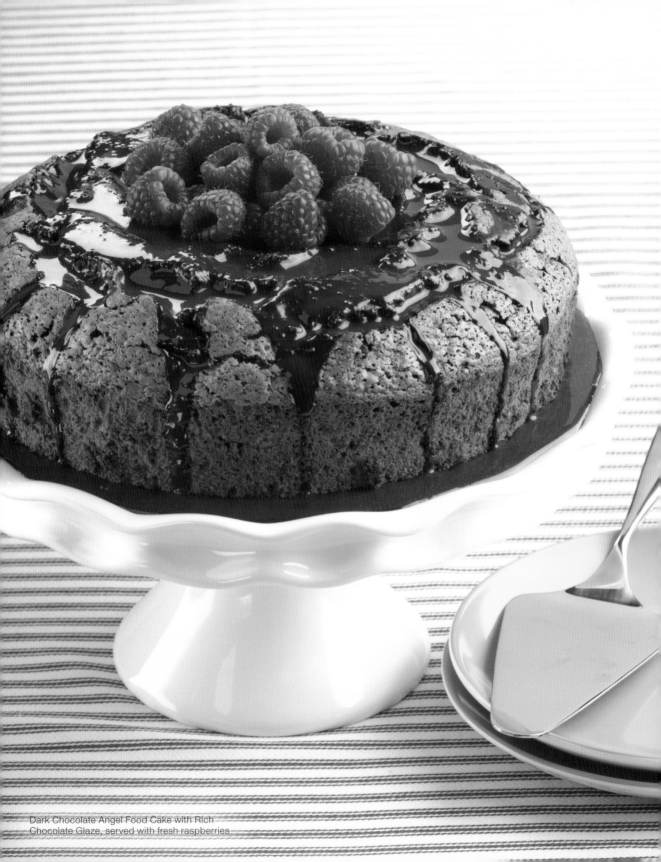

Dark Chocolate Angel Food Cake with Rich
Chocolate Glaze, served with fresh raspberries

Dark Chocolate Angel Food Cake with Rich Chocolate Glaze

SLIM IT DOWN:
Give up the glaze (25 calories).

When it comes to chocolate, there is no substitute. The darker the better, for me. So many diet plans and healthy cookbooks claim that you can have cake, eat chocolate, and so on, and then they offer a tiny sliver of cake made with sugar substitutes, little chocolate, and no flavor. Chocolate-coated cardboard would be more appealing. Here, we've created a satisfying dark-chocolate dessert that could be on the menu at any restaurant.

My inspiration for this recipe was devil's food cake. I wanted to combine the rich chocolate of that cake with the lightness of an angel food cake. I think I succeeded. It's devilishly angelic, if that's possible. Even the glaze is low in fat and calories, but high in flavor. I like to serve this cake with fresh fruit, especially raspberries or strawberries. You can also make cupcakes from this batter: just use a muffin tin with cupcake liners and change your baking time according to the package directions.

My chef's tip here is this: don't be afraid of taking help where and when you need it. You could make an angel food cake from scratch, or you could use a box, as I have here.

Makes 16 Servings:
1/16 cake per serving

50 Minutes to Prepare and Bake

1 box angel food cake mix

½ cup cocoa powder

For the Chocolate Glaze:

⅔ cup fat-free evaporated milk

½ cup cocoa powder

¼ cup confectioners' sugar

1 tsp vanilla extract

2 ounces dark chocolate (62% cacao), finely chopped

1. Preheat the oven to temperature specified on package directions.

2. In the bowl of an electric stand mixer, combine the angel food cake mix and cocoa powder. Add water according to box directions (my brand called for 1¼ cups) and beat 2 minutes on medium speed.

3. Pour the batter into an ungreased angel food cake pan and bake according to package directions (mine took 40 minutes). Let cool.

4. Make the Glaze. Warm the evaporated milk in a saucepan, then sift in the cocoa powder and sugar, whisking to avoid lumps. Stir until the mixture comes to a simmer.

5. Remove the pan from the heat and add the vanilla and chocolate. Stir until the chocolate is melted and the mixture is smooth. Drizzle the warm glaze over cooled cake.

Per Serving: 152.3 calories, 2 g total fat, 0.6 mg cholesterol, 269 mg sodium, 32.2 g total carbs, 2.5 g dietary fiber, 4.6 g protein

Dark Chocolate Cake

When you're craving chocolate cake, no substitute will do. Moist and rich, this satisfied my sweet tooth; and with half the calories, less fat, and four times the fiber of most recipes, this cake proves that nutritious ingredients yield delicious results. I used whole-wheat pastry flour and egg whites to lighten up the recipe, along with my secret ingredient—pureed canned beets.

Tip: For best results when baking, all your ingredients should be at room temperature. Place the eggs on the counter about an hour before you start baking.

Makes 8 Servings:
⅛ cake per serving

1 Hour to Prepare and Bake

4 ounces bittersweet chocolate (at least 60% cacao content), chopped

¾ cup sugar

2 whole eggs

6 egg whites

1 tsp vanilla extract

½ cup canned beets, drained, rinsed, and pureed

¼ cup flaxseeds, finely ground

½ cup whole-wheat pastry flour

¼ cup unsweetened cocoa powder

¼ tsp baking powder

1. Preheat the oven to 350° F. Prepare a 9-inch round baking pan with nonstick cooking spray.

2. Combine the chocolate, sugar, and ½ cup water in a small saucepan. Cook over low heat until the chocolate has melted, stirring occasionally. Allow to cool slightly.

3. In a mixing bowl, stir together the eggs and one of the egg whites. Add the vanilla, pureed beets, and the chocolate mixture. Whisk to combine.

4. In a separate bowl, use a fork to combine the flaxseeds, flour, cocoa powder, and baking powder. Incorporate the flour mixture into the egg mixture, stirring just until combined.

5. In a clean bowl, whisk the remaining 5 egg whites until stiff. Place 1 heaping tablespoon of the egg whites into the cake batter and stir to combine. Slowly fold the remaining egg whites into the cake batter.

6. Pour the batter into the prepared pan and bake until a toothpick inserted in the center comes out clean, 30 minutes. Remove the cake from the oven and let cool for 5 minutes before removing it from the pan.

Per Serving: 228.7 calories, 9.1 g total fat, 53.2 mg cholesterol, 105 mg sodium, 33.8 g total carbs, 4.2 g dietary fiber, 8.2 g protein

CHAPTER 12

HERBS, SPICES & SEASONINGS

Some women buy dresses. I buy spices. They're my vice.

To me, food isn't worth eating if it's bland and flavorless. Novice cooks might reach for fat, salt, or sugar for flavor; and they'll turn out some tasty food—but it won't be healthy. A good cook knows to start with wholesome food that's as close to the source as possible (as unprocessed as can be), and uses herbs and spices to impart flavor. Herbs, spices, and seasonings are a big reason why I can cook and eat what I love and still fit into my clothes!

Unfortunately, the most common seasoning in American kitchens is salt. While salt is a crucial ingredient in many recipes, it should rarely be the sole seasoning. If a food is seasoned properly—from the beginning and through every step of the cooking process—there is no need to salt or pepper your food at the table.

As you'll read in this chapter, there are plenty of tricks you can use to impart flavor with almost zero calories. When you're watching fat and calories, herbs, spices, and certain condiments are your new best friends. They add flavor and pizzazz to your cooking with little to no calories and fat. Do take care in your choice of premade spice blends and condiments, however, as many of the versions you get in the supermarket are full of salt—a big no-no when you're watching your sodium levels or you have high blood pressure.

You can buy tinned or canned spices at the grocery store, but many larger supermarkets and health-food stores have bulk spices. Buy just as much as you need and you won't be left with a tin of mace 15 years from now!

HOWMANYCATS, who has lost 27 pounds, has extolled the virtues of spices since her seventh-grade home ec class. "I fell in love with the school's spice cabinet . . . it just smelled so good and exotic when you opened the doors! My goal became having a spice cabinet like that someday and I'm happy to say, I *do* have that now!"

Let's get some terminology straight before we begin: *Herbs,* which can be used fresh or dried, are the leaves, stems, or flowers of plants used to flavor food. *Spices* are dried and come from the bark, roots, or berries of a plant. *Seasoning* is a term used for adding flavor with salt or a combination of spices and herbs, such as the blends found in this chapter.

Fresh and dried herbs are vital when preparing a healthy meal because they add flavor with virtually no calories and zero fat. The herbs can be the star or the supporting actor in a dish. When I make Tomato-Basil Vinaigrette (page 387), the basil is the star because I want to taste that grassy, piney flavor. When I make Black-Bean Burgers with Lime Cream (page 139), I want the beans and cumin to take center stage, with the cilantro adding a light lemon flavor.

In most cases, you'll want the herbs and spices to accentuate the food. Just as good lighting can make anyone look like a movie star in photos, herbs and spices can make any dish a four-star meal.

FRESH VS. DRIED HERBS

In fresh herbs, the flavor is readily available. With dried herbs, it requires some coaxing. When measuring herbs, the general rule is that you use twice as much fresh as dried.

Fresh herbs should be used:

- At the end of the cooking process. If you add fresh herbs too early, they'll lose their color.

- In an uncooked dish, such as a salad, or one that will not require much cooking. When adding herbs to uncooked dishes, allow the herbs to bloom in the food by chilling or resting the dish before serving.

- As a garnish, such as a sprinkle of fresh parsley on a dish before serving.

Dried herbs should be added at the beginning of the cooking process to extract as much flavor as possible. To release the herbs' flavorful oils, I always rub them between my hands as I add them to the dish.

SparkPeople Cooking Challenge:
Experiment with dried and fresh versions of a familiar herb. If you always use fresh basil, notice the difference when you use dried.
A fan of dried rosemary?
See how you like fresh.

HEAT UP THOSE SPICES

To unleash the full power of spices, they need to be cooked. If you add chili powder, cumin, and paprika to a pot of simmering soup, they won't really add much flavor and you probably won't even smell them. If you add them to the pot when you're sautéing onions and garlic in olive oil, they'll give off a wonderful aroma and lend their flavor to the dish right from the start.

Take a look at the Slow-Cooker White Bean Chicken Chili recipe on page 172. It's a slow-cooker recipe, but one of the first steps is to roast the chicken, vegetables, and spices in the oven for a few minutes. You might be tempted to skip that step and toss all the ingredients into the slow cooker. The chili will be much blander than if you had allowed those spices to roast. I like shortcuts in the kitchen as much as the next person, but those extra few minutes are worth it!

SparkPeople Cooking Challenge:
This week, cook your spices before adding them to a favorite family dish. Ask your family or fellow diners if they notice any difference in the flavor. I bet they will!

STORAGE

Fresh herbs should be treated like cut flowers. Pick them from the garden in the morning or purchase them as fresh as possible. Trim off the bottom of the stems, place in a glass of cool water, and loosely cover with moistened paper towels. Place them in the center of your refrigerator—except for basil, which will turn black in the cold (it prefers the counter). Always wash the herbs just before using them, and allow them to dry before chopping.

Dried herbs and spices might look pretty on the countertop, but they don't like light or warmth. Store them in opaque containers (I like tins) and keep them in a cupboard that stays cool—not in a fancy spice carousel.

Some manufacturers don't put expiration dates on herbs and spices, but that doesn't mean that the jar of poultry seasoning that's been in your pantry since 1994 is still good. It won't make you sick, but it likely doesn't have much flavor. As one member wrote: "If it's pale, it's stale."

Date all herbs and spices when you bring them home, and be sure to use up what you have before you open a new one. Six months is the average lifespan for dried herbs, whether you buy them or dry them yourself.

SparkPeople Cooking Challenge:
Clean out your spice drawer. If you can't remember when you bought it, throw it out. Date anything that's left in the drawer.

HOW DO I PAIR HERBS AND FOODS?

If you're unfamiliar with the taste of fresh herbs, visit a farmers' market and ask for a tutorial. Make shopping for herbs a tactile experience; smell them, rub them between your fingers, and, if possible, taste them. What foods come to mind? That's a good place to start.

This is a chance to be creative. We all have preferences when it comes to taste, so trust your palate and add what "sounds good" to start. You'll never know until you try. If something tastes good to you, it can't be "wrong"! If you want to be creative with herbs and spices, follow your nose. If you don't like the smell of mint and rosemary together, chances are you won't like the taste either. If cumin and cilantro smell good, go for it!

Here are some common pairings to help you get started:

- *Parsley:* cheese, eggs, seafood, vegetables, chicken, breads

- *Mint:* lamb, peas, fruit

- *Oregano:* pizza, chicken, vegetables

- *Chervil:* eggs, chicken, shellfish, summer vegetables

- *Sage:* pork, chicken, root vegetables

- *Thyme:* eggs, beef, chicken, seafood, soups, root vegetables

- *Basil:* tomatoes, pasta, olive oil, cheese, fish, green beans (I promise you, it's delicious!)

- *Rosemary:* mushrooms, roasted and grilled meats, root vegetables, breads

- *Cumin:* beans, spicy dishes, chicken, root vegetables

- *Cilantro:* spicy dishes, salads, salsas, fish, rice

GROW YOUR OWN

Herbs and spices are expensive! Even an inexperienced gardener can save some money by planting some herbs in a flowerbed or containers. Many herbs will grow indoors, even through the winter. I dry fresh herbs to save for the winter. Wash the herbs, pat them dry, and place on a cotton towel. Microwave them for 30 seconds, then crumble into jars for the pantry.

CHEF MEG'S FAVORITES

Basil The name comes from the Greek work for "royal" or "king," which is a perfect fit: it certainly reigns supreme in my garden. I dry the extra for winter and prepare pesto for freezing. Available dried or fresh, you can also find basil in cube-form in the freezer section of some supermarkets.

Chiles Most people shy away from chile peppers and chili powder because they fear the heat will burn their mouths. Just as chiles can be dark or light, they can be spicy or mild. When adding heat to a dish, it should just be enough to make the taste buds tingle and enhance other flavors—not so much that your nose is running and your eyes watering. The heat from the pepper arrives with a tingle on the tongue, then it continues with what I like to call "back heat," a warmth that continues after you chew and swallow. When choosing chili powders, know that the darker the powder, the darker the final dish will appear. Check the label of your chili powder. It should be ground chile peppers—with no added salt. Chiles go well with pork, beef, vegetables, and soups.

Cumin According to legend, cumin keeps husbands from straying. I use it almost every other day! This smoky spice can be purchased as whole seeds or ground. You can use it by itself or as part of a taco or chili seasoning (see Taco Seasoning, page 371). I use it in Latin dishes, soups, stews, bean salads, chili, salsas, and just about everything else that would benefit from its earthy, smoky flavor.

Pepper Peppercorns are the unripe fruit of a pepper plant. Known as the master spice, pepper can be purchased whole, cracked, and ground; and the peppercorns come in white and pink varieties in addition to the popular black. I prefer to buy whole and grind or crack it myself for a fresher taste. For coarsely cracked pepper, place your peppercorns in a plastic bag and spread them flat on a cutting board. Roll a heavy flat-bottomed pan or a rolling pin over them to crack. Of all spices, this is my No. 1 must-have, even before salt. Black pepper goes with any food except those with a white or light-colored sauce. In such cases, use white pepper for a more attractive finish. Almost any dish can benefit from a few twists of the pepper grinder.

Rosemary The distinctive and woodsy smell of rosemary reminds me of fall. Rosemary plants will thrive for years, so what a bargain that $2 herb plant is. I usually keep a plant close to the kitchen because it has such a lovely smell and produces a pretty flower. I love it with soups and stews, and it is perfect with roasted chicken, pork, or vegetables. More important, I use it as a condolence gift whenever someone we know loses a family member or friend. Sir Thomas More of England once described the herb as the plant of remembrance, saying " 'Tis the herb sacred to remembrance and therefore to friendship."

Thyme This herb is a charmer. I love the way it smells, so I always keep some growing in the kitchen or just outside my door. Thyme is also an easy plant to grow—it will come back each year in most climates. Its flavor can be strong, so a little will go a long way. I love to use whole sprigs in my roasting pans to impart flavor: the small leaves fall off during cooking. Thyme is wonderful in stocks, sauces, soups, pasta dishes, and with poultry.

Salt is a part of the earth and whether it is mined or pulled from the oceans, it adds flavor to foods. Use kosher salt for uncooked meats, sea salts for finishing dishes, and table salt for baking—but use none for the table! There is no salt shaker on the table at our house, and no one misses it.

> ***SparkPeople Cooking Challenge:*** Take the salt shaker off your table. Don't say anything to your family. Did they miss it?

RUBS, MARINADES, AND SAUCES

Once you've mastered herbs and spices and learned how to combine them into seasoning mixes, there's a world of low-sodium, low-fat flavoring options available to you. These mixtures can be a great help when trying to wean yourself and your family from high-fat and high-sugar condiments. Once your palate adjusts to real flavor, you'll find fatty alternatives just aren't as appealing as they used to be.

A rub is a dry mixture made up of spices, seasonings, and herbs (I prefer to omit the salt that's abundant in store-bought blends). The purpose of the rub is to add flavor to the outside of the meat; unlike a marinade, it won't penetrate beyond the surface, so use a rub for leaner cuts of meat that you will roast or grill. I like rubs because the meat will stay dry in most cases, which is perfect for a nice crispy crust.

A marinade contains acids and oil in addition to herbs and spices. If you pierce the meat, the flavor will penetrate the inside. Marinades also tenderize by breaking down some of the connective proteins in the meat, so use a marinade for tougher cuts of meat or meat that tends to be bland, like chicken breasts. How long you marinate the meat really depends on the cut of meat. Chicken will only take 30 minutes to 1 hour; beef from 1 hour up to 6 hours. When marinating fish, don't let it go any more than 20 minutes. Fish does not have much connective tissue so you run the risk of actually cooking the fish in an acid-based marinade. Marinate meats in the refrigerator.

You can easily turn any of the spice blends and rubs in the book into a marinade. For one pound of meat combine one tablespoon of rub with three tablespoons of an acid (citrus juice or vinegar) with one tablespoon of canola oil.

A note on garlic: Choose fresh garlic anytime you are going to be eating it raw, such as in a salad or dressing. Use minced jarred garlic to save time when you're going to cook it. And for rubs and marinades, look for garlic powder or dried minced garlic (not garlic salt).

SparkPeople Cooking Challenge:
The next time you're faced with a bland piece of meat or fish, mix up a marinade. The bottled varieties are full of salt and sugar, and you'll save money by making your own.

Ranch Seasoning Blend

Ranch dressing overtook Italian dressing as the nation's most popular salad dressing in 1992, and now the creamy white dressing is found on everything from vegetables to chicken wings.

The stuff that comes in a bottle is mostly salt, oil, and other fats with little flavor. I created this dried herb blend to take the place of the full-fat version. I like to mix a tablespoon of the seasoning mix with ½ cup of low-fat plain yogurt. It's still creamy and tangy but with much less fat. If you want a dressing that does not stick to the spoon, try adding ¼ cup skim milk or low-fat buttermilk to the yogurt sauce. Use fresh or dried herbs, but be sure to let the dressing sit for a few hours in the fridge to let the flavors fully develop.

This seasoning blend is great in pasta dishes, over fish or chicken, or added to soups. Compared with the packaged variety you will save up to a half-teaspoon of sodium per serving.

Makes 8 Servings:
½ tsp per serving

2 Minutes to Prepare

1 tbsp dried parsley

2 tsp dried chives

1 tsp garlic powder

½ tsp dry mustard

¼ tsp celery seed

Combine the parsley, chives, garlic, dry mustard, and celery seed in a small bowl. Store in an airtight container.

Per Serving: 3.1 calories, 0 g total fat, 0 mg cholesterol, 1 mg sodium, 0.6 g total carbs, 0.1 g dietary fiber, 0.1 g protein

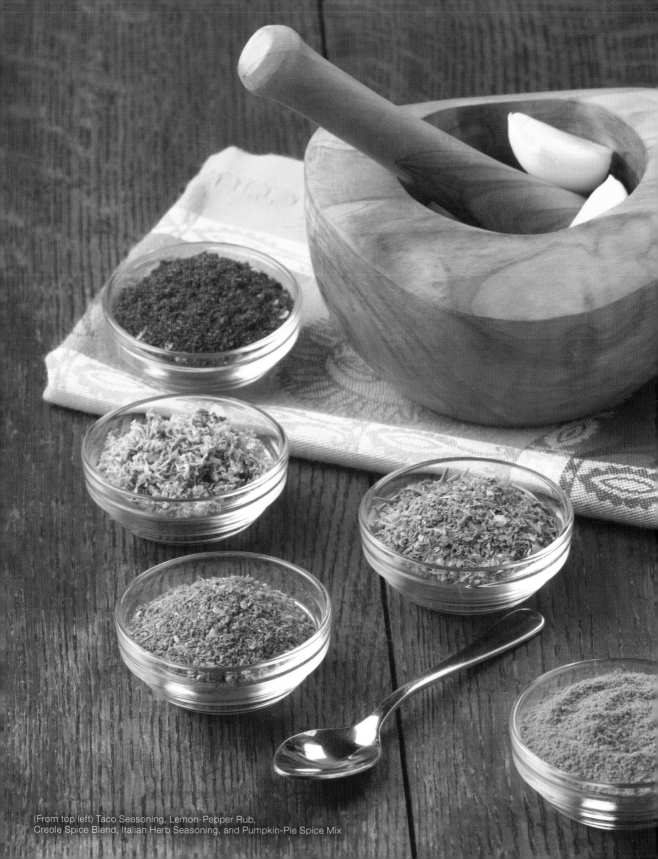

(From top left) Taco Seasoning, Lemon-Pepper Rub,
Creole Spice Blend, Italian Herb Seasoning, and Pumpkin-Pie Spice Mix

Italian Herb Seasoning

Forget buying packets of seasonings. They're expensive and often full of salt. Save sodium and money by making this easy herb blend. Use it in sauces, soups, stews, on meats . . . anywhere you want to add Italian flavor without fat or sodium!

Makes 4 Servings:
about 1 tbsp per serving

3 Minutes to Prepare

1 tbsp dried oregano

1 tbsp dried basil

1 tbsp dried sage

1 tsp dried rosemary

1 tsp red pepper flakes

In a small bowl, combine the oregano, basil, sage, rosemary, and red pepper. Store in an airtight container away from direct sunlight for up to six months. Before using, crush herbs between your fingers to release more flavor.

Per Serving: 3.9 calories, 0.1 g total fat, 0 mg cholesterol, 0.1 mg sodium, 0.7 g total carbs, 0.5 g dietary fiber, 0.1 g protein

Creole Spice Blend

Creole cooking originated in the aristocratic society of New Orleans, where the locals adapted classical European recipes to the ingredients they had on hand. Don't confuse Creole with Cajun cooking, which is based on the country-style cooking of the Acadian settlers. Creole cooking does not pack the heat that Cajun cooking does.

Makes 8 Servings:
 1 tsp per serving

5 Minutes to Prepare

2 tbsp onion flakes

2 tbsp celery seed

2 tbsp dried oregano

1 tsp hot or sweet paprika

1 tsp dried thyme

2 tsp black peppercorns

½ tsp cayenne

Combine the onion flakes, celery seed, oregano, paprika, thyme, peppercorns, and cayenne in a coffee grinder. Process until blended and peppercorns are crushed. Store for up to 6 months in a closed container and place in a dark area.

Per Serving: 17.1 calories, 0.6 g total fat, 0 mg cholesterol, 3.5 mg sodium, 3.1 g total carbs, 1.1 g dietary fiber, 0.7 g protein

Taco Seasoning

Those packets of seasoning that you buy at the grocery store add flavor to your dishes, but it mostly comes in the form of fillers and salt. Control the sodium levels of your food by making your own. You probably have all the seasonings on hand already, and you'll notice that homemade taco seasoning has a fresher taste. Making it at home is also a great way to save money!

If you prefer your taco seasoning to be milder, reduce or omit the red pepper flakes. If you want a bolder flavor, add more red pepper flakes.

Makes 3 Servings:
 1⅔ tbsp per serving

2 Minutes to Prepare

3 tbsp ground cumin

1 tbsp chili powder (see Note)

1 tbsp red pepper flakes

In a small bowl, mix together the cumin, chili powder, and red pepper flakes. Store in a closed container, away from light and heat for up to 6 months.

Note: Some commercial chili powders contain salt and other spices. Look for a version that just contains chili powder. The color of the chili powder won't affect the heat level of your dish, but it will affect the color. Look for a dark chili powder to achieve a deep reddish brown color in your finished dish.

Per Serving: 36.4 calories, 2.1 g total fat, 0 mg cholesterol, 36.3 mg sodium, 5 g total carbs, 2 g dietary fiber, 1.6 g protein

SPARK MEMBERS LOVE THEIR HERBS AND SPICES

- "I grow quite a few varieties of herbs and dry them in my kitchen," says member DOWN2SEXY. "I like a combination of sage, rosemary, and oregano for lamb, pork, or chicken. I like dill, ground black pepper, and lemon zest for mild-flavored fish. I like rosemary and garlic for trout. I like thyme, basil, and oregano for almost any poultry. I like chipotle powder, cumin, garlic, and cinnamon for Southwestern or Tex-Mex. I like paprika, garlic, and nutmeg for Stroganoff, Swedish meatballs, and just about anything with mushrooms in it (including sautéed mushrooms). I like the combination of ginger, cinnamon, nutmeg, and ground cloves with sweet fruits like berries, apples, pears, and peaches. I'm a purist when it comes to my citrus fruits, though, and don't use anything on them. I like to season summer squashes with oregano and garlic. On winter squashes I use cinnamon, nutmeg, and allspice with just little sprinkle of dark brown sugar. Spaghetti squash definitely calls for a tiny little splash of olive oil, garlic, crushed rosemary, basil, and oregano."

- SOLLAMYN says "I love herbs and spices, too, but since I live alone, I find it very convenient (and economical!) to buy mine at my local food co-op. There, I can purchase what I want in any amount that I need. That way I don't have a lot of spices on hand that I will never use more than a few times a year, and I save money by purchasing only the amount that I need. That said, I use a lot of cinnamon (I put it in my coffee every day!) and cumin. Also, I grow my own basil, thyme, oregano, and lemon balm. I can't wait to use my fresh herbs! The oregano and lemon balm are already abundant, but I'll have to be patient with the basil and thyme."

Pumpkin-Pie Spice Mix

You can easily make your own pumpkin-pie spice at home. When that first snap of autumn arrives, make up a double or triple batch of this recipe—it makes a great hostess gift for any fall event.

Makes 4 Servings
  ½ tbsp per serving

2 Minutes to Prepare

½ tsp mace

1 tbsp cinnamon

1 tsp ground ginger

½ tsp ground cloves

½ tsp allspice

½ tsp nutmeg

In a small bowl, combine the mace, cinnamon, ginger, cloves, allspice, and nutmeg. Store in an airtight container away from sunlight for up to 3 months.

Per Serving: 8.9 calories, 0.3 g total fat, 0 mg cholesterol, 1.5 mg sodium, 2.1 g total carbs, 1.2 g dietary fiber, 0.2 g protein

Low-Sodium Barbecue Rub

Use this rub on slow-cooker ribs or your favorite pork roast recipe. I prefer to use dried minced garlic rather than garlic powder (though you could substitute that) to give the rub some texture.

Makes 48 Servings:
½ tsp per serving

5 Minutes to Prepare

1 tsp celery seed

1 tsp cayenne

2 tsp granulated garlic

1 tbsp black pepper

1 tsp kosher or sea salt

1 tbsp brown sugar

1 tbsp dark chili powder

1 tbsp cumin

1 tbsp smoked paprika

In a small bowl, combine the celery seed, cayenne, garlic, black pepper, salt, brown sugar, chili powder, cumin, and paprika. Store the rub in an airtight container away from sunlight and heat for up to 6 months.

Per Serving: 2.6 calories, 0.1 g total fat, 0 mg cholesterol, 11.7 mg sodium, 0.5 g total carbs, 0.2 g dietary fiber, 0.1 g protein

Lemon-Pepper Rub

If chicken breasts are the little black dress of the culinary world (dress them up, dress them down—the possibilities are endless), then lemon pepper is the classic accessory that completes the look, or the meal, in this case. Lemon zest has an intense flavor that goes well with fish and seafood as well as chicken. Spice it up by adding paprika, pepper, and garlic for a salt-free rub. You can buy dried lemon peel, but it's flavorless and expensive. Make your own for a fraction of the cost by zesting the lemon and drying it.

Makes 4 Servings:
½ tbsp per serving

10 Minutes to Prepare

Zest of 2 lemons (about 1½ tbsp),
   minced and dried

½ tsp sweet paprika

¼ tsp black pepper

¼ tsp granulated garlic (see Note)

In a glass jar with a tight-fitting lid, combine the lemon zest, paprika, black pepper, and garlic. Shake well. Use immediately or store in the refrigerator for up to 2 weeks.

Note: Look for dried minced or granulated garlic in the spice aisle. Be sure that the ingredients list garlic and only garlic—not salt.

Per Serving: 1.7 calories, 0 g total fat, 0 mg cholesterol, 0.1 mg sodium, 0.4 g total carbs, 0.1 g dietary fiber, 0.1 g protein

CHEF MEG'S TIPS: HOW TO DRY LEMON PEEL

- Zest the lemon and place the zest on a parchment paper-lined baking sheet.

- *Short method:* Place the baking sheet in a 200° F oven for 15 to 20 minutes, shaking the pan every 5 minutes. Allow to cool before using.

- *Longer (and greener) method:* Place the baking sheet in an out-of-the-way place and allow the zest to air dry for 24 hours.

Coconut-Cilantro Pesto

If a sauce is primarily made from one herb, you can call it a pesto. While basil is most commonly used, pesto can be made from parsley, spinach, and even, in this case, cilantro. I think this is my favorite variation. Here, the cilantro replaces the basil, coconut steps in for Parmesan for mouth feel and flavor, and we punch up the flavor with a jalapeño. We conserve calories and fat by using orange juice and just a small amount of oil.

Try this on sandwiches instead of mayo or on bruschetta. Use it as a garnish for Thai-inspired dishes or simple grilled chicken or fish. It makes a great dipping sauce for the Coconut-Lime Shrimp (page 236).

Makes 12 Servings:
  1 tsp per serving

5 Minutes to Prepare

2 cups cilantro, stems trimmed

¼ cup unsweetened coconut flakes

1 jalapeño pepper, seeded and chopped

1 orange, zested and juiced

1 tbsp canola oil

In a blender or a food processor, combine the cilantro, coconut, jalapeño, orange zest and juice, and oil. Pulse until the mixture is thoroughly pureed. Use immediately or store in the refrigerator for up to 5 days. Store in the freezer for up to 3 months.

Per Serving: 26 calories, 2.4 g total fat, 0 mg cholesterol, 0.6 mg sodium, 1 g total carbs, 0.3 g dietary fiber, 0.2 g protein

Better-than-Pesto Puree

This is a great way to work more vegetables into your meals. This puree of basil, spinach, and parsley is reminiscent of pesto, with much less oil and no cheese. The fresh flavor of the herbs and spinach really shine through.

By blanching and shocking the leaves, they will keep their bright green color after being pureed. Skip this step and you'll end up with a black puree. Likewise, removing the stems from spinach and parsley is a chore, but I truly believe you end up with a smoother, tastier product in the end.

I like to use it instead of tomato sauce on pizza, but you can also add color, flavor, and almost a full serving of vegetables to any pizza, pasta, or seafood dish. For a variation, you could add a ¼ cup of toasted, cooled, and chopped walnuts.

Makes 8 Servings:
1 tbsp per serving

6 Minutes to Prepare and Cook

1 cup fresh basil leaves

1 cup spinach, washed and stems removed

½ cup flat-leaf parsley, washed and stems removed

2 tbsp minced shallots

¼ cup olive oil

½ tsp black pepper

1. Fill a medium bowl with ice water and set aside.

2. Fill a medium saucepan with water and bring to a boil over high heat. Add the basil, spinach, and parsley and cook for no more than 60 seconds. Drain and immediately transfer the leaves in the ice water to shock them; let them sit in the water for 1 minute, then drain. Wring in a clean kitchen towel to remove excess moisture.

3. Place the cooked leaves and the shallots in a food processor or blender. Puree, adding the oil in a steady stream while the blender is running. Season with pepper. This will keep in the refrigerator for 1 week or in the freezer for 6 months.

Per Serving: 65.4 calories, 6.8 g total fat, 0 mg cholesterol, 5.6 mg sodium, 1.1 g total carbs, 0.4 g dietary fiber, 0.4 g protein

Tomato Jam

You might not think of tomatoes when you think of jam, but they are a fruit, after all! The sweet and tangy flavor of the tomatoes is enhanced by the onions and garlic, then concentrated.

This pairs well with tangy goat cheese or salty feta, and it's also a nice contrast with cannellini beans (see Bruschetta with Cilantro Pesto and White Beans, page 282). Spread the jam on whole-wheat toast as an appetizer (see Creamy, Tangy Tomato Bruschetta, page 284) or as a condiment for grilled pork, fish, or beef. You could even mix this in with whole-wheat pasta topped with grilled vegetables. For a gourmet pizza, top the Quinoa-Flaxseed Pizza Dough (page 271) with a layer of Tomato Jam, a cup of goat cheese, and a drizzle of the Better-than-Pesto Puree (page 377).

Makes 24 Servings:
1 tbsp per serving

30 Minutes to Prepare and Cook

1 tbsp olive oil

1 large onion, diced (about 2 cups)

3 cloves garlic, minced

4 cups chopped grape or plum (Roma) tomatoes

2 tbsp light brown sugar

3 tbsp balsamic vinegar

1 tbsp lemon juice

¼ tsp red pepper flakes

½ tsp salt

1. Heat the oil in a large saucepan over moderate heat. Add the onions and sauté for 3 minutes. Add the garlic and continue to cook for 1 minute more just to soften them. Add the tomatoes, brown sugar, vinegar, lemon juice, red pepper, and salt. Bring the mixture to a boil, then reduce the heat and simmer on low for 25 minutes.

2. Carefully transfer the jam to a blender or a food processor. Pulse 3 to 4 times or puree slightly.

3. Cool and refrigerate. The jam will keep in the fridge for 5 days or in the freezer for several months. (To freeze, place the jam in plastic bags and squeeze the air out.)

Per Serving: 20.2 calories, 0.7 g total fat, 0 mg cholesterol, 52.3 mg sodium, 3.8 g total carbs, 0.6 g dietary fiber, 0.4 g protein

Light Lemon Sauce

Vegetables are delicious on their own, but this light lemon sauce is a great addition to roasted or steamed vegetables. I love it over Roasted Asparagus (page 318). Use this in place of Hollandaise sauce in any recipe. It has all of the tang with much less fat. If you prefer a spicier sauce, add white pepper to taste.

Makes 4 Servings:
    2 tbsp per serving

5 Minutes to Prepare

½ cup 1% milk-fat cottage cheese

2 tbsp reduced-fat sour cream

3 tbsp skim milk

2 lemons, zested and juiced

1. Combine the cottage cheese, sour cream, and milk in a food processor and pulse to a puree. (You can also use an immersion blender: just place the ingredients in a large mixing bowl.)

2. Add the lemon zest and whisk to combine, then stream in the lemon juice, whisking continuously, until the mixture is pourable. (You might not need all the lemon juice.) Serve immediately or store in the refrigerator for up to 2 days.

Per Serving: 36 calories, 1.2 g total fat, 4.3 mg cholesterol, 123.7 mg sodium, 2.3 g total carbs, 0 g dietary fiber, 4.1 g protein

Spicy Yogurt Sauce

This sauce is great with our Baked Chicken Tenders (page 194) or even our Baked Sunburst Fries (page 319). For a new twist on your grilled chicken salad, use a serving of the chicken tenders on top of a bowl of greens, with this sauce as the dressing. You can use regular plain yogurt, but the sauce will be thinner.

Makes 8 Servings:
2 tbsp per serving

5 Minutes to Prepare and Cook

3 tbsp low-sugar or all-fruit peach preserves

6 ounces plain, nonfat Greek yogurt

1 to 2 chipotle peppers in adobo sauce, seeds removed, chopped or pureed (use 2 or leave seeds if you like more heat)

1 tbsp lime juice

1. Heat the peach preserves in a saucepan until they reach a thin, syruplike consistency, about 3 minutes. (Or microwave on high for 30 seconds.) Let the preserves cool slightly, but don't let them thicken up again.

2. In a mixing bowl, combine the cooled preserves, yogurt, chipotles, and lime juice. Cover and chill for 30 minutes before serving.

Per Serving: 21.2 calories, 0 g total fat, 1.3 mg cholesterol, 27 mg sodium, 4.6 g total carbs, 0.3 g dietary fiber, 1.8 g protein

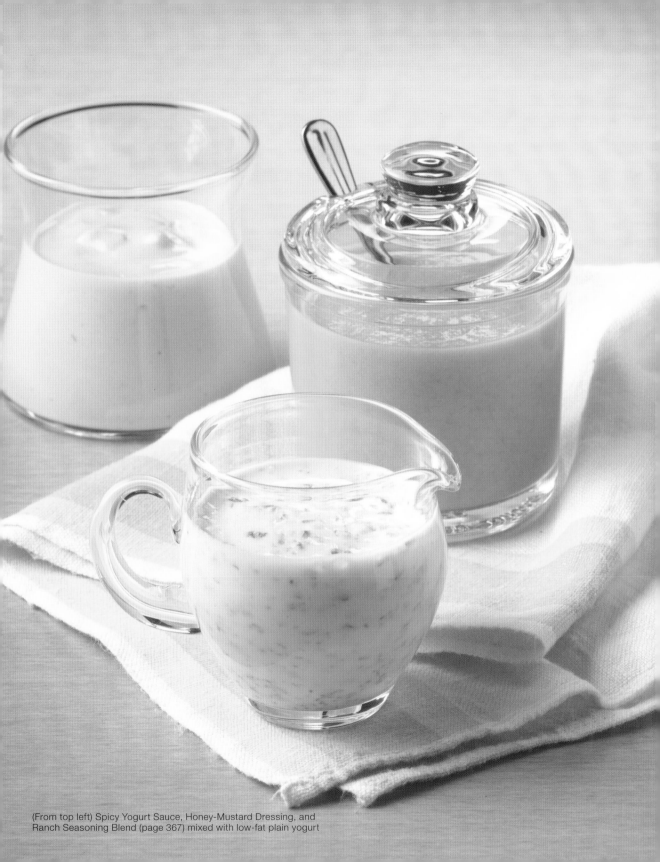

(From top left) Spicy Yogurt Sauce, Honey-Mustard Dressing, and
Ranch Seasoning Blend (page 367) mixed with low-fat plain yogurt

Honey-Mustard Dressing or Dipping Sauce

Honey mustard is a versatile condiment that's great on sandwiches and salads and, in our house, for dipping vegetables and baked chicken tenders. My kids love it! The store-bought varieties have a lengthy list of thickeners and stabilizers—and they're expensive. I was able to reduce the oil and still get a thick, rich sauce by adding just five baby carrots.

Let your kids help with this recipe—they can pour all the ingredients into the blender and help you measure. Older kids might be able to make this all on their own.

Makes 4 Servings:
2 tbsp per serving

5 Minutes to Prepare

5 baby carrots (or 1 large carrot, peeled)

1 small garlic clove, peeled and smashed

1 tbsp honey

2 tbsp rice- or white-wine vinegar

1 tbsp Dijon mustard

2 tbsp canola oil

Place the carrots, garlic, honey, vinegar, and mustard in a blender and puree. Slowly open the spout on top, and stream in the oil while the blender is running. Can be stored in the refrigerator for up to 10 days.

Per Serving: 88.5 calories, 7.1 g total fat, 0 mg cholesterol, 94.8 mg sodium, 6 g total carbs, 0.3 g dietary fiber, 0.2 g protein

Sweet and Spicy Barbecue Sauce

Barbecue sauce and grilling go hand in hand. But while grilling is a healthful cooking technique, bottled barbecue sauce is usually full of salt and sugar. Roasted vegetables are the basis for our barbecue sauce, and they add a smoky sweet flavor. We chose no-salt-added tomato paste and homemade or low-sodium stock to keep the sodium levels down. The acid in the tomatoes, vinegar, and citrus juice add flavor where we would usually rely on salt.

I like to double or triple the batch because it's just as easy to roast two pans of vegetables as it is one. I either freeze the leftovers, or I put some in a jar and take it to cookouts as a gift for the hostess.

. . . .

Chef Meg's Tip: If you don't have time to slow roast the vegetables in the oven, place them under the broiler, but watch them the entire time so that they don't burn. Under the broiler, the vegetables will cook in about 15 minutes.

. . . .

Makes 8 Servings:
¼ cup per serving

55 Minutes to Prepare and Cook

1 large red onion, quartered (about 2 cups)

2 serrano chile peppers, split in half lengthwise, stemmed and seeded (see Note)

2 bell peppers, cut into fourths lengthwise, and seeded

3 plum (Roma) tomatoes, cut into fourths lengthwise

4 cloves garlic, peeled and cut in half

1 lime, juiced

1 lemon, juiced

One 6-ounce can no-salt-added tomato paste

1 tsp chili powder

½ tsp sweet or hot paprika

1 cup apple-cider vinegar

2 cups homemade or low-sodium chicken or vegetable stock

½ cup pineapple chunks in natural juice

1. Preheat the oven to 425° F. Place the onions, peppers, tomatoes, and garlic on a sheet pan and roast for 30 minutes, stirring halfway through.

2. Transfer the roasted vegetables to a saucepan. Add the lime and lemon juice, tomato paste, chili powder, paprika, vinegar, stock, and the pineapple with its juice. Simmer for 5 minutes. Puree with an immersion blender or carefully transfer to a food processor to puree.

3. Return the pureed mixture to the saucepan and simmer for additional 10 minutes. Use immediately or transfer to a container. Refrigerate for up to 5 days or freeze for up to 3 months.

Note: A serrano chile is spicier than a jalapeño pepper. If you prefer a milder sauce, use part of the pepper or leave it out. If you prefer a spicier sauce, leave in the seeds and ribs, which contain most of the heat.

Per Serving: 69.1 calories, 0.4 g total fat, 0 mg cholesterol, 180.2 mg sodium, 15.9 total carbs, 3.1 g dietary fiber, 2.1 g protein

Spicy Garlic Oil

Oils and fats should be eaten sparingly, but when you do use them, put them to work. Infusing oil is a great way to add flavor without adding even more calories. Use this flavored oil on pizza, whole-wheat garlic bread, or even whole-wheat pasta and vegetables. A little goes a long way.

Makes 6 Servings:
½ tsp per serving

5 Minutes to Prepare and Cook

2 tbsp olive oil

4 cloves garlic, smashed and chopped

¼ tsp red pepper flakes

Place the oil, garlic, and pepper in a small saucepan over low heat. Cook until the garlic just starts to sizzle. Remove from heat and set aside to cool. Use immediately or refrigerate for up to 1 week.

Per Serving: 43 calories, 4.5 g total fat, 0 mg cholesterol, 0.4 mg sodium, 0.7 g total carbs, 0.1 g dietary fiber, 0.1 g protein

VINAIGRETTES

Vinaigrettes and families have a lot in common. Comprising two (or more) seemingly unmixable ingredients, the disparate components are either united and made stronger or they quickly go their separate ways.

What's the secret, both for family ties and an unbreakable salad dressing? The ties that bind. In the case of a vinaigrette, the oil and vinegar need a unifier, too, and that's an emulsifier.

Vinaigrettes are temporary emulsions of any variety of oil and vinegar (or another acid), plus seasonings. An emulsion is a uniform mixture of two unmixable liquids held together in suspension. These emulsified creations can be used as a salad dressing, sauce, or as a marinade to impart flavor to vegetables or proteins. The lifespan of your emulsion depends on many factors, including your ingredients, the temperature of those ingredients, and even the hands of the preparer.

When teaching about vinaigrettes, I play show and tell. I bring in a glass cruet and whip up a vinaigrette in a flash by pouring in oil, vinegar, water, and spices and giving it a shake. Not surprisingly, the oil starts to float to the top, and the spices sink to the bottom within minutes.

Then I mix mustard, spices, and vinegar in a large bowl and slowly whisk in a steady stream of olive oil. The mustard acts as a stabilizer, which keeps the oil and vinegar combined. Though it takes a few minutes longer, the result is a dressing that will stay emulsified for hours and even sometimes days. Just like people need some time to warm up to one another, so does your dressing. Room temperature ingredients will yield a stronger emulsification. In addition to mustard, you can use pureed vegetables,

anchovy paste, or no-salt-added tomato paste to bind your dressings. Regardless of what kind of vinaigrette you make, it will have between 80 and 120 calories and 9 to 14 grams of fat per tablespoon.

Once you know the basics of making a vinaigrette, the combinations are endless. Just remember the ratio of three parts oil to one part vinegar. For four servings, use three tablespoons of oil to one tablespoon of vinegar and one teaspoon of mustard or other emulsifier.

As a general rule, color coordinate your vinaigrette with what it's flavoring. Aesthetics aside, darker vinegars tend to be bolder, which makes them ideal matches for beef, mixed dark greens, and bolder flavors such as garlic and onions. Vinaigrettes made with lighter-colored vinegars pair well with fish, vegetables, and chicken, or whenever a neutral flavor is desired.

Types of Vinegar

- *Apple-Cider* Light brown and sweet

- *Balsamic* Sweet-tasting vinegar aged in wooden barrels. Younger varieties are reasonably priced, but older aged varieties can be quite expensive.

- *White- or Red-Wine* Made from aged wine, it has a lovely wine flavor. My favorite!

- *Rice-Wine* Used often in Asian dishes; I love steamed asparagus with a rice-wine vinaigrette.

- *Flavored Vinegars* Herb- or chile-infused vinegars are a great way to add flavor.

- *Distilled White* Good for cleaning and pickling, but too strong for dressings.

Additional Ingredients

Mustard is my top choice for the perfect vinaigrette. I prefer Dijon or a country-style mustard. Second is garlic, smashed and chopped! The herb varieties are endless: basil, chives, dill, tarragon, parsley, mint, thyme, or chervil. I also love to put vegetables and fruits into my vinaigrettes, such as the Tomato-Basil Vinaigrette (page 387). You can use berries, tomatoes, roasted peppers, roasted or raw garlic, shallots (a favorite!), or even carrots as the basis for your dressing (check out the Honey-Mustard Dressing on page 382).

Tomato-Basil Vinaigrette

In summertime, when your garden and the markets overflow with basil and tomatoes, this is the perfect salad dressing. It's easy, flavorful, and ready in a flash. You could swap five sun-dried tomatoes or a roasted red pepper for the cherry tomatoes in this recipe. The dressing will be thicker and have a stronger flavor. In addition to topping salads, this dressing is great on grilled chicken or in a whole-wheat pasta salad.

Makes 8 Servings:
    2 tbsp per serving

5 Minutes to Prepare

1 tsp Dijon mustard

3 tbsp red-wine vinegar

5 cherry tomatoes

¾ cup fresh basil leaves

3 tbsp olive oil

Pinch of black pepper

1 tbsp finely chopped shallot

In a blender, puree the mustard, vinegar, tomatoes, and basil. Slowly open the spout on top, and stream in the oil while the blender is running. Stir in the pepper and shallots.

Per Serving: 80.6 calories, 8.2 g total fat, 0 mg cholesterol, 26.1 mg sodium, 1.9 g total carbs, 0.4 g dietary fiber, 0.4 g protein

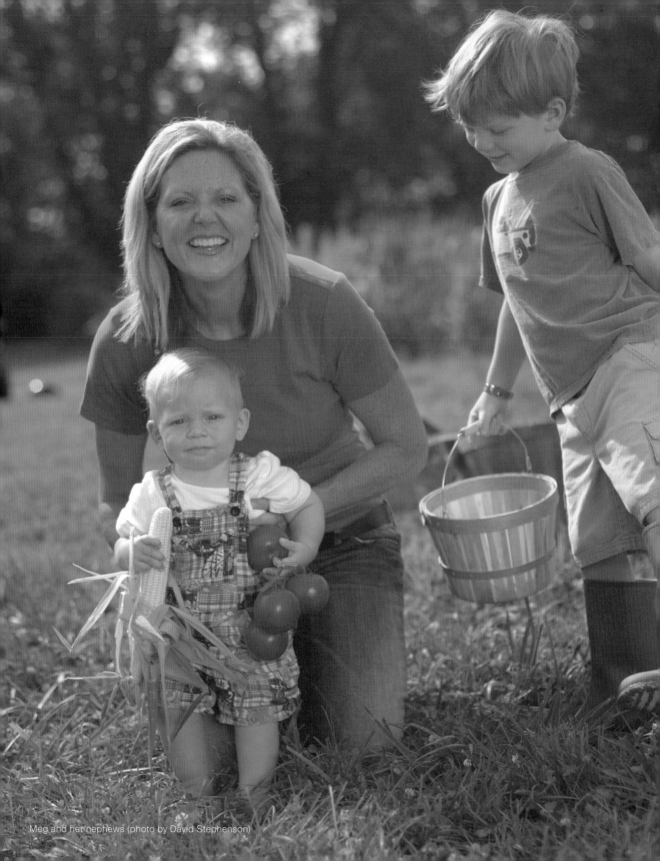

Meg and her nephews (photo by David Stephenson)

AFTERWORD

Raising Kids to Be Healthy Eaters

Once you're committed to eating right and cooking at home, it's important to get everyone else in the house on board. Healthy eating is a family affair! Teaching kids to cook sets them up for success down the line. Children who eat dinner with their families have been found to be more successful in school, less likely to get into trouble, and better able to maintain a healthy weight. Beyond all of that, eating right will help children grow and thrive.

Early in my career, I worked at the Cincinnati Shriners Hospital, which provides world-famous care—free of charge—for children and teens who have suffered burns and other skin disorders. I took one look at those kids, as I walked through the hospital foyer before my first interview, and all I wanted to do was to get to know them, comfort them, and help them get better. Food is one of the most important aspects of the healing process. To heal, the body needs large amounts of calories, but after undergoing such trauma, children often lose their appetites or find their palates have changed. So I worked with patients and their families to help the kids find

foods they liked, and I used some of the same techniques, tips, and tricks outlined in this book to make sure the food tasted good and was good for them. Getting kids, sick or well, interested in eating right and avoiding food fights at the dinner table isn't as difficult as parents think. If they're involved, they'll be interested. Throughout this book, we've concentrated on providing the tools for healthy eating. Here, we'll demonstrate how you can break the cycle of unhealthy eating and introduce your children to the kitchen. You'll also find great kid-friendly meal ideas that will make it a whole lot easier.

As a parent, you have to be involved and engaged when it comes to feeding your children and promoting emotionally healthy approaches to eating. Just as you've had to learn how to eat properly, educate yourself on your child's nutritional needs. Talk to your pediatrician first; he or she will be able to provide general guidelines as well as specific advice determined by your child's needs. We also recommend MyPyramid.gov, an interactive website developed by the United States Department of Agriculture. You can enter your child's age, gender, height, weight, and activity level and learn the recommended daily number of servings from each food group; for children older than six, you'll receive a recommended calorie count, too.

Every parent knows it takes a firm strategy when it comes to kids and food. Ellyn Satter, a registered dietitian and child psychotherapist, proposes a "division of responsibility" as a road to raising a healthy eater. Her recommendations are supported by a substantial amount of research that demonstrates that children have a healthier relationship with food, and a healthier body weight as teens and adults, when raised by caregivers who optimize their child's natural hunger cues.

Satter suggests that parents and children have distinct roles when it comes to feeding and eating responsibilities: as the parent, you are in charge of when the family eats, where the family eats, and what the family is served; the child is in charge of deciding how much (if any) food is eaten. Take a look at the following recommendations and think about where you may be crossing the lines of responsibility when feeding your child.[1]

A PARENT'S RESPONSIBILITIES

When you teach your child how to eat properly by providing good food in a healthy environment, your child will learn to make his or her own healthy-eating choices. Here are some helpful tips:

- Plan for your child to eat three meals and up to three snacks throughout the day. Do not allow eating between these planned meals and planned snack times.

- Make sure that all meals and snacks are eaten at the dining room or kitchen tables. No more eating on the couch, in front of the television or computer, in bed, or in the car. Insist that your child show up for all meals, even if the response is "I'm not hungry." Once in awhile, it's okay to serve a special family meal or snack in front of the TV, but it's important to maintain the habit of eating meals as a family at the table.

- Turn off the television and radio during snack and mealtime. Do not allow cell phones, iPods, or any other electronic devices at the table. (That also goes for you, Mom and Dad!)

- Use family mealtime to unwind and talk about highlights from the day. It is the perfect opportunity to connect with your child.

- Don't become a short-order cook. Your child should choose what to eat only from the foods offered on the table. "Cooking to order" at each meal will not foster a healthy environment in which a child will learn to be open to trying new foods.

- Never praise your child for finishing a meal and do not force your child to be a member of the clean-plate club. This will only teach your child to link food and eating with pleasing you; don't give food that emotional power.

- Likewise, do not reward, bribe, or punish your child with food. Food cannot solve relationship problems, ease loneliness, calm nerves, or relieve boredom. When adults use food to reward or punish, they may be teaching the child to become an emotional eater.

- Don't be tempted to coax or bribe a picky eater. Be patient. Establishing healthy eating habits takes a lifetime. Continue to offer your child new foods, but pair them with foods you know will be accepted. This way, your child can feel free to try the unfamiliar food, along with the favorites. Offer new foods more than once and in different forms. It may take up to 10 tries before your child accepts a new food.

Remember that you are your child's greatest example. Be a role model when it comes to exhibiting healthy eating habits and appropriate table manners.

A CHILD'S RESPONSIBILITIES

It is up to the child to decide whether to eat at all and how much to eat from the foods offered at the table. That is, kids get to select from the healthy foods offered, and then decide how much to eat. They also get to decide what to eat first. Remember, there should be absolutely no coaxing or bribing from an adult.

Keep in mind the tips offered above. If you bribe your child with the promise of dessert in return for eating vegetables, you are teaching your child that vegetables are a punishment and dessert is the ultimate reward.

We all know that children are masters at manipulation, especially with food. And parents often express the fear that their child isn't eating enough or will only eat one food—applesauce, for example. This one food becomes the power food. No matter what is prepared at mealtime the child refuses to eat it, kicking and screaming until the parents give in and the power food, applesauce, is provided. Every meal is a battleground. Situations like this are not healthy for the child or parent. Realize that a child's body will not allow starvation.

Our bodies know how much we need if we eat in a way that fosters our natural satiety. When parents hold fast to their responsibilities, there are no power struggles. The child will quickly realize that the applesauce isn't coming and he or she is no longer in control of the foods served in the home. Your child will begin to eat what you choose to serve at meal and snack times.

Make a true commitment to this strategy and you will educate your child to follow his or her natural hunger cues and develop healthy eating habits for life. Use the recipes and tips we provide in this book to plan, prepare, and serve healthy meals and snacks. Then trust your child's ability to eat and grow in the way nature intended. As with any aspect of healthy living, there is no instant cure, no magic answer. Expect some trial and error. With some patience, perseverance, and yes, a bit of cheese sauce and ranch dressing, kids can learn to like (and even love) a whole range of healthy foods.

KIDS IN THE KITCHEN: GET THEM INVOLVED

As your kids grow, get them involved in meal planning, shopping, and cooking (see Raising Junior Chefs, page 394, for advice on cooking with your kids).

When children know that all food doesn't come from a box or a takeout window, they'll become more engaged in healthier choices. Plant a garden—or some fruit trees, if you have the space. Get the children involved with watering and caring for the plants—and let them pick the fruit and vegetables during harvest and prepare treats for others. Even a small pot of herbs on the windowsill, or growing a sweet-potato vine or avocado tree from a pit will help kids understand how food comes from nature. Take your children to the local farmers' market—or to a local farm. Visit pick-your-own berry patches as part of a family outing.

Take them shopping, and make sure the visit to the supermarket isn't just about the latest sugary snack. Select a time when the store is not overly crowded and you are not rushed, and allow each child to pick out a new, healthy ingredient. It's never too early to learn about home economics: Let your children determine which brand and size is the most affordable at the supermarket. Teach them about the price tags on the supermarket shelf and what the numbers, including unit price, mean. Take calculators along and let them do the math.

Involve your children when planning meals for the week. Get them excited about trying new foods by talking about them ahead of time. The more they know about different types of foods and where they come from, the more curious and engaged they'll become.

MAKE OVER KIDS' MEALS

Exposing children to healthful meals is one of the most important things you can do to help them develop a healthy lifestyle. As adults, they'll be more likely to consume a variety of foods if new foods are routinely introduced at a young age. Here are some suggestions from real-life moms and dads to boost the nutrition of kids' menu staples.

Everyday chicken-noodle soup can be transformed by adding a serving or two of vegetables. If your kids object to "chunky" soups, bring out the blender. To give your chicken soup a makeover, sauté chopped onions, carrots, and celery in a bit of olive oil, then give them a whirl in the blender with a bit of broth before adding it to the pot of chicken, broth, and noodles. (You can also use this tactic with canned or boxed chicken soup.) Serve with whole-grain crackers in fun shapes.

The blender method can be used with many other dishes and vegetables. Try cooking minced cauliflower and broccoli and mixing them into the egg and cheese mixture you use in lasagna. Zucchini can be grated and added to a chicken and broccoli casserole.

Add a cup or two of cooked fresh or frozen pureed carrots or butternut or acorn squash to your next batch of macaroni and cheese. The texture and color resemble that of the cheesy dish while adding a serving of veggies. Our Three-Cheese Macaroni (page 265) is a lightened-up version of the classic, but don't stop there. Grilled sliced chicken or ground turkey make great additions. Experiment with finely chopped spinach, stewed tomatoes, or chopped broccoli.

Instead of minced, processed chicken nuggets, patties, and tenders, make your own. (Find our recipe on page 194.) Offer an array of dipping sauces and even try branching out to fish nuggets (use any firm, white-fleshed fish). Add herbs and spices to suit your kids' tastes, and make a large batch at a time to have them on hand for busy nights.

French fries are always a hit at the dinner table, and baking your own is an easy alternative. Experiment with different spices and potatoes. Russet, redskin, and sweet potatoes will all produce a different taste. Toss your potato slices in olive or canola oil, spread them over a baking sheet, and top with any combination of herbs and spices. For added vitamins and variety, choose sweet potatoes, butternut squash—even parsnips, carrots, and other root vegetables. Roasting adds a sweetness that will make almost any vegetable appealing to kids. (Try the Baked Sunburst Fries on page 319 or the Roasted Root Vegetables on page 315.) Offer ketchup for the kids to dip if that's what they like (choose low-sugar and reduced-sodium varieties), or try one of the sauces in Chapter 12.

Hamburgers to go with the oven-baked fries are a hit with kids! Make your burgers at home using extra-lean ground sirloin, turkey, or chicken. These types of ground meat are going to be much lower in saturated fat than anything you'd get at a drive-thru. For some variety, whip up our quick and easy homemade Black-Bean Burgers (see page 139). One of our recipe testers said her 6-year-old daughter wanted to lick the lime cream off the plate!

Grilled cheese with tomato soup is a winning combo, but this standby is usually made with processed cheese and corn syrup–laden canned soup. To save time and calories, make grilled cheese in the toaster oven or on a countertop grill. Brush whole-wheat or mixed-grain bread with just a bit of butter or spritz it with nonstick cooking spray, then swap the pre-wrapped slices for some real cheese. Reduced-fat Cheddar, Swiss, mozzarella, Havarti, Monterey Jack, and Colby are all mild enough for children. For grown-ups, add spinach, mustard, onions, or tomatoes to the grilled cheese. You can even put pear, apple, or tomato slices; halved grapes; or greens like spinach or frisée into the sandwiches. Stick to one slice of cheese per sandwich for portion control. For added creaminess, consider a thin layer of hummus. It sounds strange, but it's quite tasty.

Instead of condensed soup, pick a canned soup with no added sweeteners. Add canned tomatoes to boost the nutrition and cut the richness of a creamy soup. (Use an immersion blender to smooth the chunky bits.) Make your own cream of tomato soup by mixing two 15-ounce cans of canned tomatoes and a pint of fat-free half-and-half or a cup of skim milk. Heat until simmering, season with salt and pepper, and puree in the blender. Top with fresh basil. (Kids also love the Minestrone Soup and Lifesaving Lentil Soup in chapter 6. Puree the soups for picky eaters.)

The more variety you offer, the more likely your kids will eat a variety of foods. One way I make this possible with my kids is that once a week we have a "Build Your Own Night." Whether it is tacos, sandwiches, or salads, we pull together as many healthy ingredients as we can find in the kitchen, which results in as much variety as possible.

Our favorite is Pasta Night. I prepare whole-grain pasta, and we steam broccoli, carrots, and asparagus—really anything that is in season. I sauté chopped tomatoes, mushrooms, and onions and grate hard cheese (like Parmesan or

Romano). You can even add chopped, cooked chicken breasts, browned lean ground beef or turkey, or even lean sausage. Then everyone jumps in to create their own "pasta à la me" dish! (This is a great way to make one meal into two—the next morning you can make a vegetable-stuffed omelet or create a quick vegetable puree that you can use in soups or spreads for sandwiches.)

We left the best for last: pizza. I think the reason we love it so much is because it often represents downtime, celebrations, and cooks' nights off. My kids beg for a Pizza Night because they love working with the dough, they get to choose their own topping, and they each get an individual pie. And the smell from the oven is irresistible.

Raising Junior Chefs

With all the talk of how we should help kids stay healthy, my mind keeps returning to the same thought: teach them to cook! In my home, the kitchen is an extension of the family room, and my three teen boys have helped me cook since they were small. Teaching your kids to cook doesn't mean that you have to turn them loose on their own. It just means letting them play an active role in meal planning, preparation—and cleanup. Training little chefs is easy. Here are some tips to get you started:

- *Keep it clean.* Teach good sanitation habits early, like basic hand-washing techniques using warm water and soap. I always tell my culinary school students to sing two rounds of "Happy Birthday" while washing their hands.

- *Mix it up.* Start them with mixing and kneading tasks. Herb blends and spice rubs (see Chapter 12) are a great idea as a first mixing experience—just make sure they wash their hands when finished and keep hands away from eyes and mouths if any hot spices are involved.

- *Savor the experience.* I would encourage you to start with savory ingredients and save the sweet recipes for later. Remember when you started feeding your infant real food and the pediatrician suggested starting with vegetables? It's the same principle. A good junior-chef recipe is Tuna Noodle Casserole on page 231.

- *Sweeten the deal.* Once you are ready to move to sweet recipes, I would start with smoothies (see page 81) and let them experiment with different flavors. Try adding some protein and fiber to the mixes by including yogurt, ground flaxseed, or wheat germ. Encourage seasonal eating when selecting the fruits and vegetables.

- *Herbal remedy.* Bits of unidentified green objects on a plate can be intimidating to a child. Purchase herb clippers and ask your petite chef to help with the meal by cutting fresh herbs. If you don't have the clippers, just use a clean pair of kitchen scissors. Encourage them to taste each herb and tell them which flavors pair well with which foods. (See Chapter 12 for more info on herbs and spices.)

- *Start chopping.* When your chef is ready to cut vegetables with a knife, choose a small, non-serrated paring knife. Start with semi-soft vegetables and fruits like cucumbers, tomatoes, summer squash, bananas, and peaches. Once they feel comfortable with these, move to harder vegetables like carrots or potatoes. I would reserve any very hard winter root vegetables such as butternut squash or yams for adult hands only.

- *Make it a teaching moment.* Make the experience an extension of the classroom. One of my fondest memories of cooking with my mother was during International Week at my grade school. I chose France and asked my mother to help me make chocolate éclairs. The basic éclairs are made with pâte à choux pastry dough—a big undertaking for an 11-year-old, but with her help they were a success. I remember how she helped me multiply the recipe so that we tripled the ingredients to make enough for the whole class. I did not know it at the time, but it was a valuable lesson in math. I have taken that same concept and applied it at home. We let our kids pick a foreign country and have them research the native dishes. We make a field trip to an international grocery store and explore. Pad Thai (page 246) or Chicken Kebob Pitas (page 140) are great beginner's recipes—though they'll need some help from Mom or Dad.

Tips from Our Members

Here, some of our members and employees share their best advice for raising healthy eaters.

- "My one-dish tuna noodle dinner is a hit with my teens. I boil whole-grain noodles, add a family-size packet of tuna, mix in a can of reduced-sodium cream of mushroom soup, and sprinkle with spices. While the water boils, I heat frozen peas in the microwave, then add them to the tuna. Then we have fruit for dessert and a glass of milk for a balanced meal."

- "We love grilled chicken and vegetables with rice. Toss the chicken and seasonal vegetables in two separate bags and coat with olive oil and Italian seasoning. It takes about 10 minutes to grill the chicken and vegetables. I keep premade rice in the freezer that can be heated up in the microwave. Our family favorite is a mixture of brown and white rice."

- "For my 3-year-old and 1-year-old, I make brown rice with black beans and a little cheese on top, or quesadillas (whole-wheat tortillas, veggies, beans, cheese, and salsa)."

- "We love whole-wheat pasta with cheese and broccoli; heat-and-serve brown rice with kidney beans and tomatoes; and spinach and turkey omelets."

- "Biggest mistake parents can make: Not walking the walk. If Mom and Dad aren't eating healthy foods, kids won't either."

- "Don't forget that you have the whole day to get them to eat a well-rounded diet—don't try to force everything into one meal."

- "Let them enjoy sweets now and again, in moderation. Many families take these away completely, which leads to their kids overindulging at birthday parties or on play dates."

- "Ultimately, your preferences will set the tone in your home. I'm amazed that my kids ask for many of the foods that I eat every day, even though they aren't packaged, sweet, or fattening. They avoid sugary drinks and love to drink water because their grandparents preach this fact and make it fun to find other options. They love high-fiber cereal because their aunt always has a bowl with them when she visits."

- "I tried to start healthy habits from the very beginning so that's all they have ever known. I always serve vegetables with lunch and dinner. They don't always get eaten and the things I serve aren't always perfect, but I try to make good choices for our family most of the time."

- "Be prepared! I make a few batches of meals I know they like (one is lentils with cauliflower, apples, carrots, and onion over noodles) so that if I'm serving something I don't think they will like, I have a healthy backup for them that doesn't require me to cook two meals."

- "Be careful that you don't let impatience and schedules get in the way of age-appropriate learning. Mistakes, drops, and spills are all part of learning to measure, pour, and mix. Keep the pace slow and encouraging so they enjoy the time in the kitchen—before, during, and after the meal."

- "Institute 'no, thank you' helpings. Insist everyone at the table try at least one bite of every food presented. After that, allow them to say 'no, thank you.' "

- "Give them fruits and vegetables in creative and unconventional ways. Try putting fruit cubes on skewers, serve carrot and celery sticks in a coffee mug, and cut the food however they request it. If your daughter will only eat cucumbers in rounds not sticks, so be it! She's eating them, isn't she?"

APPENDIX A

Weekly Meal Plan

Just as this cookbook isn't a diet book—we've banned the "D" word—this meal plan isn't meant to be a diet plan. The two weeks of meals laid out here show you how you can integrate our recipes into your busy life. You can eat our food every day, for all three meals plus two snacks, and still lose weight. You won't go hungry. You won't feel deprived. You won't get bored.

Our meal plans have between 1,400 and 1,600 calories, with balanced amounts of protein, carbohydrates, and fat, plus adequate fiber and a moderate amount of sodium to keep you satisfied and nourished. You can consult Spark People.com to determine the program that fits your specific needs, but these meals will fit comfortably into whatever plan you choose.

Unless otherwise noted, meals represent one serving of a recipe. Recipes printed in blue are accompanied by a photo.

We can reorganize these plans into meal types: breakfast, lunch, dinner, and snacks. Full nutrition info is listed below.

WEEK 1	SUNDAY	MONDAY	TUESDAY
BREAKFAST	Skinny Eggs Florentine 1 cup skim milk 1 banana 453 calories • 11 g fat 23 g protein • 6 g fiber 454 mg sodium	Muesli 1 cup skim milk 1 cup strawberries 371 calories • 14 g fat 19 g protein • 14 g fiber 133 mg sodium	Egg-White Omelet 1 cup grapes 1 Multigrain Roll 252 calories • 3 g fat 22 g protein • 4 g fiber 363 mg sodium
SNACK 1	Nutty Fruity Granola ½ cup plain, low-fat yogurt 311 calories • 11 g fat 17 g protein • 3 g fiber 172 mg sodium	1 serving whole-wheat crackers 1 ounce reduced-fat cheddar cheese 169 calories • 5 g fat 10 g protein • 3 g fiber 334 mg sodium	Nutty Fruity Granola ½ cup plain, low-fat yogurt ½ cup sliced strawberries 256 calories • 10 g fat 11 g protein • 5 g fiber 87 mg sodium
LUNCH	Three-Cheese Macaroni 3 ounces grilled chicken 1 cup grapes 413 calories • 10 g fat 33 g protein • 6 g fiber 484 mg sodium	2 slices whole-wheat bread Lemon Herb-Roasted Chicken Lettuce, tomato, and pickles 1 tbsp Honey Mustard Dressing 1 cup skim milk 1 small orange 429 calories • 12g fat 33 g protein • 7 g fiber 361 mg sodium	Slow-Cooker Salsa Chicken 1 ounce shredded reduced-fat Cheddar ½ cup brown rice ½ cup broccoli 1 cup skim milk 436 calories • 6 g fat 47 g protein • 6 g fiber 587 mg sodium
SNACK 2	Avocado Cherry-Tomato Salsa ½ cup carrot sticks ½ cup celery sticks 161 calories • 7 g fat 4 g protein • 9 g fiber 494 mg sodium	1 small apple 1 tbsp peanut butter 158 calories • 8 g fat 5 g protein • 4 g fiber 0 mg sodium	Blueberry Flaxseed Muffin 1 tbsp peanut butter 244 calories • 10 g fat 7 g protein • 4 g fiber 320 mg sodium
DINNER	Barbecue Chicken Pizza 1 cup skim milk 293 calories • 5 g fat 24 g protein • 4 g fiber 518 mg sodium	Slow-Cooker Salsa Chicken 2 cups mixed spring greens 1 whole-wheat tortilla ½ cup pineapple 353 calories • 6 g fat 33 g protein • 9 g fiber 668 mg sodium	Minestrone Soup with Parmesan Crisp 1 slice whole-wheat bread 1 cup skim milk 411 calories • 8 g fat 23 g protein • 12 g fiber 510 mg sodium
DAILY TOTALS	1,631 calories • 44 g fat 101 g protein • 28 g fiber 2,122 mg sodium	1,479 calories • 45 g fat 100 g protein • 37 g fiber 1,495 mg sodium	1,599 calories • 37 g fat 110 g protein • 32 g fiber 1,868 mg sodium

WEDNESDAY	THURSDAY	FRIDAY	SATURDAY
1 whole-wheat English muffin 1 tsp heart-healthy margarine PB&J Smoothie	Blueberry Flaxseed Muffin 1 cup skim milk ½ ounce sunflower seeds	1 cup high-fiber cereal 1 cup skim milk 1 cup raspberries	Nutty Fruity Granola Coach Nicole's Simple Blackberry Smoothie
451 calories • 12 g fat 18 g protein • 11 g fiber 511 mg sodium	287 calories • 9 g fat 14 g protein • 4 g fiber 402 mg sodium	279 calories • 2 g fat 12 g protein • 12 g fiber 381 mg sodium	385 calories • 12 g fat 18 g protein • 11 g fiber 172 mg sodium
Sweet and Spicy Pecans 2 tbsp raisins	Lemon Herb-Roasted Chicken, Honey-Mustard Dressing	Fruit Salad with Poppy Seed Dressing 1 ounce unsalted peanuts	1 piece low-fat string cheese 1 serving whole-wheat crackers
162 calories • 10 g fat 2 g protein • 2 g fiber 6 mg sodium	201 calories • 8 g fat 27 g protein • 0 g fiber 132 mg sodium	170 calories • 8 g fat 5 g protein • 6 g fiber 4 mg sodium	202 calories • 8 g fat 9 g protein • 1 g fiber 392 mg sodium
Farro-Arugula Salad with Walnut Vinaigrette 3 ounces grilled chicken 1 apple	Minestrone Soup with Parmesan Crisp 1 Multigrain Roll 1 pear	Garlic Chicken Slaw in Lettuce Cups 1 orange Baked Lemon-Spiced Rice	2 cups baby spinach 1 hard-boiled egg ½ cup carrots ½ cup red bell pepper Tomato-Basil Vinaigrette 1 slice whole-wheat bread
397 calories • 14 g fat 31 g protein • 8 g fiber 451 mg sodium	263 calories • 6 g fat 13 g protein • 12 g fiber 300 mg sodium	424 calories • 10 g fat 33 g protein • 8 g fiber 438 mg sodium	342 calories • 16 g fat 13 g protein • 7 g fiber 342 mg sodium
½ cup raisin bran cereal 1 cup soy milk	1 banana 1 tbsp peanut butter 1 cup skim milk	½ whole-wheat pita 2 tbsp salsa 1 ounce shredded, reduced-fat cheddar	½ cup skim milk Dark Chocolate Angel Food Cake with Rich Chocolate Glaze
221 calories • 8 g fat 9 g protein • 7 g fiber 300 mg sodium	289 calories • 9 g fat 14 g protein • 4 g fiber 129 mg sodium,	143 calories • 3 g fat 10 g protein • 3 g fiber 483 mg sodium	238 calories • 2 g fat 13 g protein • 2 g fiber 396 mg sodium
Slow-Cooker White Bean Chicken Chili 1 cup skim milk 1 cup broccoli 1 ounce baked tortilla chips	Three-Cheese Macaroni 3 ounces Beef Roast 1 cup grapes	Spinach and Mushroom-Stuffed Pork Tenderloin 1 cup skim milk Wheat Berry and Broccoli Salad 1 plum	Bluegrass Jambalaya
353 calories • 4 g fat 26 g protein • 13 g fiber 375 mg sodium	511 calories • 16 g fat 42 g protein • 6 g fiber 491 mg sodium	524 calories • 20 g fat 50 g protein • 7 g fiber 408 mg sodium	386 calories • 9 g fat 18 g protein • 7 g fiber 371 mg sodium
1,584 calories • 47 g fat 86 g protein • 41 g fiber 1,642 mg sodium	1,552 calories • 48 g fat 111 g protein • 26 g fiber 1,454 mg sodium	1,540 calories • 42 g fat 110 g protein • 37 g fiber 1,713 mg sodium	1,554 calories • 47 g fat 70 g protein • 28 g fiber 1,674 mg sodium

WEEK 2	SUNDAY	MONDAY	TUESDAY
BREAKFAST	1 serving low-fat Greek yogurt Warm and Spicy Banana Waffle ½ cup sliced strawberries 426 calories • 9 g fat 25 g protein • 7 g fiber 443 mg sodium	Tomato-Cheese Frittata 1 slice whole-wheat toast 1 cup skim milk 441 calories • 9 g fat 26 g protein • 7 g fiber 594 mg sodium	½ cup blueberries 1 cup skim milk Stepfanie's Oatmeal Mix 456 calories • 16 g fat 18 g protein • 11 g fiber 133 mg sodium
SNACK 1	Cucumber-Melon Cups with Mint Dressing 68 calories • 1 g fat 1 g protein • 2 g fiber 7 mg sodium	1 slice whole-wheat bread 1 tbsp low-sodium almond butter 194 calories • 9 g fat 9 g protein • 4 g fiber 288 mg sodium	1 serving shredded wheat crackers 1 hard-boiled egg 198 calories • 8 g fat 9 g protein • 3 g fiber 222 mg sodium
LUNCH	Salad Niçoise with Crispy Capers 475 calories • 14 g fat 23 g protein • 11 g fiber 173 mg sodium	Baby Spinach Salad with Strawberries and Toasted Almonds Multigrain Roll 1 string cheese 319 calories • 21 g fat 13 g protein • 6 g fiber 289 mg sodium	Black Bean and Corn Salad 1 ounce shredded pepper Jack cheese 1 whole-wheat tortilla 1 cup fresh spinach 327 calories • 14g fat 14 g protein • 8 g fiber 683 mg sodium
SNACK 2	Lunch Box Carrot Slaw with Apples 90 calories • 1 g fat 3 g protein • 4 g fiber 87 mg sodium	1 serving low-fat Greek yogurt 1 peach Spring Cupcake with Citrus Icing 268 calories • 5 g fat 18 g protein • 4 g fiber 175 mg sodium	1 cup skim milk Spring Cupcake with Citrus Icing 232 calories • 5 g fat 11 g protein • 2 g fiber 242 mg sodium
DINNER	Spinach and Mushroom-Stuffed Pork Tenderloin Wild Rice with Roasted Shallots and Garlic 1 cup skim milk 483 calories • 15 g fat 48 g protein • 4 g fiber 433 mg sodium	Maple-Glazed Roasted Salmon Quick Herbed Couscous with Vegetables 407 calories • 15 g fat 33 g protein • 5 g fiber 220 mg sodium	1 slice Italian bread Skimpy Shrimp Scampi 1 cup green beans 430 calories • 17 g fat 36 g protein • 9 g fiber 581 mg sodium
DAILY TOTALS	1,542 calories • 41 g fat 100 g protein • 28 g fiber 1,143 mg sodium	1,628 calories • 59 g fat 100 g protein • 26 g fiber 1,565 mg sodium	1,642 calories • 60 g fat 89 g protein • 33 g fiber 1,862 mg sodium

WEDNESDAY	THURSDAY	FRIDAY	SATURDAY
1 whole-wheat English muffin 1 poached egg 1 ounce reduced-fat Swiss cheese ½ tomato, sliced 1 cup skim milk ½ cup cantaloupe balls	½ grapefruit 1 cup skim milk 1 cup raisin bran cereal	1 serving low-fat Greek yogurt 1 tsp honey 1 banana Raspberry Streusel Muffin	1 cup sliced strawberries Light Spinach and Mushroom Quiche 1 cup skim milk
428 calories • 13 g fat 30 g protein • 6 g fiber 739 mg sodium	321 calories • 2 g fat 14 g protein • 14 g fiber 429 mg sodium	360 calories • 6 g fat 20 g protein • 6 g fiber 243 mg sodium	386 calories • 12 g fat 20 g protein • 5 g fiber 412 mg sodium
1 mini whole-wheat bagel 1 ounce low-fat cream cheese	1 whole-wheat pita 1 tbsp strawberry all-fruit preserves	2 slices canned pineapple 1 cup nonfat cottage cheese	1 serving low-fat Greek yogurt ½ cup blueberries
184 calorie • 8 g fat 8 g protein • 3 g fiber 293 mg sodium	195 calories • 2 g fat 6 g protein • 5 g fiber 345 mg sodium	220 calories • 1 g fat 30 g protein • 1 g fiber 790 mg sodium	151 calories • 0 g fat 16 g protein • 2 g fiber 64 mg sodium
Baked Chicken Tenders Multigrain Roll Sautéed Cumin Carrots	1 pear Mushroom-Cheese Frittata Quinoa with Pea Pods and Peppers	Chicken Kebob Pitas with Creamy Cucumber Sauce 1 cup snap peas Ranch Yogurt Sauce	1 cup broccoli with Lemon-Pepper Rub Slimmer Sloppy Joes
300 calories • 7 g fat 33 g protein • 6 g fiber 467 mg sodium	431 calories • 11 g fat 0 g protein • 9 g fiber 205 mg sodium	374 calories • 12 g fat 36 g protein • 6 g fiber 450 mg sodium	416 calories • 7 g fat 31 g protein • 13 g fiber 632 mg sodium
Stepfanie's Oatmeal Mix (made with water)	Banana Honey Cake 1 cup skim milk	SparkGuy's Best Trail Mix	1 banana 1 tbsp peanut butter
165 calories • 8 g fat 4 g protein • 4 g fiber 1 mg sodium	222 calories • 4 g fat 10 g protein • 1 g fiber 251 mg sodium	158 calories • 7 g fat 4 g protein • 4 g fiber 107 mg sodium	183 calories • 8 g fat 4 g protein • 3 g fiber 1 mg sodium
Better-for-You Beef Stroganoff Easy Steamed Vegetable Packets 1 cup skim milk	Baked Sunburst Fries Crunchy Cod Sandwich with Tartar Sauce	Grilled Shrimp with Jicama-Grapefruit Slaw 1 serving baked tortilla chips	Spinach Salad with Cherries and Pomegranate Vinaigrette Meg-herita Pizza
506 calories • 10 g fat 46 g protein • 10 g fiber 364 mg sodium	421 calories • 9 g fat 12 g protein • 10 g fiber 708 mg sodium	429 calories • 14 g fat 28 g protein • 14 g fiber 334 mg sodium	419 calories • 23 g fat 12 g protein • 6 g fiber 287 mg sodium
1,582 calories • 45 g fat 121 g protein • 29 g fiber 1,864 mg sodium	1,590 calories • 28 g fat 62 g protein • 39 g fiber 1,938 mg sodium	1,596 calories • 47 g fat 121 g protein • 27 g fiber 1,828 mg sodium	1,554 calories • 49 g fat 82 g protein • 29 g fiber 1,139 mg sodium

APPENDIX B

Healthy Pantry Checklist

One of the easiest ways to start on the path to healthy cooking and eating is to have the right ingredients at hand. Use our Healthy Pantry Checklist to get started. You don't have to buy everything at once, but refer to this checklist when making your weekly meal plans and shopping lists, as we demonstrate in Appendix D (page 413).

Fruits and Vegetables	
Fresh	
Apples	Herbs (parsley, cilantro, basil)
Bananas	Lemons and Limes
Bell Peppers	Mushrooms
Berries	Oranges
Broccoli	Potatoes
Carrots (shredded, whole, baby)	Shallots
Celery	Squash (butternut, zucchini, summer)
Cucumbers	Sweet potatoes
Garlic	Tomatoes
Ginger	Varieties of Lettuce (Baby Spinach, Romaine, Bibb, Mixed Baby Greens)
Green beans	White or Yellow Onions
Frozen	
Berries	Green beans
Broccoli	Mixed vegetables (for stir-fries and quick dinners)
Edamame (shelled)	

Fruits and Vegetables, cont'd.

Canned/Dried

Petite Diced Tomatoes (no salt added)

Raisins or other dried fruit (no sugar added)

Roasted red peppers (in water)

Sun-dried tomatoes (not packed in oil)

Tomato Paste (no salt added)

Tomato Sauce (no salt added)

Dairy

Cheddar (reduced-fat)

Feta

Goat cheese

Milk (skim)

Parmesan

Swiss (reduced-fat)

Yogurt (plain—low-fat or Greek)

Grains

Bread (whole-wheat)

Couscous (whole-wheat)

Oats (old-fashioned or steel-cut)

Pasta (whole-wheat)

Quinoa

Rice (brown)

Tortillas (whole-wheat or corn)

Protein

Fresh/Frozen

Beef (ground—at least 93% lean)

Chicken (whole or boneless, skinless breasts)

Eggs/egg whites

Pork tenderloin

Salmon fillets (preferably wild-caught)

Shrimp (raw, deveined, and shelled)

Turkey (bacon, breasts, or ground—at least 93% lean)

White-fleshed fish (tilapia, cod, etc.)

Canned/Dried

Beans (black or Northern/cannellini)

Chicken and Vegetable Stock (low-sodium)

Chickpeas

Lentils (brown or green)

Tuna (low-sodium, packed in water)

Spices, Seasonings, and Flavorings

Basil, dried

Bay leaf

Black and white peppercorns

Cayenne

Chili powder

Cinnamon

Cloves

Cumin

Curry powder

Honey

Nutmeg

Oregano

Paprika

Red pepper flakes

Rosemary

Salt (sea and kosher)

Tarragon

Thyme

Vanilla extract

Baking Needs

Baking powder	Cream of tartar
Baking soda	Flour (all-purpose or whole-wheat)
Cocoa powder (dark)	

Condiments/Dry Goods

Flaxseeds (whole or ground)	Oil (olive, canola, and peanut)
Mustard (brown or Dijon)	Vinegar (Balsamic, and red- or white-wine)
Nuts (raw almonds, pecans, or walnuts)	

APPENDIX C

Choosing a Cooking Oil

Cooking oils, and the fats they contain, are not created equal, and there are a few aspects to consider before you pull a bottle off the grocery-store shelf—primarily the fat's culinary abilities and its nutritional benefits. That said, there are plenty of oils that, when used in the right quantities, can add flavor *and* nutritional benefits to your diet.

We turned to Becky and the experts at SparkPeople, MyPyramid.gov, and the Cleveland Clinic for information on the various types of fats and how they affect your health, then took their advice to the kitchen.

THE SKINNY ON FATS

One of the quickest and healthiest ways to reduce calories and lose weight is to cut back on fat, which is what we've done in recipes throughout the cookbook. Eating a diet low in fat is an important step in keeping your heart and arteries healthy, too. Remember that all fats and oils are not created equal; however, all fats and oils are still high in calories. Keep in mind:

- Mono-unsaturated fats help to lower the LDL (lazy/bad cholesterol) while NOT lowering the HDL (healthy/good cholesterol). These fats are the most heart friendly.

- Polyunsaturated fats help lower the LDL (lazy/bad cholesterol) but they also lower the HDL (healthy/good cholesterol). So they are somewhat heart healthy.

- Saturated fats raise the LDL (lazy/bad cholesterol) and increase the risk of heart disease. Therefore, they are not heart healthy.

- Trans fatty acids can raise the LDL (lazy/bad cholesterol) and triglycerides levels, and lower the HDL (healthy/good cholesterol). They are not heart healthy.

- Research indicates that omega-3 fatty acids, a type of polyunsaturated fat, reduce inflammation, helping to prevent inflammatory diseases like heart disease and arthritis. In addition to warding off inflammation, omega-3s are also essential to the brain, impacting behavior and cognitive function, and are especially necessary during fetal development.

IT'S NOT JUST THE OIL, IT'S THE PROCESS

The way an oil is processed, stored, and used impacts its healthfulness, too. There are a variety of ways of obtaining oil. For the healthiest products, look for oils that have been extracted physically rather than chemically. They should be labeled "expeller-pressed," or "cold-pressed," as the heat used to chemically process oils can degrade them.

Besides heat, light and air are the other enemies of oil stability and freshness, so keep these tips in mind:

- Buy oil packaged in dark glass, as opposed to clear glass or plastic.

- Buy small bottles.

- Keep the lid tightly closed between uses.

- Store oil in a cool, dark place. See the accompanying chart for specific storage guidelines.

CAN YOUR OIL TAKE THE HEAT?

After carefully selecting your oil, the last thing you'll want to do is to expose it to high heat in your own kitchen. Since high heat can damage oils, stick to the following guidelines when cooking:

- Know the smoke point of the oil you're working with (see the charts below). The smoke point is the temperature to which an oil can be heated before it starts to smoke. Never heat oil to the smoking point, as this will certainly damage its fatty-acid content (and give your food a burnt flavor).

- Lessen the length of time the oil will be in contact with heat by adding the oil just before adding the food. (Remember: heat the pan, heat the oil, then heat the food.)

Keep in mind that fat is the most concentrated form of energy and contains 9 calories per gram, or about 120 calories per tablespoon—whether it's lard, olive oil, or sesame oil. In other words, a little goes a long way. To keep portions in check, use a measuring spoon, a bottle with a pour spout, or a pump bottle, which allows more flow control.

Cooking Oils Comparison

Oil	Smoke point	Primary type of fat	Notes on cooking
Canola	Medium-high	Mono-unsaturated	An almost flavorless cooking oil (which makes it good for baking) that is low in artery-clogging saturated fats and rich in mono-unsaturated fats with small levels of omega-3. Store in a dark pantry. Canola oil is the best choice nutritionally.
Corn	Medium	Polyunsaturated	Although this oil is only slightly higher in saturated fats than healthy oils, corn oil is often hydrogenated. Use it sparingly as a cooking oil. Store in the refrigerator.
Flavored	Do not heat	Varies, depending on the base oil used	Use for garnish or flavoring, not for cooking. Store in the refrigerator.
Grapeseed	Medium-high	Polyunsaturated	Light green and slightly sweet, it's lovely for salads. Store in the refrigerator.
Nuts or seeds	Do not heat (see exception with peanut oil)	Mono-unsaturated if sourced from almonds, cashews, hazelnuts, macadamia, pecans, peanuts, pistachios; polyunsaturated if sourced from flax, hemp, pumpkin, or sunflower seeds, or walnuts	Hemp and flaxseed oils are great in smoothies; nut oils are flavorful and good for salads. Store in the refrigerator.

Cooking Oils Comparison, cont'd.

Oil	Smoke point	Primary type of fat	Notes on cooking
Olive (extra-virgin)	Medium-high	Mono-unsaturated	My favorite oil for its fruity flavor, heart-healthy nutrition profile, and greenish color. It's great in dishes where you want a stronger flavor, such as salads or pasta, and is good for sautéing. Store in a dark pantry.
Peanut	Medium-high	Mono-unsaturated	A flavorful oil that is best used in dishes that can stand up to its strong flavor. Store in a dark pantry.
Sesame	Do not heat	Mono-unsaturated	Use it as a seasoning. Only use a drizzle, or dilute it with a more neutral oil; otherwise, it will overpower your dish! Store in the refrigerator.
Soybean	Medium	Polyunsaturated	Another neutral cooking oil, but it is often highly refined and hydrogenated, so there are better choices out there. Store in a dark pantry.
Sunflower and Safflower	High	Polyunsaturated	Inexpensive and mild in taste, excellent all-purpose oils with long shelf lives. Store in the refrigerator.

- *Oils to avoid:* Cottonseed, Coconut, Palm

- *High Smoke Point Oils:* use for high-heat cooking techniques like searing and browning.

- *Medium-High Smoke Point Oils:* use for cooking techniques using moderate to high heat, like roasting and stir-frying.

- *Medium Smoke Point Oils:* use for cooking techniques using medium to low heat, like sautéing and low-temperature roasting

- *No Heat Oils:* used in dressing, dips, seasonings, or marinades. Homemade versions only last a few days due to the low acid content and will turn rancid quickly.

APPENDIX D

Create a Healthy Grocery List
in 4 Easy Steps

Without a shopping list, a casual trip to the grocery store can be a recipe for disaster. Sometimes, even with a list in hand, we still find ourselves in a state of confusion as we meander through the store. Organizing your shopping list can smooth out your grocery-shopping experience and make shopping and cooking more efficient.

Whether you're shopping for one meal or seven, yourself or a house full of people, the process is the same. SparkPeople.com experts have put together the following steps to help you plan healthful meals, create an organized list, and save time and money.

4 STEPS TO A HEALTHY AND ORGANIZED SHOPPING LIST

Step 1: Keep a pad of paper and pen posted in your kitchen at all times.

A small chalkboard or dry-wipe board will also work. When you run out of something in the kitchen, jot it down. This will prevent you from starting a recipe only to discover that you're out of garlic or nutmeg, and it will save you the hassle of searching through the cupboards to try to find out what's missing. Don't worry about making a neat, organized list—just get the missing items recorded. Make this a habit for everyone in your house; even kids can help. Don't throw a package into the recycling bin or garbage until you've written the item on your running list. You can also refer to Appendix B, our Healthy Pantry Checklist, as a guide.

Step 2: Plan your meals.

We all plan our meals differently, depending on how many people we're feeding and how often we go to the store or farmers' market. However, this step should always precede shopping. Set aside some time at least once a week to plan your meals for the days ahead. Here are some basic things to keep in mind:

Your schedule: Look at your calendar for the week or days ahead. Do you have a busy week coming up? How much time do you have to cook on each night of the week (it may vary day to day, especially if you manage a larger household or have children). Sit down with your calendar and plan meals based on how much time you have available. Choose a variety of quick recipes, dishes that yield leftovers, and meals that require more time so that cooking always fits into your schedule. Don't forget about slow-cooker meals for nights when cooking isn't an option.

Tip: "Our family always plans an additional quick meal for the week," explains Tanya Jolliffe, a healthy-eating expert for SparkPeople.com. "Something is always bound to come up and put a wrench in your meal plan for the week, so think about one extra quick-fix meal you can prepare and add that to your shopping every week." That way, you don't have to resort to fast food or pay a premium for a restaurant meal just because you're short on time.

Company: Do you have people coming to visit soon? You may need to buy special items at the store or plan for a larger dinner. Also, be sure to consider any special food preferences or allergies.

Coupons, sales, and deals: Some people prefer to look at coupons and sale flyers during the meal-planning stage so they can create meals around lower-cost ingredients. Others prefer to plan their meals and then look for coupons or deals on the items they need to make those meals. Decide which method works best for you. Just make sure whatever you buy can be worked into your meal plan and that you're not just buying something because it's on sale—if you buy it and don't use it, you haven't saved any money. Keep in mind that many coupon deals are for highly processed, often unhealthy foods that you probably shouldn't be buying anyway, so keep both health and cost in mind.

The season: What you cook and eat should change according to what's in season and what you like, but remember that fruits and vegetables in season are going to be cheaper and more readily available. Save money by planning your meals around produce at its peak taste and lowest price!

Step 3: Gather your recipes.

Now that you've planned your meals based on time, taste, season, and coupons, assemble your recipes. We've made this easy for you by collecting our best recipes in this one volume—and we hope that many of them will become a regular part of your meal plan. For the rest of those recipes that have been passed on from friends and family, or cut from the pages of newspapers and magazines, try using a basic template for all recipes (or enter them on SparkRecipes.com). When you come across a great recipe, grab a blank template from your stash, jot it down in your own writing and place it in a binder organized by time, season, cuisine, or another parameter. To streamline your planning process, include a mini grocery list on the recipe template so you can quickly see what ingredients you need to make the dish. You can also highlight specialty ingredients (such as certain herbs or special cheeses) that you don't typically keep on hand.

Step 4: Create your master grocery list.

Next, sit down with your running list of staples (from Step 1), your weekly meal plan, and your recipes to create one organized list that will help you navigate the store. You can avoid walking back and forth across the store by separating your list into grocery store departments: produce items, bulk foods, bakery, deli/meat/poultry, frozen foods, dry goods, dairy, beverages, home goods, and miscellaneous. Set up your list based on your preferences and the layout of your supermarket. Don't forget to attach your coupons to the list before you head to the store!

As you did for your recipes, creating one master shopping list template will save you time and keep your list organized. Include a section where you can list the meals you planned for the week and then the groceries you need, organized by department. SparkPeople's Weekly Grocery Shopping List template (page 416) makes it easy (you'll find it available for download on SparkPeople.com, too).

When you arrive at the store, stick to your list and don't get distracted by the various supermarket promotions. Once you're home from the store, put your groceries away systematically to streamline cooking in the days ahead. Keep your pantry and refrigerator organized, storing similar items together. When every item has its place, cooking will become more efficient.

No more excuses about not being able to create healthy meals! Staying organized, saving money, and finding the time to cook healthful meals each night boils down to meal planning and a good shopping list. The time you spend in this planning phase will more than pay off when it's time to cook, so make it a habit to start each week with a plan.

SPARKPEOPLE'S WEEKLY SHOPPING LIST

Start by planning your meals each day, taking into account how much time you have available to cook.

This Week's Meals			
Sunday	Monday	Tuesday	Wednesday
Thursday	Friday	Saturday	

Grab your recipes, coupons, and running grocery list and combine it all onto this master list.

Shopping List	
Bread/Bakery	Bulk Foods
Dairy/Refrigerated	Deli, Meat, Poultry
Dry/Canned Goods	Fresh Produce
Frozen Foods	Herbs/Spices/Baking
Household/Misc.	

APPENDIX E

How to Keep Fruits and Veggies Fresh

Eating more fruits and vegetables is a requirement for every healthy eater. But when you buy fresh produce, do you end up throwing away more than you eat? You're not alone. According to the U.S. Environmental Protection Agency, Americans throw away nearly 31.6 million tons of food every year. And a recent University of Arizona study found that the average family tosses 1.28 pounds of food a day, for a total of 470 pounds a year! That's like throwing away $600!

Storing fresh produce is a little more complicated than you might think. If you want to prevent spoilage, certain foods shouldn't be stored together at all, while others that we commonly keep in the fridge should actually be left on the countertop. To keep your produce optimally fresh (and cut down on food waste), use this handy guide developed by Stepfanie.

COUNTERTOP STORAGE TIPS

There's nothing as inviting as a big bowl of crisp apples on the kitchen counter. To keep those apples crisp and all countertop-stored produce fresh, keep them out of direct sunlight, either directly on the countertop, in an uncovered bowl, or inside a perforated plastic bag.

REFRIGERATOR STORAGE TIPS

For produce that is best stored in the refrigerator, remember the following guidelines:

- Keep produce in perforated plastic bags in the produce drawer of the refrigerator. (To perforate bags, punch holes in the bag with a sharp object, spacing them about as far apart as the holes you see in supermarket apple bags.) Or consider the reusable cotton produce bags that are becoming more available; bring them to the market with you to cut down on plastics.

- Keep fruits and vegetables separate, in different drawers, because ethylene can build up in the fridge, causing spoilage.

- When storing herbs (and interestingly, asparagus, too), snip off the ends, store upright in a glass of water (like flowers in a vase), and cover with a plastic bag.

Food is expensive, and most people can't afford to waste it. Keep this handy chart in your kitchen so you can refer to it after every shopping trip (you can download a copy from SparkPeople.com). Then you'll be able to follow through with your good intentions to eat your five to nine servings a day, instead of letting all of that healthy food go to waste.

WHAT TO STORE WHERE

Use this color-coded key along with the chart below:

- Store unwashed and in a single layer

- Store unwashed and in a plastic bag

- Store in a paper bag

- Ethylene producers (keep away from other fruits and vegetables, see Note)

Store in Refrigerator	
Apples (storage >7 days)	Green onions
Apricots	Herbs (except basil)
Artichokes	Honeydew
Asparagus	Leafy vegetables
Beets	Leeks
Blackberries	Lettuce
Blueberries	Lima beans
Broccoli	Mushrooms
Brussels sprouts	Okra
Cabbage	Peas

Store in Refrigerator, cont'd.	
Cantaloupe	Peppers
Carrots	Plums
Cauliflower	Radishes
Celery	Raspberries
Cherries	Spinach
Corn	Sprouts
Cucumbers	Strawberries
Figs	Summer squash
Grapes	Yellow squash
Green beans	Zucchini

Store on Countertop	
Apples (storage < 7 days)	Mangoes
Bananas	Oranges
Basil	Papayas
Eggplant	Persimmons
Garlic	Pineapple
Ginger	Plantains
Grapefruit	Pomegranates
Jicama	Tomatoes
Lemons	Watermelon
Limes	

Ripen on Counter, Then Refrigerate	
Avocados	Peaches
Kiwi	Pears
Nectarines	Plums

Store in a Cool, Dry Place	
Acorn squash	Pumpkins
Butternut squash	Spaghetti squash
Onions (away from potatoes)	Sweet potatoes
Potatoes (away from onions)	Winter squash

Note: All fruits and vegetables emit an odorless, harmless, and tasteless gas called ethylene after they're picked, but some foods produce it in greater quantities. When ethylene-producing foods are kept in close proximity with ethylene-sensitive foods, especially in a confined space (like a bag or drawer), the gas will speed up the ripening process of the other produce. Use this to your advantage if you want to speed up the ripening process of an unripe fruit, for example, by putting an apple in a bag with an unripe avocado. But if you want your already-ripe foods to last longer, remember to keep them away from ethylene-producing foods, as designated in the chart above.

THE SHELF LIFE OF FRUITS AND VEGETABLES

In addition to storing your fruits and veggies properly, it's good to know approximately how long the fresh stuff will last. Plan your trip to the grocery or farmers' market accordingly so that your foods are at the peak of freshness when you plan to prepare them, and you're not throwing away food that's gone bad before you get a chance to use it.

Once you've brought it home and stored it properly, you can prioritize your produce. First, eat the things that will spoil quickly, such as lettuce and berries. Save the longer-lasting foods (like eggplant and oranges) for later in the week.

1–2 Days	2–4 Days
Artichokes	Arugula
Asparagus	Avocados
Bananas	Cucumbers
Basil	Eggplant
Broccoli	Grapes
Cherries	Lettuce
Corn	Limes
Dill	Pineapple
Green beans	Zucchini
Mushrooms	
Strawberries	
Watercress	

4–6 Days	7+ Days
Apricots	Apples
Blueberries	Beets
Brussels sprouts	Cabbage
Cauliflower	Carrots
Grapefruit	Celery
Leeks	Garlic
Lemons	Hard Squash
Oranges	Onions
Oregano	Potatoes
Parsley	
Peaches	
Pears	
Peppers	
Plums	
Spinach	
Tomatoes	
Watermelon	

APPENDIX F

25 Good, Cheap Foods

We hope we've dispelled the myth that eating healthy is expensive! The cost benefits of cooking at home far outweigh the money you'll save by cutting processed and takeout foods from your family's diet. We surveyed a major East Coast metropolitan grocery chain to determine these prices. Costs will vary according to where you live, but this list represents foods that traditionally offer great health value while being kind to your wallet.

PROTEIN

1. *Canned salmon:* $2.89 for 14.75 ounces (59 cents per serving)—Get your omega-3s for less. Salmon is full of these healthy fats, which help lower cholesterol and prevent heart attacks. Swap canned salmon for tuna in Salad Niçoise with Crispy Capers (page 115).

2. *Chicken breasts:* $3.49 per pound (87 cents per serving)—Easy-to-prepare and versatile, chicken is full of lean protein, which helps keep you fuller longer.

3. *Natural peanut butter:* $3.39 for 16 ounces (42 cents per serving)—Skip the sugary, processed varieties and spread the real stuff on whole-grain bread. Throw a tablespoon in smoothies or yogurt, use it as a dip for carrots and pretzels, or mix it with a bit of low-sodium soy sauce, brown sugar and garlic, then thin with water for a quick sauce. We use it in our vegetarian Pad Thai (page 246).

4. *Canned beans:* 84 cents for 15 ounces (22 cents per serving)—Bulk up soups and stews while getting protein and fiber. Try chickpeas or black beans if you're not a fan of kidneys or pintos. Drain,

rinse, and puree with lemon juice, garlic, cumin, and a bit of vegetable broth for a quick dip. Try our Black Bean and Corn Salad (page 121).

5. *Eggs:* $1.99 for a dozen large (17 cents per serving)—Not just for breakfast, eggs are among the easiest foods to cook. If you're watching your cholesterol, scramble one egg and two egg whites. Add onion and spinach and you've got a great omelet. Our Tomato-Cheese Frittata (page 92) is great for any meal of the day.

6. *Dried lentils:* 79 cents per pound (20 cents per serving)—Full of protein and fiber, lentils cook in just 15 minutes! Throw some in soups and stews or cook with curry powder for a quick, spicy meal. We mean it when we call it Lifesaving Lentil Soup (page 157).

7. *Almonds:* $3.99 for 9 ounces (44 cents per serving)—Get vitamin E, fiber, and protein while satisfying a crunchy craving. Nuts are rich in an amino acid that could be linked to heart benefits. Chop up a few raw ones and throw them on yogurt, or add them to a salad, like Baby Spinach Salad with Strawberries and Toasted Almonds (page 111).

FRUITS

8. *Frozen fruit and berries:* $2.99 to $5.99 per pound (75 cents to $1.50 per serving)—Since fruit is frozen at the peak of freshness, frozen fruit is a great way to get the health benefits of summer's bounty all year round. Berries are very low in calories, but full of vitamins and antioxidants. Frozen berries can be used in oatmeal or drained and baked into muffins and quick breads. Throw some in the blender with milk or yogurt for a healthy treat. See Superior Smoothies (pages 81) for some great ideas.

9. *Apples:* 68 cents each—They might not keep the doctor away, but apples are actually full of antioxidants, which help slow the progression of age-related diseases. Lunch Box Carrot Slaw with Apples (page 112) is a kid-pleasing way to get that apple a day.

10. *Bananas:* 35 cents each—Slice one on your morning yogurt or oatmeal for some added fiber and only 100 calories or so. Snack on a potassium-rich banana to prevent cramps after a workout. Warm and Spicy Banana Waffles (page 98) make a perfect Sunday breakfast dish.

11. *Grapes:* $2.99 per pound (75 cents per serving)—Freeze grapes for a low-calorie dessert or snack.

Grapes—especially the dark purple ones—contain plenty of antioxidants that are known to help heart health. We add them to our Crunchy Chicken Salad (page 217).

VEGETABLES

12. *Romaine or other hearty lettuce:* $1.99 per head (66 cents per serving)—Banish the iceberg and choose sturdy Romaine for your salads. It will give you more fiber and nutrients, plus a satisfying crunch. Try it for Garlic Chicken Slaw in Lettuce Cups (page 129).

13. *Carrots:* $2.79 for 3 pounds (23 cents per serving)—Mom was right. Carrots are good for your eyes, thanks to the antioxidants they contain, including beta-carotene. (That's what makes them orange!) Dip them in hummus (made from canned beans), natural peanut butter, or low-fat dressings—or make our Chilled Curry-Carrot Soup with Citrus Yogurt (page 153).

14. *Frozen spinach:* $2 for 16 ounces (50 cents per serving)—Thaw and drain this good-for-you green, then toss it in omelets, soups, stir-fries, and pasta sauces. Spinach is full of vitamins A, C, and K; plus fiber and even calcium. It's delicious in our Spinach Stuffed Chicken with Cheese Sauce (page 196).

15. *Canned tomatoes:* $1 for 14.5 ounces (28 cents per serving)—Choose low-sodium or no-salt-added varieties and throw a can in pasta sauces or chili to stretch a meal. Puree a can with a cup of skim milk and season to taste for your own tomato soup. You'll get a dose of vitamins A, B, and C and lycopene, an antioxidant known to prevent cancer. Our Weeknight Spaghetti (page 256) is sure to become a family favorite.

16. *Garlic:* 50 cents per head (5 cents per serving)—Ditch the bottled and powdered stuff if you want to reap more of the myriad health benefits. Pungent and tasty, garlic can help lower cholesterol and prevent blood clots, plus it can have a small effect on high blood pressure. Crush or chop it to release more of the antioxidants. Spicy Garlic Oil (page 384) adds a kick of flavor to any dish.

17. *Sweet potatoes:* $1.49 per pound (37 cents per serving)—Aside from being sweet and delicious, these bright root vegetables are a great source of fiber and antioxidants. Bake, mash, or roast them—you'll forget about those other, paler potatoes. Baked Sunburst Fries (page 319) will change your idea of French fries forever!

18. *Onions:* 97 cents each (32 cents per serving)—Like garlic, this

pungent vegetable is full of health benefits. Onions have been proven to lower risks for certain cancers, and they add lots of flavor with few calories. Try roasting them to bring out their sweetness and cut their harsh edge. (If you well up while cutting them, store onions in the fridge for a tear-free chop.) French Onion Soup with Whole-Wheat Croutons (page 162) is our healthy take on the classic comfort fare.

19. *Broccoli:* $2.49 per pound (63 cents per serving)—Broccoli is a superstar in the nutrition world: full of fiber, it will provide you with vitamins A and C, and a host of antioxidants. Wheat Berry and Broccoli Salad (page 298) makes for a filling lunch or side dish.

WHOLE GRAINS

20. *Whole-grain pasta:* $1.50 for 13.25 ounces (45 cents per serving)—With a nutty flavor and a subtle brown color, whole-wheat pasta perks up any meal. Start with half regular, half whole-wheat pasta, then gradually add more wheat pasta for a burst of fiber and nutrients. Ratatouille with Whole-Wheat Pasta (page 258) is a great make-ahead meal.

21. *Popcorn kernels:* $2.39 for 32 ounces (30 cents per serving)—Air-popped popcorn has just 30 calories and a trace of fat. Pop a few cups, spritz with olive oil or butter spray, and sprinkle on your favorite seasonings for a guilt-free treat. For an extra-sweet treat, try Caramel Popcorn (page 337).

22. *Brown rice:* $1.49 for 16 ounces (19 cents per serving)—Brown rice is a great side dish, but you can also use it to help stretch your ground meat. Mix a cup of cooked rice with 8 ounces of lean ground beef next time you make meatloaf to save 45 calories and 5 grams of fat (and some money) per serving. Our Spanish Rice (page 287) is a flavorful way to get your whole-grain goodness.

23. *Oats:* $3.19 for 42 ounces (15 cents per serving)—Oatmeal is a hearty breakfast, but you can also cook sturdy steel-cut oats in chicken broth for a savory side dish. Or, mix oats with ground turkey to stretch your meatballs. Stepfanie's Oatmeal Mix (page 79) adds dried fruit and nuts for extra flavor.

DAIRY

24. *Quarts of low- or fat-free yogurt:* $2.49 for 32 ounces (47 cents per serving)—Buy large containers of plain or vanilla yogurt, then add real fruit. You'll save money and calories by not buying fancy, single-serve cups. Spicy Yogurt Sauce (page 380) is a tasty alternative to high-fat condiments.

25. *Gallon of skim milk:* $3.04 (19 cents per serving)—It really does a body good. Full of calcium and protein, milk can help stretch a meal. Pair an 8-ounce cup with a piece of fruit or a granola bar for a filling snack.

APPENDIX G

Metric Equivalent Charts

The recipes in this book use the standard United States method for measuring liquid and dry or solid ingredients (teaspoons, tablespoons, and cups). The information on this chart is provided to help cooks outside the U.S. successfully use these recipes. All equivalents are approximate.

METRIC EQUIVALENTS FOR DIFFERENT TYPES OF INGREDIENTS

A standard cup measure of a dry or solid ingredient will vary in weight depending on the type of ingredient. A standard cup of liquid is the same volume for any type of liquid. Use the following chart when converting standard cup measures to grams (weight) or milliliters (volume).

Standard Cup	Fine Powder (e.g., flour)	Grain (e.g., rice)	Granular (e.g., sugar)	Liquid Solids (e.g., butter)	Liquid (e.g., milk)
1	140 g	150 g	190 g	200 g	240 ml
¾	105 g	113 g	143 g	150 g	180 ml
⅔	93 g	100 g	125 g	133 g	160 ml
½	70 g	75 g	95 g	100 g	120 ml
⅓	47 g	50 g	63 g	67 g	80 ml
¼	35 g	38 g	48 g	50 g	60 ml
⅛	18 g	19 g	24 g	25 g	30 ml

Useful Equivalents for Liquid Ingredients by Volume

¼ tsp				1 ml	
½ tsp				2 ml	
1 tsp				5 ml	
3 tsp	1 tbsp		½ fl oz	15 ml	
	2 tbsp	⅛ cup	1 fl oz	30 ml	
	4 tbsp	¼ cup	2 fl oz	60 ml	
	5⅓ tbsp	⅓ cup	3 fl oz	80 ml	
	8 tbsp	½ cup	4 fl oz	120 ml	
	10⅔ tbsp	⅔ cup	5 fl oz	160 ml	
	12 tbsp	¾ cup	6 fl oz	180 ml	
	16 tbsp	1 cup	8 fl oz	240 ml	
	1 pt	2 cups	16 fl oz	480 ml	
	1 qt	4 cups	32 fl oz	960 ml	
			33 fl oz	1000 ml	1 l

Useful Equivalents for Dry Ingredients by Weight

(To convert ounces to grams, multiply the number of ounces by 30.)

1 oz	¹⁄₁₆ lb	30 g
4 oz	¼ lb	120 g
8 oz	½ lb	240 g
12 oz	¾ lb	360 g
16 oz	1 lb	480 g

Useful Equivalents for Cooking/Oven Temperatures

Process	Fahrenheit	Celsius	Gas Mark
Freeze Water	32° F	0° C	
Room Temperature	68° F	20° C	
Boil Water	212° F	100° C	
Bake	325° F	160° C	3
	350° F	180° C	4
	375° F	190° C	5
	400° F	200° C	6
	425° F	220° C	7
	450° F	230° C	8
Broil			Grill

Useful Equivalents for Length

(To convert inches to centimeters, multiply the number of inches by 2.5.)

1 in			2.5 cm	
6 in	½ ft		15 cm	
12 in	1 ft		30 cm	
36 in	3 ft	1 yd	90 cm	
40 in			100 cm	1 m

APPENDIX H

Nutritional Guidelines Chart

Choose Often (daily)	Limit (no more than 3–4 times/week)	Avoid (special occasions only)
Meat and Protein 2–4 servings/day		
Lean cuts of beef and pork (fat trimmed off), poultry (chicken and turkey) without skin, dried beans and peas, lentils, tofu, egg whites, egg substitutes, fish and shellfish, tuna canned with water	Egg yolks, fish sticks, tuna canned in oil, poultry with skin, chicken nuggets, turkey hot dogs, turkey bologna, nuts, peanut butter	Prime-grade meats, duck, goose, dark poultry meat, bacon, sausage, bologna, salami, hot dogs, ribs, organ meats, fried meats
Dairy and Calcium-rich Foods 2–3 servings/day		
Skim milk, 1% milk, 1% buttermilk, nonfat yogurt, nonfat frozen yogurt, fat-free cheese, low-fat cottage cheese, soy milk, soy cheese, other dairy-free milk substitutes	2% milk, 4% cottage cheese, ice milk, light cream cheese, light sour cream, low-fat yogurt, sherbet, low-fat cheese	Whole milk, regular cheese, cream, half-and-half, most nondairy creamers, real and nondairy whipped cream, cream cheese, sour cream, ice cream, custard-style yogurt
Fruits and Vegetables 5–9 servings/day		
Fresh, frozen, canned, or dried fruits and vegetables of all kinds	Olives, avocados, coconut	Fruits and vegetables prepared in butter or cream sauce, fried fruits and vegetables, vegetables with high-fat salad dressing
Grains 6–11 servings/day		
100% whole-grain breads, bagels, pasta, and cereals; oats; brown rice; bulgur; baked corn tortillas; low-fat crackers; air-popped popcorn; sprouted-grain bread; quinoa	White-flour breads; bagels; pasta; and cereals; angel-food cake; crackers; fat-free cakes and cookies; biscuits; fig bars; oatmeal-raisin cookies; pancakes; waffles; packaged mixes; white rice; granola	Croissants; pastry; pies; doughnuts; sweet rolls; snack crackers (with trans fats); grain products prepared with cream, butter, or cheese sauce

Choose Often (daily)	Limit (no more than 3–4 times/week)	Avoid (special occasions only)
Fats and Oils 1–3 servings/day		
Olive oil, canola oil, peanut oil	Safflower, corn, soybean, sesame, sunflower oils, margarine, mayonnaise, lower-fat salad dressings, margarine that does not contain hydrogenated oil	Butter; lard; beef tallow; bacon fat; shortening; palm, palm kernel, and coconut oils; margarine or shortening made with hydrogenated oil

ENDNOTES

Chapter 2: The Science of Satisfaction

1. David A. Kessler, M.D., *The End of Overeating: Taking Control of the Insatiable American Appetite* (New York: Rodale, 2009).

2. Survey of Income and Program Participation, 2004 Panel, Wave 8.

3. *The National Center on Addiction and Substance Abuse at Columbia University: The Importance of Family Dinners VI* (September 2010). http://www.casacolumbia.org/templates/Publications_Reports.aspx.

4. Sarah E. Anderson, Ph.D. and Robert C. Whitaker, M.D., M.P.H., "Household Routines and Obesity in US Preschool-Aged Children," *Pediatrics* 125, No. 3 (March 2010): 420–428. http://pediatrics.aappublications.org/cgi/content/abstract/125/3/420.

5. *F as in Fat: How Obesity Policies are Failing in America.* July 2009 report: Trust for America's Health, Robert Wood Johnson Foundation. http://healthyamericans.org/reports/obesity2009/Obesity2009Report.pdf.

6. Julia A. Ello-Martin, et al., "Dietary Energy Density in the Treatment of Obesity: A Year-long Trial Comparing 2 Weight-loss Diets," *American Journal of Clinical Nutrition* 85, No. 6 (June 2007): 1465–1477.

Chapter 9: Whole Grains

1. Nadine R. Sahyoun, et al., "Whole-Grain Intake is Inversely Associated with the Metabolic Syndrome and Mortality in Older Adults" *The American Journal of Clinical Nutrition* 83, No. 1 (January 2006): 124–131.

2. Majken K Jensen, et. al, "Whole Grains, Bran, and Germ in Relation to Homocysteine and Markers of Glycemic Control, Lipids, and Inflammation," *American Journal of Clinical Nutrition* 83, No. 2 (February 2006): 275–283.

Chapter 11: Snacks & Desserts

1. *F as in Fat: How Obesity Policies are Failing in America.* July 2009 report: Trust for America's Health, Robert Wood Johnson Foundation. http://healthyamericans.org/reports/obesity2009/Obesity2009Report.pdf.

Afterword: Raising Kids to Be Healthy Eaters

1. *Divisions of Responsibility.* Copyright © 2010 by Ellyn Satter. Published at www.EllynSatter.com.

RECIPE CATEGORY INDEX

MULTIPLE SERVINGS OF FRUITS AND VEGETABLES

Baby Spinach Salad with Strawberries and Toasted Almonds (3), 111

Baked Sunburst Fries (2), 319

Better-for-You Beef Stroganoff (2), 214

Black Bean and Corn Salad (2), 121

Bluegrass Jambalaya (2), 169

Braised Mexican Beef with Crispy Corn Tortillas (2), 219

Braised Spinach with Pine Nuts (2), 329

Braised Swiss Chard with Beans (2), 324

Broccoli and Spaghetti Squash with Lemon Pepper (4), 243

Chicken Creole (2), 170

Chilled Curry-Carrot Soup with Citrus Yogurt (3½), 153

Chocolate-Covered Cherry Smoothie (3), 82

Coach Nicole's Simple Blackberry Smoothie (2), 83

Creamy Broccoli-Cheese Soup (2), 161

Cucumber-Melon Cups with Mint Dressing (2), 123

Easy Steamed Vegetable Packets (3), 323

Egg-White Omelet with Spinach and Mushrooms (2), 89

Farro-Arugula Salad with Walnut Vinaigrette (2), 297

Fruit Salad with Poppy Seed Dressing (2), 346

Grapefruit-Pear Salad with Fennel (3), 124

Green Bean Casserole (2), 327

Grilled Vegetable Pizza (2), 275

Grilled Veggie Sandwiches with Fresh Mozzarella (2), 145

Herbed Mushrooms with Bacon (1½), 321

Light and Creamy Crab Chowder (2), 166

Minestrone Soup with Parmesan Crisps (2½), 154

Miso Vegetable Soup (1½), 165

Pad Thai (1½), 246

Parmesan Chicken with Tomato-Basil Salad (2), 186

PB&J Smoothie (2), 83

Potato Salad with Veggies and Bacon (2), 322

Pumpkin-Pie Smoothie (2), 82

Quick Herbed Couscous with Vegetables (2), 293

Quinoa with Pea Pods and Peppers (2), 296

Ratatouille with Whole-Wheat Pasta (2½), 258

Roasted Beet and Apple Salad (2), 116

Salad Niçoise with Crispy Capers (2½), 115

HIGH FIBER

30 MINUTES OR LESS

MEMBER MAKEOVERS

GREAT FOR COMPANY

VEGETARIAN

INDEX

PHOTO CREDITS

ACKNOWLEDGMENTS

The authors would like to thank:

SparkPeople founder, CEO, and resident motivation expert Chris Downie, for his unbridled enthusiasm and devotion to SparkPeople and its mission to make healthy living a reality for everyone. Without his passion and commitment to SparkPeople, none of this would be possible. Chris has helped us all learn how a small team of people can "spark" a grassroots movement that's changed tens of millions of lives along the way. This cookbook fully reflects the philosophy he has created in the last decade. And, Karina Downie, who gave us valuable input early on and inspires us with her passion for and commitment to "real food."

Our President, Tami Corwin, for getting this book idea kicked off and for her expert guidance and keen eye over the entire project. Her legendary insight transformed this manuscript into the healthy cooking "bible" you're reading today.

SparkPeople Head Dietitian Becky Hand for reading every chapter multiple times and for her entertaining and educational spin on nutrition. Her effervescent personality and positive attitude are contagious.

SparkPeople healthy-eating expert Tanya Jolliffe, for reviewing nutritional content and guidance with meal plans.

Editor Marisa Bulzone, for her attention to detail and help throughout the project. Her tremendous experience was much appreciated.

Other SparkPeople team members past and present who directly worked on the cookbook: Kelly Berger, Beth Cavanaugh, Nicole Nichols, and Jenny Uhlmansiek.

The rest of the SparkPeople team, without whom none of this would be possible: Dominic Acito, Anne Allen, Kevin Carroll, Bruce Corwin, Catherine Cram, Samantha Donohue, Paul Elfers, Andy Cougs Firsich, Brian Franklin, Elliott Giles, Angie Heilmann, Dave Heilmann, Nancy Howard, Tom

Kennedy, Josh Knepfle, Jeremy Martin, Sean McCosh, Tim Metzner, Jen Mueller, Natalie Nichols, Jeff Rezer, Denise Tausig, and Rachel Von Nida.

Every SparkPeople member working hard to reach goals and spread the spark around the world.

A special thanks to our editor, Patty Gift, for her flexibility and guidance throughout the process.

Our gifted team at Hay House, led by Louise Hay and Reid Tracy. Others on the Hay House Team include Margarete Nielsen, Laura Koch, Sally Mason, Tricia Breidenthal, and Christy Salinas.

Stephanie Tade, our agent, for continuing to believe in us. From the proposal through the final recipe testing and beyond, she rolled up her sleeves and helped us in every way imaginable.

Photographer Randy Hoover, who took all the beautiful, mouthwatering food photos throughout the book, along with his incredible team: studio manager Sarah Diebold; food stylist Lynne Morris and her team, Gail Gattas and Jessica Baesel; hair and makeup artist Diane Amon; and assistant Allison McAdams. We spent plenty of long days putting together the photos for the book, and what fun it was! Set stylist Nora Martini assisted with the shots at Meg's house.

Photojournalist David Stephenson, who spent a day on the Barton family farm shooting Meg and her family. He captured amazing images of her in "real life." That same day, Chris Higginbotham and Tim Cantrell, our awesome video team, patiently worked around photo shoots to tape videos for the web.

Our Success Story photographers—Sarah Diebold, Adam Wiggall, Michele Kranik, Elma Blum, Harrington Photography, and Limelite Studios, along with food stylist and blogger Julie Fagan, and hair and makeup team Jennifer Ramos and Annette Cobos—ensured our hard-working members' "after" photos looked great!

The participants in our "Ditch the Diet" taste test and follow-up cooking class. Thanks for letting us show you that you can love the food you eat!

Mark Krumme and his team at Prestige AV & Creative Services, for their help with the "Ditch the Diet" followup.

The Galvin and Barton families for all the support and use of your beautiful homes.

The faculty, staff, and students of the Midwest Culinary Institute at Cincinnati State Technical and Community College for the use of their facilities and their name, along with their tremendous support.

Meg would like to thank:

My family: husband, Mark; and boys, Noah, Ian, and Josh. The book would not be possible without you. Thank you for all the nights of experimentation, evaluation, and clean-up. It sure did make for some fun dinner conservations.

Stepfanie, "the voice of the SparkPeople," for all her help with a new venture of writing a book. We did it!

My neighbor, Amy Kindt, for being the official guinea pig who was sworn to secrecy.

Chef-in-training Peggy Neal, as the tester for every recipe in the book. Her meticulous documentation was amazing.

My Aunt Margaret "Cissy" Williams and my oldest brother, John, for their work on making the farmhouse and garden picture perfect.

My mother, Jill, my first culinary instructor. She taught me to love food and embrace the experience of the meal.

My dad, James W. Barton, for all the years of life lessons on ethics, farming, cooking, and most importantly the art of storytelling! He taught me to write as I would speak—letting my voice tell the story. And the story begins . . .

Stepfanie would like to thank:

Tami Corwin, for her unwavering faith in me, her tremendous experience, and her amazing advice. You trusted me to wear so many hats during the writing and production of this book, and it represents a real-life education that is infinitely valuable to me. Thanks to you, I'm an author!

My talented, generous, and incredibly humble co-author, Meg, for her hard work and ever-present smile. We did it! What are we going to do now?

My Papa, Jim Romine, for teaching me to show love through food and my Gramma Willie Pfeiffer for passing along her love for baking.

My mother, Janet Buechner, for always welcoming me into the kitchen, and raising me to become the woman I am today. She taught me that, even from 7,000 miles away, foods can bring the people you love into your life.

All the friends and family scattered across three continents who welcomed me into their kitchens, handed me an apron, and taught me their native cuisines.

Chris Downie, Dave Heilmann, and the entire SparkPeople team for creating such a wonderful work environment. I love waking up and coming to work each morning.

Randy Hoover and his entire team for helping me learn the ropes of art direction and set styling. You all taught me so much!

Sam, for his endless support and confidence in me.

ABOUT THE AUTHOR

MEG GALVIN

At SparkPeople.com, Chef Meg Galvin develops healthy recipes, tests member-submitted dishes, and teaches the fundamentals of cooking through informative and entertaining videos and articles. A World Master Chef since 2005, Chef Meg was the host of the regional television show *The Dish,* which aired on a local CBS affiliate and online. Meg now hosts cooking videos on the local FOX affiliate.

Galvin earned a bachelor's degree in business administration from Eastern Kentucky University and a certificate of culinary arts from Le Cordon Bleu in London. She is certified as an executive chef by the American Culinary Federation and is working toward her court of master sommeliers wine certification.

Galvin is a faculty member at Cincinnati State Technical and Community College, home of the Midwest Culinary Institute (MCI), an American Culinary Federation certified college. In addition, she oversees one of a handful of programs in the country that allows culinary students to transfer to earn a four-year degree in the culinary arts.

Raised on a large family farm in central Kentucky, Galvin now lives in northern Kentucky with her husband and three teenage sons—including twins. On any given day, she can be found hitting the pavement on long runs or cheering on her sons at their numerous sporting events. She balances her busy schedule by incorporating her home life and career, bringing her kids into the kitchen and testing recipes on—and with—her family.

STEPFANIE ROMINE

Stepfanie Romine is editor of SparkRecipes.com and dailySpark.com, SparkPeople's healthy living blog, where she writes about topics such as cooking, yoga, and stress relief. A vegetarian and runner, Romine has studied ethnic cuisines on three continents. She is a longtime practitioner of Ashtanga yoga and became a certified yoga teacher in 2009.

With degrees in French and journalism from Ohio University, Romine started her career in newspapers, first as a copy editor, then as a business reporter, food blogger, and columnist. She joined SparkPeople in 2008, thus marrying her passions for writing and healthy living.

Romine lives in Cincinnati, where she and her boyfriend fuel long runs and bike rides with healthy homemade meals.

SPARKPEOPLE.COM

SparkPeople.com is one of the leading diet, fitness, and healthy living destinations on the web, with more than 10 million members; free weight loss, nutrition, and fitness tracking tools; and a positive community of people who are committed to reaching their goals and supporting one another along the way. SparkPeople combines the science of nutrition and fitness with the science of motivation and the power of social networking. The company has seven websites, including SparkReci pes.com, with more than 300,000 healthy and delicious recipes.

Join us online! Use special code SparkBook2 to get your SparkPoints.

NOTES

NOTES

NOTES

NOTES

NOTES

NOTES

NOTES

NOTES

HAY HOUSE TITLES OF RELATED INTEREST

YOU CAN HEAL YOUR LIFE, *the movie,* starring Louise L. Hay & Friends
(available as a 1-DVD program and an expanded 2-DVD set)
Watch the trailer at: **www.LouiseHayMovie.com**

THE SHIFT, the movie,
starring Dr. Wayne W. Dyer
(available as a 1-DVD program and an expanded 2-DVD set)
Watch the trailer at: **www.DyerMovie.com**

• •

***THE CORE BALANCE DIET: 4 Weeks to Boost Your Metabolism
and Lose Weight for Good,*** by Marcelle Pick, MSN, OB/GYN NP

***A COURSE IN WEIGHT LOSS: 21 Spiritual Lessons for Surrendering
Your Weight Forever,*** by Marianne Williamson

FULL: A Life Without Dieting, by Michael A. Snyder, M.D., F.A.C.S.

***HEALTH BLISS: 50 Revitalizing NatureFoods & Lifestyle Choices
to Promote Vibrant Health,*** by Susan Smith Jones, Ph.D.

JUST 10 LBS: Easy Steps to Weighing What You Want (Finally), by Brad Lamm

All of the above are available at your local bookstore,
or may be ordered by contacting Hay House (see next page).

• •

We hope you enjoyed this Hay House book. If you'd
like to receive our online catalog featuring additional information
on Hay House books and products, or if you'd like to find out
more about the Hay Foundation, please contact:

Hay House, Inc., P.O. Box 5100, Carlsbad, CA 92018-5100
(760) 431-7695 or (800) 654-5126
(760) 431-6948 (fax) or (800) 650-5115 (fax)
www.hayhouse.com® • **www.hayfoundation.org**

• •

Published and distributed in Australia by: Hay House Australia Pty. Ltd., 18/36 Ralph St.,
Alexandria NSW 2015 • *Phone:* 612-9669-4299 • *Fax:* 612-9669-4144 • www.hayhouse.com.au

Published and distributed in the United Kingdom by: Hay House UK, Ltd., 292B Kensal Rd.,
London W10 5BE • *Phone:* 44-20-8962-1230 • *Fax:* 44-20-8962-1239 • www.hayhouse.co.uk

Published and distributed in the Republic of South Africa by: Hay House SA (Pty), Ltd.,
P.O. Box 990, Witkoppen 2068 • *Phone/Fax:* 27-11-467-8904 • www.hayhouse.co.za

Published in India by: Hay House Publishers India, Muskaan Complex, Plot No. 3, B-2, Vasant Kunj,
New Delhi 110 070 • *Phone:* 91-11-4176-1620 • *Fax:* 91-11-4176-1630 • www.hayhouse.co.in

Distributed in Canada by: Raincoast, 9050 Shaughnessy St., Vancouver, B.C. V6P 6E5
Phone: (604) 323-7100 • *Fax:* (604) 323-2600 • www.raincoast.com

• •

Take Your Soul on a Vacation

Visit **www.HealYourLife.com**® to regroup, recharge,
and reconnect with your own magnificence.Featuring blogs,
mind-body-spirit news, and life-changing wisdom
from Louise Hay and friends.

Visit **www.HealYourLife.com** today!

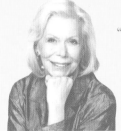